BRADY

PARAMEDIC CARE: PRINCIPLES & PRACTICE

MEDICAL EMERGENCIES

Workbook

Robert S. Porter

BRYAN E. BLEDSOE, D.O., F.A.C.E.P., F.A.A.E.M., F.A.E.P., EMT-P
Emergency Department Staff Physician
Baylor Medical Center—Ellis County
Waxahachie, Texas
and
Clinical Associate Professor of Emergency Medicine
University of North Texas Health Sciences Center
Fort Worth, Texas

ROBERT S. PORTER, M.A., NREMT-P
Senior Advanced Life Support Educator
Madison County Emergency Medical Services
Canastota, New York
and
Flight Paramedic
AirOne, Onondaga County Sheriff's Department
Syracuse, New York

RICHARD A. CHERRY, M.S., NREMT-P
Clinical Assistant Professor of Emergency Medicine
Director of Paramedic Training
SUNY Upstate Medical University
Syracuse, New York

Prentice Hall

Upper Saddle River, New Jersey 07458

D1299570

Dedication

To Kris and sailing: Pleasant distractions from writing about and practicing prehospital emergency medicine.

PUBLISHER: *Julie Alexander*
EXECUTIVE EDITOR: *Greg Vis*
MANAGING DEVELOPMENT EDITOR: *Lois Berlowitz*
DEVELOPMENT EDITOR: *Dan Zinkus*
MARKETING MANAGER: *Tiffany Price*
DIRECTOR OF MANUFACTURING & PRODUCTION: *Bruce Johnson*
SENIOR PRODUCTION MANAGER: *Ilene Sanford*
MANAGING PRODUCTION EDITOR: *Patrick Walsh*
PRODUCTION EDITOR: *Jeanne Molenaar*
PRODUCTION SUPERVISION: *Navta Associates, Inc.*
PRINTER/BINDER: *Banta Harrisonburg*

Printed in the United States of America
10 9 8 7 6 5 4

ISBN 0-13-021637-2

Prentice-Hall International (UK) Limited, *London*
Prentice-Hall of Australia Pty. Limited, *Sydney*
Prentice-Hall Canada Inc., *Toronto*
Prentice-Hall Hispanoamericana, S.A., *Mexico*
Prentice-Hall of India Private Limited, *New Delhi*
Prentice-Hall of Japan, Inc., *Tokyo*
Prentice-Hall (Singapore) Pte Ltd
Editora Prentice-Hall do Brasil, Ltda., *Rio de Janeiro*

NOTICE ON CARE PROCEDURES

It is the intent of the authors and publisher that this workbook be used as part of a formal EMT-Paramedic program taught by qualified instructors and supervised by a licensed physician. The procedures described in this workbook are based upon consultation with EMT and medical authorities. The authors and publisher have taken care to make certain that these procedures reflect currently accepted clinical practice; however, they cannot be considered absolute recommendations.

The material in this workbook contains the most current information available at the time of publication. However, federal, state, and local guidelines concerning clinical practices, including, without limitation, those governing infection control and universal precautions, change rapidly. The reader should note, therefore, that the new regulations may require changes in some procedures.

It is the responsibility of the reader to familiarize himself or herself with the policies and procedures set by federal, state, and local agencies as well as the institution or agency where the reader is employed. The authors and the publisher of this workbook disclaim any liability, loss, or risk resulting directly or indirectly from the suggested procedures and theory, from any undetected errors, or from the reader's misunderstanding of the text. It is the reader's responsibility to stay informed of any new changes or recommendations made by any federal, state, and local agency as well as by his or her employing institution or agency.

CONTENTS

Self-Instructional Workbook

Paramedic Care: Principles & Practice

MEDICAL EMERGENCIES

INTRODUCTION
To the Self-Instructional Workbook
Paramedic Care: Principles & Practice

Welcome to the self-instructional workbook for *Paramedic Care: Principles & Practice*. This workbook is designed to help guide you through an educational program for initial or refresher training that follows the guidelines of the 1998 U.S. Department of Transportation EMT-Paramedic National Standard Curriculum. The workbook is designed to be used either in conjunction with your instructor or as a self-study guide you use on your own.

This workbook features many different ways to help you learn the material necessary to become a paramedic, including those listed below.

FEATURES

Review of Chapter Objectives
Each chapter of *Paramedic Care: Principles & Practice* begins with objectives that identify the important information and principles addressed in the chapter reading. To help you identify and learn this material, each workbook chapter reviews the important content elements addressed by these objectives as presented in the text.

Case Study Review
Each chapter of *Paramedic Care: Principles & Practice* includes a case study, introducing and highlighting important principles presented in the chapter. The workbook reviews these case studies and points out much of the essential information and many of the applied principles they describe.

Content Self-Evaluation
Each chapter of *Paramedic Care: Principles & Practice* presents an extensive narrative explanation of the principles of paramedic practice. The workbook chapter (or chapter section) contains between 10 and 90 multiple-choice questions to test your reading comprehension of the textbook material and to give you experience taking typical emergency medical service examinations.

Special Projects
The workbook contains several projects that are special learning experiences designed to help you remember the information and principles necessary to perform as a paramedic. Special projects include crossword puzzles, personal benchmarking activities, and a variety of other exercises that develop and refine your skills of assessing patients and caring for their illnesses.

Chapter Sections
Several chapters in *Paramedic Care: Principles & Practice* are long and contain a great deal of subject matter. To help you grasp this material more efficiently, the workbook breaks these chapters into sections with their own objectives, content review, and special projects.

Content Review
The workbook provides a comprehensive review of the material presented in this volume of *Paramedic Care: Principles & Practice*. After the last text chapter has been covered, the workbook presents an extensive content self-evaluation component that helps you recall and build upon the knowledge you have gained by reading the text, attending class, and completing the earlier workbook chapters.

National Registry Practical Evaluation Forms

Supplemental materials found at the back of the workbook include the National Registry Practical Evaluation Forms. These or similar forms will be used to test your practical skills throughout your training and, usually, for state certification exams. By reviewing them, you have a clearer picture of what is expected of you during your practical exam and a better understanding of the type of evaluation tool that is used to measure your performance.

Patient Scenario Flash Cards

This workbook contains 3″ × 5″ cards, each of which presents a patient scenario with signs and symptoms. On the reverse side is the appropriate field diagnosis and the care steps you should consider providing for the patient. These cards will help you recognize and remember common serious medical emergencies, their presentation, and the appropriate care that should be given.

ACKNOWLEDGMENTS

Contributors

We wish to acknowledge the extraordinary talents and efforts of the following people who contributed chapters to this workbook. In developing study guides, questions, and activities, they have upheld the highest standards of EMS instruction.

Beth Lothrop Adams, M.A., R.N., NREMT-P
ALS Coordinator
EHS Programs
Adjunct Assistant Professor
Emergency Medicine
The George Washington University
Fairfax, Virginia

Elizabeth Coolidge-Stolz, M.D.
Medical Writer, Health Educator
North Reading, Massachusetts

Reviewers

The reviewers listed below provided many excellent suggestions for improving this workbook. Their assistance is greatly appreciated.

Edward B. Kuvlesky, NREMT-P
Battalion Chief
Indian River County EMS
Indian River County, Florida

K. Lee Watson, NREMT-P
Martinsville-Henry County Rescue Squad
Martinsville, Virginia

HOW TO USE

The Self-Instructional Workbook

Paramedic Care: Principles & Practice

The self-instructional workbook accompanying *Paramedic Care: Principles & Practice* may be used as directed by your instructor or independently by you during your course of instruction. The recommendations listed below are intended to guide you in using the workbook independently.

- Examine your course schedule and identify the appropriate text chapter or other assigned reading.

- Read the assigned chapter in *Paramedic Care: Principles & Practice* carefully. Do this in a relaxed environment, free of distractions, and give yourself adequate time to read and digest the material. The information presented in *Paramedic Care: Principles & Practice* is often technically complex and demanding, but it is very important that you comprehend it. Be sure that you read the chapter carefully enough to understand and remember what you have read.

- Carefully read the Review of Chapter Objectives at the beginning of each workbook chapter (or section). This material includes both the objectives listed in *Paramedic Care: Principles & Practice* and narrative descriptions of their content. If you do not understand or remember what is discussed from your reading, refer to the referenced pages and reread them carefully. If you still do not feel comfortable with your understanding of any objective, consider asking your instructor about it.

- Reread the case study in *Paramedic Care: Principles & Practice,* and then read the Case Study Review in the workbook. Note the important points regarding assessment and care that the Case Study Review highlights, and be sure that you understand and agree with the analysis of the call. If you have any questions or concerns, ask your instructor to clarify the information.

- Take the Content Self-Evaluation at the end of each workbook chapter (or section), answering each question carefully. Do this in a quiet environment, free from distractions, and allow yourself adequate time to complete the exercise. Correct your self-evaluation by consulting the answers at the back of the workbook, and determine the percentage you have answered correctly (the number you got right divided by the total number of questions). If you have answered most of the questions correctly (85 to 90 percent), review those that you missed by rereading the material on the pages listed in the answer key and be sure you understand which answer is correct and why. If you have more than a few questions wrong (less than 85 percent correct), look for incorrect answers that are grouped together. This suggests that you did not understand a particular topic in the reading. Reread the text dealing with that topic carefully, and then retest yourself on the questions you got wrong. If incorrect answers are spread throughout the chapter content, reread the chapter and retake the Content Self-Evaluation to ensure that you understand the material. If you don't understand why your answer to a question is incorrect after reviewing the text, consult with your instructor.

- In a similar fashion, complete the exercises in the Special Projects section of the workbook chapters (or sections). These exercises are specifically designed to help you learn and remember the essential principles and information presented in *Paramedic Care: Principles & Practice*.

- When you have completed this volume of *Paramedic Care: Principles & Practice* and its accompanying workbook, prepare for a course test by reviewing both the text in its entirety and your class notes. Then take the Content Review examination in the workbook. Again, review your score and any questions you have answered incorrectly by referring to the text and rereading the page or pages where the material is presented. If you note groupings of wrong answers, review the entire range of pages or the full chapter they represent.

If, during your completion of the workbook exercises, you have any questions that either the textbook or workbook doesn't answer, write them down and ask your instructor about them. Prehospital emergency medicine is a complex and complicated subject, and answers are not always black-and-white. It is also common for different EMS systems to use differing methods of care. The questions you bring up in class, and your instructor's answers to them, will help you expand and complete your knowledge of prehospital emergency medical care.

The authors and Brady Publishing continuously seek to ensure the creation of the best materials to support your educational experience. We are interested in your comments. If, during your reading and study of material in *Paramedic Care: Principles & Practice*, you notice any error or have any suggestions to improve either the textbook or workbook, please use the comment form at the back of this workbook. Alternatively, you can direct your comments via the Internet at the following address:

harrier@localnet.com

You can also visit the Brady website at:
www.bradybooks.com/paramedic

GUIDELINES TO BETTER TEST-TAKING

The knowledge you will gain from reading the textbook, completing the exercises in the workbook, listening in your paramedic class, and participating in your clinical and field experience will prepare you to care for patients who are seriously ill or injured. However, before you can practice these skills, you will have to pass several classroom written exams and your state's certification exam successfully. Your performance on these exams will depend not only on your knowledge but also on your ability to answer test questions correctly. The following guidelines are designed to help your performance on tests and to better demonstrate your knowledge of prehospital emergency care.

1. Relax and be calm during the test.

A test is designed to measure what you have learned and to tell you and your instructor how well you are doing. An exam is not designed to intimidate or punish you. Consider it a challenge and just try to do your best. Get plenty of sleep prior to the examination. Avoid coffee or other stimulants for a few hours before the exam and be prepared.

Reread the text chapters, review the objectives in the workbook, and review your class notes. It might be helpful to work with one or two other students and ask each other questions. This type of practice helps everyone better understand the knowledge presented in your course of study.

2. Read the questions carefully.

Read each word of the question and all the answers slowly. Words such as "except" or "not" may change the entire meaning of the question. If you miss such words, you may answer the question incorrectly even though you know the right answer.

EXAMPLE:
The art and science of Emergency Medical Services involves all of the following EXCEPT:

    A. sincerity and compassion.
    B. respect for human dignity.
    C. placing patient care before personal safety.
    D. delivery of sophisticated emergency medical care.
    E. none of the above

The correct answer is C, unless you miss the "EXCEPT."

3. Read each answer carefully.

Read each and every answer carefully. While the first answer may be absolutely correct, so may the rest, and thus the best answer might be "all of the above."

EXAMPLE:
Indirect medical control is considered to be:

    A. treatment protocols.
    B. training and education.
    C. quality assurance.
    D. chart review.
    E. all of the above

While answers A, B, C, and D are correct, the best and only acceptable answer is "all of the above," E.

4. Delay answering questions you don't understand and look for clues.

When a question seems confusing or you don't know the answer, note it on your answer sheet and come back to it later. This will ensure that you have time to complete the test. You will also find that other questions in the test may give you hints to answer the one you've skipped over. It will also prevent you from being frustrated with an early question and letting it affect your performance.

EXAMPLE:
Upon successful completion of a course of training as an EMT-P, most states will

    A. certify you. (correct)
    B. license you.
    C. register you.
    D. recognize you as a paramedic.
    E. issue you a permit.

Another question, later in the exam, may suggest the right answer:

The action of one state in recognizing the certification of another is called:

    A. reciprocity. (correct)
    B. national registration.
    C. licensure.
    D. registration.
    E. extended practice.

5. Answer all questions.

Even if you do not know the right answer, do not leave a question blank. A blank question is always wrong, while a guess might be correct. If you can eliminate some of the answers as wrong, do so. It will increase the chances of a correct guess.

EXAMPLE:
When a paramedic is called by the patient (through the dispatcher) to the scene of a medical emergency, the medical control physician has established a physician/patient relationship.

    A. True
    B. False

A true/false question gives you a 50 percent chance of a correct guess.

The hospital health professional responsible for sorting patients as they arrive at the emergency department is usually the:

    A. emergency physician.
    B. ward clerk.
    C. emergency nurse.
    D. trauma surgeon.
    E. both A and C (correct)

A multiple-choice question with five answers gives a 20 percent chance of a correct guess. If you can eliminate one or more incorrect answers, you increase your odds of a correct guess to 25 percent, 33 percent, and so on. An unanswered question has a 0 percent chance of being correct.

Just before turning in your answer sheet, check to be sure that you have not left any items blank.

CHAPTER 1
*
Pulmonology

With each chapter of the Workbook, we identify the objectives and the important elements of the text content. You should review these items and refer to the pages listed if any points are not clear.

Because Chapter 1 is lengthy, it has been divided into parts to aid your study. Read the assigned text pages, then progress through the objectives and self-evaluation materials as you would with other chapters. When you feel secure in your grasp of the content, proceed to the next part.

Part 1, pp. 2–35

Review of Chapter Objectives

After reading this part of the chapter, you should be able to:

1. Discuss the epidemiology of pulmonary diseases and pulmonary conditions. **p. 4**

Respiratory emergencies are among the most common EMS calls—up to 28 percent, according to one study. Respiratory emergencies lead to over 200,000 deaths per year. Because of the frequency of such calls, it is critical that you be knowledgeable about diseases that affect the respiratory system.

2. Identify and describe the function of the structures located in the upper and lower airway. **pp. 5–11**

The airway is functionally divided into the upper airway and the lower airway. The upper airway is comprised of the nasal cavity, pharynx, and larynx. The lower airway is comprised of the trachea, bronchi, alveoli, and lungs. The ability to take in oxygen and excrete carbon dioxide via the airway is essential to life. Therefore, it is critical that you be able to identify and understand the function of each structure of the airway and of the airway as a whole.

3. Discuss the physiology of ventilation and respiration. **pp. 11–18**

The major function of the respiratory system is the exchange of gases between the person and the environment. Three processes allow the gas exchange to take place: ventilation, diffusion, and perfusion. Ventilation is the movement of air in and out of the lungs. Diffusion is the movement of gases between the lungs and the pulmonary capillaries (oxygen from the lungs into the bloodstream; waste carbon dioxide from the bloodstream into the lungs) as well as between the systemic capillaries and the body tissues (oxygen from the bloodstream into the cells; waste carbon dioxide from the cells into the bloodstream). Perfusion is the circulation of blood through the capillaries. Adequate perfusion is critical to adequate gas exchange in the lungs and body tissues. These three processes—ventilation, diffusion, and perfusion—together provide for respiration.

4. Identify common pathological events that affect the pulmonary system. **pp. 18–21**

Any disease state that affects the pulmonary system will ultimately disrupt ventilation, diffusion, or perfusion, or a combination of these processes. Ventilation may be disrupted by diseases that cause obstruction of any part of the airway, disrupt the normal function of the chest wall, or impair nervous system control of breathing. Diffusion can be disrupted by a change in concentration of atmospheric oxygen or by any disease that affects the structure or patency of alveoli, the thickness of the respiratory membrane, or the permeability of the capillaries. Perfusion will be affected by any disease that limits blood flow through the lungs and the body or reduces the volume of the oxygen-carrying red blood cells or hemoglobin. Understanding how different diseases and conditions may affect the processes of respiration is important to your ability to choose appropriate emergency care for a respiratory emergency.

5. **Compare various airway and ventilation techniques used in the management of pulmonary diseases.** p. 36

Two principles govern the overall management of respiratory emergencies. (1) Give first priority to the airway. (2) Always provide oxygen to patients with respiratory distress or the possibility of hypoxia, including those with chronic obstructive pulmonary disease (COPD). (To review airway and ventilation techniques used in the management of specific diseases, see text pages 35–59, which are covered in the workbook pages for part 2 of this chapter.)

6. **Review the use of equipment utilized during the physical examination of patients with complaints associated with respiratory diseases and conditions.** pp. 29–30, 32–34

You should be familiar with the use of equipment that is available for physical examination of patients with respiratory complaints. These include the stethoscope, the pulse oximeter, handheld devices for measuring peak expiratory flow rate (PEFR), and end-tidal carbon dioxide detection devices.

CASE STUDY REVIEW

It is important to review each emergency response you participate in as a paramedic. Similarly, we will review the case study that precedes each chapter. We will address the important points of the response as addressed by the chapter. Often, this will include the scene size-up, patient assessment, patient management, patient packaging, and transport.

Reread the case study on pages 3 and 4 in Paramedic Care: Medical Emergencies *before reading the discussion below.*

This case study demonstrates how paramedics can reach a field diagnosis and choose appropriate emergency treatment in a respiratory emergency. On this call, Tony and Lee gather critical information from the patient history.

All Tony and Lee know from the dispatch is that their patient is a male who is having difficulty breathing. They learn slightly more from the First Responder on the scene: The patient is 55 years old and is already being given oxygen.

They grab the equipment they think they may need, enter the house (checking for safety), and approach the patient, who is seated at the kitchen table, obviously short of breath. They avoid leaping to conclusions and begin their systematic assessment. The initial assessment confirms that the patient has a patent airway, is moving a little air, and has a strong pulse. They replace the nasal cannula the First Responder had provided with a nonrebreather mask and continue the assessment.

The physical exam reveals diminished breath sounds, rhonchi, use of accessory muscles of respiration, and cyanosis around the mouth. These findings confirm the original complaint: breathing difficulty. But since this is a medical patient (no mechanism of injury was noted during the scene size-up), Tony and Lee know that the most critical information is likely to come from the history.

In fact, they learn that the patient has been diagnosed with emphysema (and has an ongoing 60 pack/year smoking history), and some worsening or exacerbation of this condition is the most likely cause of the patient's current emergency.

Tony and Lee know that emphysema results in bronchoconstriction, alveolar collapse, and a decrease in pulmonary capillaries, which interfere with ventilation and diffusion. The constricted bronchi and destruction of the walls of the small bronchioles make exhalation difficult, causing the rhonchi heard on auscultation of this patient, and also prevent oxygen from reaching the alveoli. The patient no longer has enough healthy alveoli nor pulmonary capillaries to provide for adequate oxygen diffusion into the bloodstream. This, they understand, is why the patient's pulse oximetry reading is only 90 percent, even though he is receiving supplemental oxygen.

The two paramedics know that emergency treatment must be aimed at relief of the patient's hypoxia and bronchoconstriction. They continue administration of supplemental oxygen to compensate for the decreased diffusion the patient's diseased alveoli and capillaries are providing. In consultation with medical direction, they start an IV of normal saline, knowing that the fluid may counter any dehydration present and may help to loosen any excess mucus that may be blocking the bronchioles. Additionally, medical direction orders nebulizer administration of albuterol to relieve bronchoconstriction, as well as methylprednisolone by IV push to relieve inflammation.

Monitoring of the patient en route to the hospital shows the effectiveness of these interventions. The patient's respirations slow to a normal rate and his oxygen saturation increases to 94 percent.

CONTENT SELF-EVALUATION

Each of the chapters in this Workbook includes a short content review. The questions are designed to test your ability to remember what you read. At the end of this Workbook, you can find the answers to the questions as well as the pages where the topic of the question was discussed in the text. If you answer the question incorrectly or are unsure of the answer, review the pages listed.

MULTIPLE CHOICE

_____ 1. Which of the following is considered an intrinsic risk factor for respiratory disease?
   A. smokestack pollutants
   B. polluted water
   C. genetic predisposition
   D. cigarette smoking
   E. stress

_____ 2. Which of the following is NOT part of the upper airway?
   A. nasal cavity
   B. oropharynx
   C. laryngopharynx
   D. trachea
   E. larynx

_____ 3. Which of the following IS part of the lower airway?
   A. esophagus
   B. ileum
   C. tonsils
   D. hypopharynx
   E. bronchi

_____ 4. Most of the exchange of oxygen and carbon dioxide takes place in the:
   A. trachea.
   B. bronchi.
   C. pulmonary ducts.
   D. bronchioles.
   E. alveoli.

_____ 5. The three processes that allow gas exchange to occur in the lungs and body tissues are:
   A. ventilation, diffusion, perfusion.
   B. inspiration, expiration, ventilation.
   C. resistance, compliance, perfusion.
   D. ventilation, inspiration, expiration.
   E. inspiration, compliance, diffusion.

_____ 6. The mechanical process of moving air in and out of the lungs is:
   A. ventilation.
   B. diffusion.
   C. perfusion.
   D. inspiration.
   E. inhalation.

_____ 7. The process by which gases move between the alveoli and the pulmonary capillaries is:
   A. infusion.
   B. perfusion.
   C. respiration.
   D. diffusion.
   E. permeation.

_____ 8. Lung perfusion is dependent on three factors—adequate blood volume, efficient pumping by the heart, and intact:
   A. alveoli.
   B. respiratory membrane.
   C. bronchioles.
   D. goblet cells.
   E. pulmonary capillaries.

_____ 9. Any of the following can disrupt ventilation EXCEPT:
   A. obstruction of the upper airway.
   B. obstruction of the lower airway.
   C. blockage of the pulmonary arteries.
   D. impairment of normal function of the chest wall.
   E. abnormalities of the nervous system's control of breathing.

_____ 10. Which of the following abnormal breathing patterns is characterized by long, deep breaths that are stopped during the inspiratory phase and separated by periods of apnea?
   A. ataxic (Biot's) respirations (seen with increased intracranial pressure)
   B. central neurogenic hyperventilation (seen with stroke or brainstem injury)
   C. Kussmaul's respirations (seen with metabolic acidosis)
   D. apneustic respirations (seen with stroke or severe central nervous system disease)
   E. Cheyne-Stokes respirations (seen with terminal illness or brain injury)

_____ 11. Which of the following is NOT likely to cause hypoxia (a supply of oxygen inadequate to meet the needs of the body's cells)?
   A. ascension to a high altitude
   B. esophageal ulceration
   C. black lung disease
   D. left-sided heart failure
   E. asbestos inhalation

_____ 12. Pulmonary shunting results from:
   A. alveolar collapse.
   B. blockage of pulmonary capillaries.
   C. bronchoconstriction.
   D. excess mucus production.
   E. airway obstruction.

_____ 13. The most important action when you arrive on scene and discover that a hazardous material is present is to:
   A. have supplemental oxygen available.
   B. remove the patient from the environment.
   C. search for additional patients.
   D. put on self-contained breathing apparatus.
   E. call for a hazardous materials team.

_____ 14. You are dispatched to a patient with difficulty breathing. Which of the following should be part of the scene size-up?
   A. Establish a patent airway.
   B. Look for clues to the possible cause.
   C. Evaluate AVPU mental status.
   D. Determine respiration rate.
   E. Ready the oxygenation equipment.

_____ 15. During the initial assessment, your general impression of the patient's respiratory status should include all of the following elements EXCEPT:
   A. pulse.
   B. position.
   C. color.
   D. mental status.
   E. ability to speak.

16. Which of the following is NOT a classic sign of respiratory distress?
    A. pursed lips
    B. tracheal tugging
    C. diaphoresis
    D. nasal flaring
    E. cyanosis

17. Which of the following is TRUE with regard to assessing the airway?
    A. Noisy breathing usually indicates a complete obstruction.
    B. Obstructed breathing is not always noisy breathing.
    C. If the airway is blocked, artificial respiration must be started immediately.
    D. If the airway is blocked, endotracheal intubation must be established.
    E. If the airway is open, the patient is breathing.

18. Which of the following is the MOST ominous sign of possible life-threatening respiratory distress?
    A. altered mental status
    B. audible stridor
    C. 1- to 2-word dyspnea
    D. tachycardia
    E. use of accessory muscles

19. Orthopnea is:
    A. dizziness when rising from a supine position.
    B. dyspnea that occurs while lying supine.
    C. short attacks of dyspnea that interrupt sleep.
    D. apnea that occurs while in an upright position.
    E. pleuritic pain that occurs during breathing.

20. Many respiratory complaints result from worsening of a long-standing disease the patient knows he has and can tell you about during the history. All of the following are such long-term respiratory diseases EXCEPT:
    A. pneumonia.
    B. emphysema.
    C. chronic bronchitis.
    D. asthma.
    E. lung cancer.

21. Which of the following medications would be of LEAST significance if found in the home of a patient with a respiratory complaint?
    A. oxygen
    B. bronchodilator
    C. vitamin C tablets
    D. corticosteroid
    E. antibiotic

22. Cardiac patients often present with dyspnea.
    A. True
    B. False

23. Allergic reaction to a medication may be the cause of a respiratory complaint.
    A. True
    B. False

24. A patient with significant respiratory distress may breathe through pursed lips. Breathing through pursed lips helps to:
    A. prevent tracheal collapse.
    B. force air past a bronchial obstruction.
    C. bring up excess mucus.
    D. close the epiglottis.
    E. keep the alveoli open.

25. Pink or bloody sputum is commonly seen with any of the following EXCEPT:
    A. pulmonary edema.
    B. lung cancer.
    C. tuberculosis.
    D. allergic reaction.
    E. bronchial infection.

_____ 26. Asymmetrical chest movement is most likely to be found during:
   A. auscultation.
   B. capnometry.
   C. oximetry.
   D. inspection.
   E. percussion.

_____ 27. Subcutaneous emphysema is most likely to be found during:
   A. oximetry.
   B. percussion.
   C. capnometry.
   D. palpation.
   E. inspection.

_____ 28. Wheezing is most likely to be detected during:
   A. oximetry.
   B. auscultation.
   C. percussion.
   D. capnometry.
   E. palpation.

_____ 29. Rattling sounds in the larger airways associated with excess mucus are called:
   A. stridor.
   B. wheezing.
   C. crackles.
   D. snoring.
   E. rhonchi.

_____ 30. A harsh, high-pitched sound heard on inspiration, associated with upper airway obstruction, is called:
   A. snoring.
   B. stridor.
   C. crackles.
   D. rhonchi.
   E. rales.

_____ 31. In general, tachycardia is a nonspecific finding seen, for example, with fear, anxiety, or fever. In a patient with a respiratory complaint, however, tachycardia may also indicate:
   A. hypothermia.
   B. hypertrophy.
   C. hypotension.
   D. hyperopia.
   E. hypoxia.

_____ 32. Drugs that may cause an elevation in both heart rate and blood pressure include:
   A. diuretics such as furosemide.
   B. analgesics such as morphine sulfate.
   C. tranqulizers such as diazepam.
   D. sympathomimetics such as albuterol.
   E. beta blockers such as labetalol.

_____ 33. An elevated respiratory rate in a patient with dyspnea is most likely caused by:
   A. bradycardia.
   B. dysuria.
   C. hypoxia.
   D. anemia.
   E. tachycardia.

_____ 34. In a patient with dyspnea, a persistently slow respiratory rate:
   A. indicates impending respiratory arrest.
   B. is less critical than a persistently rapid rate.
   C. is a common symptom of asthma.
   D. indicates cardiac involvement.
   E. is commonly associated with pneumonia.

_____ 35. Which of the following measures end-expiratory carbon dioxide?
   A. spirometry
   B. sphygmomanometry
   C. capnometry
   D. oximetry
   E. tomography

LABEL THE DIAGRAMS

Supply the missing labels for the drawing of the upper airway by writing the appropriate letters in the spaces provided.

A. Cricoid cartilage
B. Cricothyroid membrane
C. Epiglottis
D. Esophagus
E. Glottic opening
F. Thyroid cartilage
G. Tongue
H. Tonsils and adenoids

I. Trachea
J. Turbinates
K. LARYNGOPHARYNX
L. LARYNX
M. NASAL CAVITY
N. NASOPHARYNX
O. OROPHARYNX

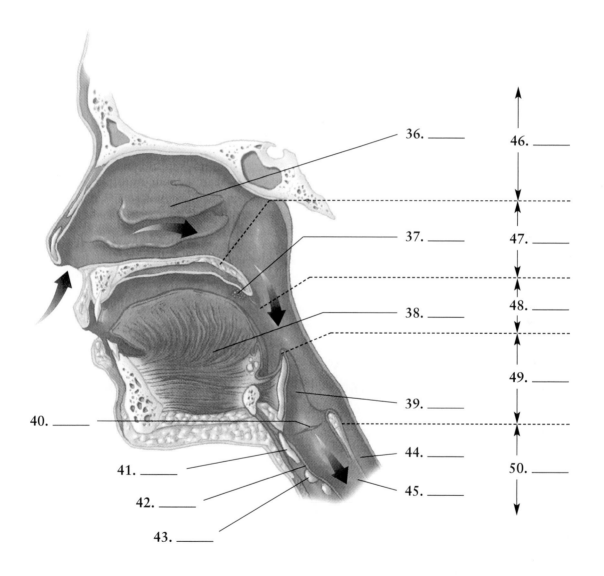

36. _____

46. _____

37. _____

47. _____

48. _____

38. _____

49. _____

39. _____

40. _____

44. _____

41. _____

50. _____

42. _____

45. _____

43. _____

Supply the missing labels for the drawing of the lower airway by writing the appropriate letters in the spaces provided.

A. Carina
B. Larynx
C. Left mainstem bronchus
D. Right mainstem bronchus
E. Trachea

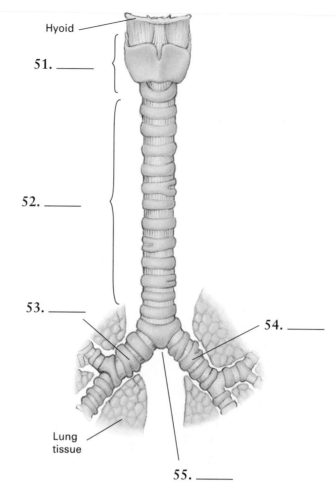

Hyoid

51. _____

52. _____

53. _____

54. _____

Lung tissue

55. _____

SPECIAL PROJECT

Evaluating Abnormal Breathing Patterns

On the line provided, write the name of each abnormal breathing pattern illustrated below. Review the illustration on page 20 of the text to check your answers.

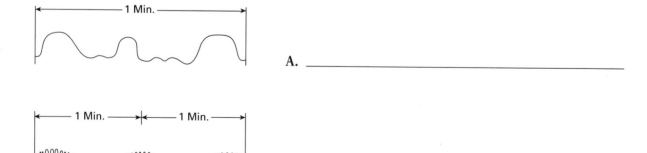

1 Min.

A. _____

1 Min. ⟶⟵ 1 Min.

B. _____

C. _____

D. _____

E. _____

Read the following three scenarios about patients who present with abnormal breathing patterns. On the lines—on the basis of the brief information given—write the name of the breathing pattern the patient seems to display and the condition (or conditions, if you think there is more than one possibility) you think is most likely causing the abnormal breathing pattern. (You must decide which three of the five patterns illustrated above are represented in the scenarios.) Review the text, pages 19–21, for help in completing your answers.

Scenario 1: You are called to the home of an elderly woman who is unresponsive. Her family tells you she had her ninetieth birthday last month but has been bedridden for two weeks and has "not been doing very well." Today, they have not been able to rouse her. On assessment, you find that the patient is breathing in a pattern of progressively increasing tidal volume, followed by progressively declining volume, separated by periods of apnea.

Breathing pattern: _____ **Probable cause:** _____

_____

_____

Scenario 2: You are called to a local fitness center where a middle-aged man who was participating in an exercise class suddenly complained of a terrible headache. He lurched sideways, then sat down hard on the exercise mat. By the time you arrive, he has lost consciousness. When you assess his breathing, you find repeated sets of gasping ventilations separated by periods of apnea.

Breathing pattern: _____ **Probable cause:** _____

_____

_____

Scenario 3: You are dispatched to a downtown office where the billing manager has fallen ill. You find her slumped on a sofa in the women's restroom. She has an altered mental status and is barely coherent. A medical ID bracelet identifies her as a diabetic. A co-worker says that she has been diabetic since childhood and takes insulin by injection but has lately been neglecting to take her injections regularly. Her respirations are deep and rapid.

Breathing pattern: _____ **Probable cause:** _____

_____

_____

CHAPTER 1
✳
Pulmonology

Part 2, pp. 35–59

Review of Chapter Objectives

After reading this part of the chapter, you should be able to:

7. **Identify the epidemiology, anatomy, physiology, pathophysiology, assessment findings, and management (including prehospital medications) for the following respiratory diseases and conditions:**

a. **Adult respiratory distress syndrome**   **pp. 36–38**

Adult respiratory distress syndrome (ARDS) is characterized by pulmonary edema caused by fluid accumulation in the interstitial spaces in the lungs. The mortality rate is 70 percent. ARDS occurs as a result of increased vascular permeability and decreased fluid removal from the lungs. A variety of lung insults can cause this inability to maintain proper fluid balance, including sepsis, pneumonia, inhalation injuries, emboli, tumors, and others noted in the text chapter. ARDS interferes with diffusion, causing hypoxia. In addition to evaluating the degree of the patient's respiratory distress, assessment is aimed at discovering symptoms and history that point to the underlying condition. Prehospital management is supportive (oxygen supplementation is essential to compensate for diffusion defects); in-hospital care is aimed at treatment of the underlying condition.

b. **Bronchial asthma**   **pp. 38–39, 43–48**

Asthma is an obstructive lung disease that causes abnormal ventilation. While deaths from other respiratory diseases are decreasing, deaths from asthma have been on the increase, with 50 percent of those deaths occurring before the patient reaches the hospital. Asthma is thought to be caused by a combination of genetic predisposition and environmental triggers that differ from individual to individual. These include allergens, cold air, exercise, stress, and certain medications. Exposure to a trigger causes release of histamine which, in turn, causes both bronchial constriction and capillary leakage that leads to bronchial edema. The result is a significant decrease in expiratory airflow, which is the essence of an "asthma attack." In the early phase of an attack, inhaled bronchodilator medications such as albuterol will help. In the late phase, inflammation sets in and anti-inflammatory drugs are required to alleviate the condition. Assessment must focus first on evaluation and support of the airway and breathing. Most patients will report a history of asthma. The physical exam should focus on the chest and neck to assess breathing effort. The respiratory rate is the most critical of the vital signs. EMS systems should also be able to measure the peak expiratory flow rate. Treatment is aimed at correction of hypoxia (oxygen administration) and relief of bronchospasm and inflammation. A special case is status asthmaticus, a severe, prolonged attack that does not respond to bronchodilators. It is a serious emergency requiring prompt recognition, treatment, and transport. Another special case is asthma in children, which is treated much as for adults but with altered medication dosages and some special medications.

c. Chronic bronchitis   pp. 38–39, 41–43

Chronic bronchitis is classified, along with emphysema, as a chronic obstructive pulmonary disease (COPD). COPD affects 25 percent of adults, with chronic bronchitis affecting one in five adult males. Chronic bronchitis reduces ventilation as a result of increased mucus production that blocks airway passages. It is often caused by cigarette smoking but also occurs in nonsmokers. There may be a history of frequent respiratory infections. Chronic bronchitis is usually associated with a productive cough and copious sputum. Patients tend to be overweight and often become cyanotic, so they are sometimes called "blue bloaters." Auscultation of the airway often reveals rhonchi due to mucus occlusion. The goals of treatment are relief of hypoxia and reversal of bronchoconstriction. Because these patients may be dependent on a hypoxic respiratory drive (low oxygen levels stimulate respiration), respiratory effort may become depressed when oxygen is administered. Needed oxygen should not be withheld, but the patient's respirations must be carefully monitored. IV fluids may help loosen mucous congestion. Medical direction may also order administration of a bronchodilator, such as albuterol, metaproterenol, or ipratropium bromide, and may also recommend corticosteroid administration.

d. Emphysema   pp. 38–43

Like chronic bronchitis, emphysema is classified as a chronic obstructive pulmonary disease (COPD). Alveolar walls are destroyed by exposure to noxious substances such as cigarette smoke or other environmental toxins. The disease also causes destruction of the walls of the small bronchioles, which contributes to a trapping of air in the lungs. The result is a decrease in both ventilation and diffusion. Patients tend to breathe through pursed lips, which creates a positive pressure that helps to prevent alveolar collapse. A developing decrease in PaO_2 leads to a compensatory increase in red blood cell production (polycythemia). Emphysema patients are more susceptible to acute respiratory infections and cardiac dysrhythmias. They become dependant on bronchodilators and corticosteroids and, in the final stages, supplemental oxygen. In contrast to chronic bronchitis sufferers, emphysema patients often lose weight and seldom have a cough except early in the morning. Because of the habit of breathing through pursed lips and the color produced by polycythemia, they are sometimes called "pink puffers." Clubbed fingers are common. Auscultation may reveal diminished breath sounds and, at times, wheezes and rhonchi. There may also be signs of right-sided heart disease. As a result of severe respiratory impairment, COPD patients may exhibit confusion, agitation, somnolence, 1-to-2-word dyspnea, and use of accessory muscles to assist respiration.

e. Pneumonia   pp. 49–51

Pneumonia, or lung infection, is a leading cause of death in the elderly and those with HIV infection and is the fifth leading cause of death in the U.S. overall. It is an infection most commonly caused by bacterial or viral infection, rarely by fungal and other infections. Risk factors center on conditions that cause a defect in mucus production or ciliary action that weaken the body's natural defenses against invaders of the respiratory system. Common signs and symptoms include an ill appearance, fever and shaking chills, a productive cough, and sputum. Many cases involve pleuritic chest pain. Auscultation usually reveals crackles in the involved lung segments, or sometimes wheezes or rhonchi, and occasionally egophony (change in spoken "E" sound to "A"). Percussion produces dullness over the affected areas. Some forms of pneumonia do not produce these distinctive symptoms, presenting instead with systemic complaints such as headache, malaise, fatigue, muscle aches, sore throat, nausea, vomiting, and diarrhea. Diagnosis in the field is unlikely and treatment is supportive. Place the patient in a comfortable position and administer high-flow oxygen. In severe cases, ventilatory assistance and possibly endotracheal intubation may be necessary. Medical direction may recommend administration of a beta agonist. Antipyretics may be given to reduce a high fever.

f. Pulmonary edema   pp. 36–38

Pulmonary edema (fluid in the interstitial spaces of the lungs) is often associated with ineffective cardiac pumping action, as in left-sided ventricular heart disease. (Pulmonary edema associated with heart disease is discussed in Chapter 2, "Cardiology.") Non-cardiogenic pulmonary edema was discussed above under the objective for adult respiratory distress syndrome (ARDS).

g. Pulmonary thromboembolism pp. 54–56

A pulmonary embolism is a blood clot (thrombus) that lodges in an artery in the lungs. One in five cases of sudden death is caused by pulmonary thromboembolism. It is a life-threatening condition because it can significantly reduce pulmonary blood flow (perfusion), causing hypoxemia (lack of oxygen in the blood). Immobilization, such as recent surgery, a long bone fracture, or being bedridden, increases the risk of developing an embolism. Other risk factors for clot formation include pregnancy, oral birth control medications, cancer, and sickle cell anemia. The classic symptom of pulmonary embolism is a sudden onset of severe dyspnea, which may or may not be accompanied by pleuritic pain. The physical exam may reveal other signs including labored breathing, tachypnea, and tachycardia. In severe cases, there may be signs of right-sided heart failure, including jugular vein distention and possibly falling blood pressure. Auscultation may reveal no significant findings. In 50 percent of cases, examination of the extremities will reveal signs suggesting deep venous thrombosis (warm, swollen extremity with thick cord palpated along the medial thigh and pain on palpation or when extending the calf). Because a large embolism may cause cardiac arrest, be prepared to perform resuscitation. Primary care is aimed at support of the airway, breathing, and circulation. As necessary, assist ventilations and provide supplemental oxygen. Endoctracheal intubation may be required. Establish IV access, monitor vital signs and cardiac rhythms, and transport expeditiously to a facility that can care for the patient's critical needs.

h. Neoplasms of the lung pp. 51–52

Lung cancer (neoplasms, literally "new growths" or tumors) is the leading cause of cancer-related death in the U.S. in both men and women. The primary problems are disruption of diffusion and, if the bronchioles are involved, of ventilation as well. The primary risk factor is cigarette smoking. Inhalation of other environmental toxins is also a risk factor. Less commonly, lung cancer can result from the spread of cancer from another part of the body. EMS calls to patients with lung cancer may involve a variety of complaints related to the disease, including cough, hoarseness, chest pain, and bloody sputum. There may be fever, chills, and chest pain if the patient has developed pneumonia. There can be weakness, numbness of the arm, shoulder pain, and difficulty swallowing. The physical exam may reveal weight loss, crackles, wheezes, rhonchi, and diminished breath sounds in the affected lung. There may be venous distention of the arms and neck. Your primary responsibility is to identify and address signs of respiratory distress. Assist ventilation and administer supplemental oxygen as needed. Establish IV access and consult medical direction about possible administration of bronchodilators and corticosteroids. Transport, but be alert for any DNR (do not resuscitate) orders.

i. Upper respiratory infections (URI) pp. 48–49

Infections of the upper airways of the respiratory tract are among the most common infectious conditions for which patients seek medical assistance, and you will see them in the field. Even though these infections are rarely life-threatening, they can produce considerable discomfort. At-home management is usually symptomatic, with treatment for pain and fever, as needed, as well as appropriate antibiotic therapy if the infection is bacterial. However, a URI in a person with pre-existing pulmonary disease can trigger severe problems and you should pay particularly close attention to airway and ventilation in patients with asthma or COPD. Be sure to monitor the condition with pulse oximetry and ECG during transport to a treatment facility.

j. Spontaneous pneumothorax pp. 56–57

Spontaneous pneumothorax, which occurs in the absence of trauma, is a relatively common condition, occurring in roughly 18 persons per 100,000 population. It is relatively likely to recur as well (with 50% recurrence rate at two years). Significant risk factors include male gender, age 20 to 40 years, tall, thin stature, and history of cigarette smoking. Presentation is marked by sudden onset pleuritic chest or shoulder pain, often precipitated by a bout of coughing or by heavy lifting. The loss of negative pressure in the affected hemithorax prevents proper chest expansion, and the patient may report dyspnea. In individuals who do NOT have significant underlying pulmonary disease, a pneumothorax of up to 15 to 20% of the chest cavity can be tolerated fairly well. Monitor symptoms and pulse oximetry readings during transport. Be especially attentive in your ongoing assessment of patients who require positive-pressure ventilation. These patients are at higher risk for development of tension pneumothorax, which is marked by increasing resistance to ventilation, along with hypoxia, cyanosis, and possible hypotension. Exam will reveal tracheal deviation away from the affected side of the chest and distention of the jugular vein. Needle decompression of a tension pneumothorax may be required.

k. Hyperventilation syndrome   pp. 57–58

Hyperventilation, with rapid breathing, chest pain, and numbness in the extremities, is often associated with anxiety, and it is called hyperventilation syndrome in this setting. However, you should remember that a number of significant and common medical conditions can cause hyperventilation, including cardiovascular and pulmonary conditions such as acute myocardial infarction and pulmonary thromboembolism, sepsis, pregnancy, liver failure, and several metabolic and neurologic disorders. Be conservative and consider hyperventilation to be a sign of a serious medical problem until proven otherwise. Management centers on reassurance and assisting the patient to consciously decrease rate and depth of breathing, maneuvers that will increase PCO_2.

8. Given several preprogrammed patients with nontraumatic pulmonary problems, provide the appropriate assessment, prehospital care, and transport.   pp. 4–59

The airway is functionally divided into the upper airway and the lower airway. The upper airway is comprised of the nasal cavity, pharynx, and larynx. The lower airway is comprised of the trachea, bronchi, alveoli, and lungs. The ability to take in oxygen and excrete carbon dioxide via the airway is essential to life. Therefore, it is critical that you be able to identify and understand the function of each structure of the airway and of the airway as a whole.

CONTENT SELF-EVALUATION

MULTIPLE CHOICE

_____ 1. Two conditions in which respiration is frequently dependent on hypoxic respiratory drive and use of supplemental oxygen may induce respiratory depression are:
  A. asthma and pneumonia.
  B. spontaneous pneumothorax and pneumonia.
  C. asthma and emphysema.
  D. asthma and adult respiratory distress syndrome.
  E. chronic bronchitis and emphysema.

_____ 2. The pulmonary edema characteristic of adult respiratory distress syndrome (ARDS) is caused by:
  A. left-sided cardiac ventricular failure.
  B. right-sided cardiac ventricular failure.
  C. accumulation of fluid in the pulmonary interstitial spaces.
  D. obstruction of pulmonary capillaries by thrombi.
  E. chronic constriction of terminal airways and alveoli.

_____ 3. Factors that commonly cause acute aggravation of symptoms due to chronic obstructive pulmonary disease (COPD) include all of the following EXCEPT:
  A. progression of lung cancer.
  B. exertion, including heavy lifting and exercise.
  C. allergens such as foods and dust.
  D. tobacco smoke.
  E. occupational airborne pollutants such as chemical fumes.

_____ 4. Common physical attributes of a person with emphysema include all of the following EXCEPT:
  A. chronic cough.   D. pinkish tone to skin.
  B. barrel chest.   E. thin build.
  C. clubbing of the fingers.

_____ 5. Common physical attributes of a person with chronic bronchitis include all of the following EXCEPT:
A. chronic cough.
B. thin build.
C. bluish, cyanotic tone to skin.
D. cough producing large amounts of sputum.
E. ankle edema.

_____ 6. The epidemiology of asthma includes all of the following EXCEPT:
A. an increase in mortality rate over the past decade.
B. a death rate in whites that is roughly twice that in blacks.
C. the fact that it is a common disorder in both males and females.
D. mortality change seen mostly in persons over age 45 years.
E. the fact that half of asthma deaths occur in the prehospital setting.

_____ 7. Medications commonly used by persons with asthma include all of the following EXCEPT:
A. beta agonists administered via inhaler.
B. oral doses of aspirin.
C. anticholinergics administered via inhaler.
D. oral doses of corticosteroid.
E. cromolyn sodium administered via inhaler.

_____ 8. The chief management goals for an acute asthma attack involve improvement in:
A. blood pH (acidosis), hypoxia, and wheezing.
B. hypoxia, bronchospasm, and wheezing.
C. blood pH (acidosis), hypoxia, and local inflammation.
D. hypoxia, bronchospasm, and local inflammation.
E. hypoxia, wheezing, and local inflammation.

_____ 9. Be prepared for which of the following when caring for a patient with status asthmaticus?
A. respiratory acidosis with electrolyte imbalance
B. dehydration with early signs of renal failure
C. respiratory depression when administered supplemental oxygen
D. respiratory arrest requiring endotracheal intubation
E. tracheal inflammation causing airway obstruction

_____ 10. Upper respiratory infections can affect all of the following EXCEPT:
A. the sinuses.
B. the lungs.
C. the middle ear.
D. the nose.
E. the pharynx.

_____ 11. Pleuritic chest pain associated with pneumonia is:
A. dull and aching in character.
B. sharp or tearing in character.
C. cramplike and hard to localize.
D. likely to radiate to the jaw or left arm.
E. only present on deep inspiration.

_____ 12. Major risk factors for pneumonia are HIV infection, very young or old age, and immunosuppressive therapy.
A. True
B. False

_____ 13. Standard management of lung cancer includes all of the following EXCEPT:
A. checking for instructions such as DNR (do not resuscitate) orders.
B. placement of ECG leads for cardiac monitoring.
C. administration of supplemental oxygen.
D. airway and ventilatory support as needed.
E. emotional support of patient and family.

_____ 14. Roughly one in five cases of sudden death is due to pulmonary emboli.
   A. True
   B. False

_____ 15. The mortality rate for pulmonary emboli is greater than 50%.
   A. True
   B. False

_____ 16. Risk factors for pulmonary emboli include all of the following EXCEPT:
   A. obesity.
   B. pregnancy.
   C. prolonged immobilization.
   D. deep vein thrombophlebitis.
   E. use of oral contraceptives, especially in smokers.

_____ 17. The ventilation-perfusion mismatch characteristic of pulmonary embolism is due to loss of blood flow to a ventilated segment of lung tissue.
   A. True
   B. False

_____ 18. Common physical findings in pulmonary embolism include all of the following EXCEPT:
   A. evidence suggestive of deep venous thrombosis.
   B. labored, painful breathing.
   C. tachypnea and tachycardia.
   D. cardiac dysrythmias.
   E. normal chest auscultation.

_____ 19. Which of the following statements about spontaneous pneumothorax is FALSE?
   A. Most patients have acute onset pain in the chest or shoulder region.
   B. Onset of pain often follows coughing or heavy lifting.
   C. Spontaneous pneumothorax is much more common in women than in men.
   D. Spontaneous pneumothorax is more common among smokers and persons with COPD.
   E. Supplemental oxygen is sufficient therapy for the majority of patients with spontaneous pneumothorax.

_____ 20. The respiratory alkalosis of hyperventilation syndrome often results in:
   A. cramping of the muscles of the hands and feet.
   B. slowing of cardiac electrical conduction, causing bradycardia.
   C. cramping of facial muscles causing characteristic grimace.
   D. one of several cardiac dysrhythmias.
   E. altered mental status, specifically, lethargy and depression.

_____ 21. Respiratory emergencies due to central nervous system (CNS) dysfunction are relatively rare.
   A. True
   B. False

_____ 22. Numerous peripheral nervous system conditions can cause respiratory compromise, including the diseases of polio and amyotrophic lateral sclerosis, as well as Guillian-Barré syndrome.
   A. True
   B. False

_____ 23. The processes of ventilation, diffusion, and perfusion allow gas exchange to occur efficiently in the lungs and other body tissues. The derangement in pulmonary embolism is principally of:
  A. ventilation.
  B. diffusion.
  C. perfusion.
  D. a combination of ventilation and diffusion.
  E. a combination of diffusion and perfusion.

_____ 24. Carbon monoxide exposure is potentially life threatening because carbon monoxide displaces oxygen from hemoglobin in red blood cells.
  A. True
  B. False

_____ 25. The most common auscultation finding in a patient with pneumonia is:
  A. stridor over the involved segment.
  B. decreased or absent breath sounds over the involved segment.
  C. expiratory wheezing over the involved segment.
  D. crackles (rales) over the involved segment.
  E. pleural friction rub over the involved segment.

MATCHING

Match each respiratory emergency with its key prehospital management steps by writing the letter of the steps in the space provided next to the emergency.

_____ 26. adult respiratory distress syndrome (ARDS)

_____ 27. chronic obstructive pulmonary disease (COPD), either emphysema or chronic bronchitis

_____ 28. asthma

_____ 29. childhood epiglottitis

_____ 30. lung cancer

_____ 31. inhalation of a toxic substance

_____ 32. pulmonary embolism

  A. correct hypoxia, reverse bronchospasm, and reduce inflammation
  B. assure safety of rescue personnel, remove patient for transport, maintain open airway, and deliver humidified, high-concentration oxygen
  C. maintain airway and ventilation as needed, deliver oxygen, establish IV access, cardiac monitoring, and pulse oximetry, and transport to facility for care of underlying condition
  D. maintain airway, ventilation, and circulation as needed, deliver oxygen, establish IV access, cardiac monitoring, and pulse oximetry, and check extremities during transport to appropriate facility
  E. maintain airway and ventilation as needed with exception that examination of the throat should be avoided
  F. relieve hypoxia, reverse bronchoconstriction, assist ventilations as needed
  G. deliver oxygen, support ventilation as allowed by orders or advance directive, correct hypoxia as possible, and provide emotional support

SPECIAL PROJECT

Assessing Respiratory Emergencies

Read the assessment written for each of three patients evaluated in a prehospital setting and identify the probable cause for each emergency. Check the Assessment section of the textbook for each disorder to refamiliarize yourself with characteristic findings on history and physical examination.

Scenario 1: You are called to an elementary school where a student has become "suddenly ill" during a class birthday party. You find a distressed 7-year-old child who is breathing rapidly and shallowly and whose skin tone is becoming dusky. The use of accessory muscles to breathe is evident. The school nurse offers you a box containing an inhaler that she says the child uses on an "as needed" basis and states she isn't sure what ingredients were in the cupcakes brought for the party. She adds that the boy has several severe food allergies.

Probable cause: _____

Scenario 2: You are called to a home where an elderly man is "short of breath." On arrival, you find a thin, elderly man with a broad chest whose breathing is labored despite use of a home supplemental oxygen setup. His daughter tells you that he has had a cold recently, and he suddenly became "shorter of breath" this morning. On exam, the man has a fever of 101 degrees, is somewhat confused in answering your questions, and can say only 2–3 words before needing to breathe again. Breath sounds are diminished bilaterally and rales are present at the right base.

Probable cause for acute emergency: _____

Probable underlying disorder: _____

Scenario 3: You are called to a home where a visitor has fallen ill. The man's son tells you that his father had just arrived after a two-day car trip to visit the family and had seemed fine until after dinner. Then the older man complained of a sudden inability "to catch his breath" and "awful pain in the shoulder like a knife." The patient is standing over a couch, breathing rapidly and shallowly. Tachycardia is present but rhythm is even. Blood pressure is normal and chest auscultation is within normal limits.

Probable cause: _____

CHAPTER 2
Cardiology

Because Chapter 2 is lengthy, it has been divided into three parts to aid in your study. Read the assigned text pages, then progress through the objectives and self-evaluation materials as you would with other chapters. When you feel secure in your grasp of the content, proceed to the next part.

Part 1, pp. 68–157

Review of Chapter Objectives

After reading this part of the chapter, you should be able to:

1. Describe the incidence, morbidity, and mortality of cardiovascular disease. pp. 68, 258

Cardiovascular disease (CVD) is serious and extremely common, with more than 60 million Americans affected. Morbidity is considerable: An American has a nonfatal heart attack (myocardial infarction, MI) roughly every 29 seconds. Coronary heart disease (CHD), one type of CVD, is the single largest killer of Americans and Canadians. Roughly 466,000 Americans die annually from CHD, half of them before reaching a hospital. Many deaths from CHD are sudden and involve lethal cardiac dysrhythmias. Many deaths from MI occur within the first 24 hours, frequently within the first hour.

2. Discuss prevention strategies that may reduce the morbidity and mortality of cardiovascular disease. p. 68

There are two public health prevention strategies. The first is to educate people about the risk factors for CVD and encourage lifestyle modifications to minimize the potential impact of risk factors. The second strategy is to teach signs and symptoms of a heart attack so patients can receive medical intervention as soon as possible. As you will see, the likelihood of success with thrombolytic therapy for a heart attack in evolution (treatment with a clot-buster drug to dissolve the clot causing myocardial ischemia/hypoxia) is highest when care is instituted very early in the course of the attack.

3. Identify the risk factors most predisposing to coronary artery disease. p. 68

Factors proven to increase the risk of CVD include (1) smoking, (2) older age, (3) family history of cardiac disease, (4) hypertension, (5) hypercholesterolemia, (6) diabetes mellitus, (7) cocaine use, and (8) male gender. Factors that are thought to increase risk include (1) diet, (2) obesity, (3) oral contraceptives, (4) sedentary lifestyle, (5) Type A personality (competitive and aggressive), and (6) psychosocial tension (stress).

4. **Describe the anatomy of the heart, including the position in the thoracic cavity, layers of the heart, chambers of the heart, and location and function of the cardiac valves.** pp. 70–75

The adult heart is roughly the size of a clenched fist, and it lies in the center of the mediastinum posterior to the sternum and anterior to the spine. Roughly two-thirds of the heart lies to the left of midline, with roughly one-third to the right. The bottom of the heart, the apex, lies just above the diaphragm, whereas the top of the heart, or base, lies at roughly the level of the second rib. The heart's connections with the great vessels are at the base. The heart is made up of three tissue layers: The innermost is the endocardium, which has the same type of cells as the endothelial lining of blood vessels and is continuous with the linings of the vessels entering and leaving the heart. The thickest layer is the middle layer of muscle cells, the myocardium. These unique muscle cells physically resemble skeletal muscle but have electrical properties similar to smooth muscle cells. The outermost layer of the heart is the pericardium, a protective sac made of connective tissue arranged in two layers, the visceral pericardium (also called the epicardium) and the parietal pericardium. Normally, about 25 mL of pericardial fluid is contained between the two layers of pericardium, and the heart moves freely within the pericardial sac.

The heart is made up of two side-by-side pumps, the left side and the right side. Each side has an upper chamber, the atrium, which receives blood, and a lower chamber, the ventricle, which pumps blood into other blood vessels. The atria are separated by an interatrial septum, and the ventricles are separated by an interventricular septum. The atrial walls are thin in contrast with the ventricular walls, and almost all of the heart's pumping force is generated by the ventricles. The left ventricle, which pumps blood into the aorta, has a much thicker wall than the right ventricle, which pumps blood into the pulmonary artery (see Figures 2-2 to 2-5).

The heart contains two sets of valves that help to keep blood flowing properly through the chambers and into the aorta and pulmonary artery: The atrioventricular valves lie between each atrium and ventricle. The left atrioventricular valve is called the mitral valve, and it has two characteristic leaflets. The right atrioventricular valve is called the tricuspid valve, and it has three characteristic leaflets. When the papillary muscles that connect the valves to the walls of the heart relax, the leaflets open and blood flows from the atria into the ventricles. Special fibers called the chordae tendoneae connect the leaflets of a valve to the papillary muscles, and these fibers prevent the leaflets from prolapsing back into the atrium when the valve is open. The semilunar valves lie between the ventricles and the artery into which each empties. The left semilunar valve, or aortic valve, lies between the left ventricle and the aorta. The right semilunar valve, or pulmonic valve, lies between the right ventricle and the pulmonary artery. When these valves open, blood flows in a one-way path from the ventricles into the arteries, and backflow into the ventricles is prevented.

The superior and inferior vena cavae carry deoxygenated blood from the body to the right atrium. Blood flows through the right atrium and ventricle before entering the pulmonary artery, which carries it to the lungs. Oxygenated blood leaves the lungs through the pulmonary veins and enters the left atrium. The left ventricle pumps the blood into the aorta, which feeds the oxygenated blood into peripheral arteries to flow to the rest of the body. Pressure within the heart is markedly higher on the left than on the right because resistance to flow is higher in the peripheral circulation than it is in the pulmonary circulation. Consequently, the myocardium of the left ventricle thickens as an infant ages to the point that the adult left ventricle is markedly thicker than the right.

5. **Identify the major structures of the vascular system, the factors affecting venous return, the components of cardiac output, and the phases of the cardiac cycle.** pp. 76–78

In the pulmonary circulation, blood enters the lungs via the pulmonary arteries and their smaller branches, the arterioles. It eventually flows through capillaries that form networks over alveoli, and gas exchange (movement of oxygen into the blood and carbon dioxide from the blood) takes place here. The oxygenated blood then flows into the pulmonary venules and larger pulmonary veins and enters the left atrium. The peripheral circulation begins with the aorta, which receives oxygenated blood from the left ventricle. The aorta has numerous branches. These arteries and the smaller arterioles ensure oxygenated blood flows to all parts of the body. Oxygenated blood eventually enters capillary beds and oxygen exchange between blood and tissues occurs. Deoxygenated blood enters smaller venules, which empty into the larger veins that return blood to the right atrium. Gas exchange occurs in capillaries because their walls are only one cell thick. This same cell layer, the endothelium, is the innermost layer of arteries and veins.

Although the heart acts effectively as two side-by-side pumps, the contraction of the myocardium takes place as if the heart is one unit. The two atria contract at the same time, and the ventricles contract together. The atrioventricular valves open and close together, as do the two semilunar valves. The sequence of events that occurs between the end of one ventricular contraction and the next is called the cardiac cycle. Diastole, or relaxation phase, is the first part of the cycle. During diastole, blood enters the ventricles through the mitral and tricuspid valves. The aortic and pulmonic valves are closed, so the ventricles fill and no blood flows into the great vessels. During systole, the second phase, the heart contracts. First, the atria contract quickly, pumping the last of their blood into the ventricles. Then, when the pressure within the ventricles becomes greater than the pressure in the aorta and pulmonary artery, the semilunar valves open, the ventricles contract, and blood is pumped into the great arteries. This same pressure event closes the atrioventricular valves, eliminating backflow through the heart.

Under normal conditions, about two-thirds of the blood in the left ventricle at the end of diastole is pumped into the aorta during systole. This ratio of blood pumped to blood contained is called the cardiac ejection fraction. The amount of blood pumped by the left ventricle in one contraction is called the stroke volume, and it varies between roughly 60 and 100 mL, with an average of 70 mL. Cardiac output is defined as the amount of blood pumped in one minute. It is a function of stroke volume and heart rate: stroke volume (mL/beat) × heart rate (beats/minute) = cardiac output (mL/minute). Under average conditions, the heart rate is 60–100 bpm. Thus, average cardiac output = 70 mL × 70 bpm = 4,900 mL/minute, or almost 5L every minute.

6. Define preload, afterload, and left ventricular end-diastolic pressure and relate each to the pathophysiology of heart failure. **p. 78**

Stroke volume (the volume of blood pumped in one heartbeat) depends on three factors: preload, cardiac contractility, and afterload. The heart can only pump out the blood it receives during diastole. The pressure in the filled ventricle at the end of diastole is termed preload, or end-diastolic volume. Starling's law states that as the stretch on cardiac muscle increases (that is, as preload increases), the greater will be the force of the subsequent contraction. When preload increases, contraction pressure increases. Because the major factor determining preload is venous return from the body (or the lungs), the greater the venous return, the greater the preload and the greater the ventricular contraction pressure. Obviously, this only applies to a range of normal return volumes. If an excessive volume flows into the atrium, the atrium will become overly stretched and eventually weaken. For the left ventricle, which pumps blood to the body (including the vital brain, myocardium, and kidneys), preload is determined by venous return from the lungs. Afterload is the pressure against which the ventricles must contract to pump blood into the aorta and pulmonary arteries. An increase in afterload (peripheral resistance) decreases stroke volume. Conversely, a decrease in afterload eases the work of the ventricles and increases stroke volume.

Cardiac output (the amount of blood pumped into the aorta per minute) depends on left ventricular end-diastolic volume, myocardial contractility, and peripheral vascular resistance as measured at the origin of the aorta. Heart failure, the inability of the left ventricle to pump a physiologically adequate supply of blood, can result from a preload (ventricular end-diastolic volume) that is too low to allow effective pumping (a clinical example is shock), a reduction in cardiac contractility such that effective pumping is impossible (a clinical example is loss of myocardium through one or more MIs), or a significant increase in systemic vascular resistance (hypertension). In many cases, more than one factor (preload, contractility, afterload) may be chronically disturbed.

7. Identify the arterial blood supply to any given area of the myocardium. **p. 75**

The left coronary artery supplies the left ventricle, the interventricular septum, part of the right ventricle, and the heart's electrical conduction system. It has two main branches, the anterior descending artery and the circumflex artery. The right coronary artery supplies a portion of the right atrium and ventricle and part of the conduction system. It has two main branches, the posterior descending artery and the marginal artery. (Note that anatomic variants do exist.). There are normally numerous anastomoses, or connections, among the coronary arteries and their branches. Most of the blood drains from the coronary circulation through the anterior great cardiac vein and the lateral marginal veins into the coronary sinus. The right coronary artery empties directly into the right atrium via smaller cardiac veins.

8. Compare and contrast the coronary arterial distribution to the major portions of the cardiac conduction system. pp. 75, 78–80

Objective 7 explains the distribution of blood through the coronary artery system.

The pacemaker cells (those with the highest level of automaticity, and thus the drivers for all of the other conductive cells) are generally in the sinoatrial (SA) node, which is located high in the right atrium (an area supplied by the right coronary artery). One branch of the conduction system leads to the left atrium. Most of the conductive cells run in one of the internodal atrial pathways through the right atrial wall to meet at the atrioventricular (AV) node. The left coronary artery typically supplies these tissues.

The conduction system then passes through the bundle of His into the interventricular septum, where the right and left bundle branches become apparent as feeders of conduction branches into the walls of the right and left ventricles. The right bundle branch delivers the electrical impulse to the apex of the right ventricle. From there, the fibers of the Purkinje system spread it across the myocardium. The interventricular septum is typically supplied by the left coronary artery, as are the conduction fibers in the wall of the left ventricle. Some fibers in the right ventricular wall may be supplied by the right coronary artery.

9. Identify the structure and course of all divisions and subdivisions of the cardiac conduction system. pp. 78–84

The cardiac conduction system, which carries the electrical impulse that causes depolarization and contraction of myocardial cells, is shown in Figure 2-12. The pacemaker cells are normally found in the sinoatrial (SA) node, which is located high in the right atrium, and this is the usual origin of the electrical impulse that triggers each heartbeat. Several internodal atrial pathways carry the impulse from the SA node through the wall of the right atrium to the atrioventricular (AV) node. The impulse is carried to the left atrium via another pathway. At the AV junction, the conduction of the impulse is slowed (which allows adequate time for the ventricles to fill). The impulse moves from the AV junction via the AV fibers to the bundle of His, located high in the interventricular septum. The impulse then moves down the right and left bundle branches. The right bundle branch delivers the impulse to the apex of the right ventricle, and the fibers of the Purkinje system deliver it from there across the myocardium. The left bundle branch delivers the impulse to the thicker myocardium of the left ventricle. The left bundle branch does so via the anterior and posterior fascicles, both of which eventually terminate in the Purkinje system. Repolarization, which electrically readies the myocardial cells for the next heartbeat, proceeds in the opposite direction.

10. Identify and describe how the heart's pacemaking control, rate, and rhythm are determined. pp. 78–84

The cells with the highest degree of automaticity act as the heart's pacemakers, and these cells are usually found in the SA node, located high in the right atrium. On average, these cells generate impulses at the rate of 60–100 bpm. The cells of the AV node typically generate impulses at the lower rate of 40–60 bpm, and the cells of the Purkinje system, which also demonstrate automaticity, fire at roughly 15–40 bpm. Impulses generated in the SA node and conducted normally through the heart produce the ECG patterns characteristic of normal atrial rhythm.

Heart rate is controlled in part by the nervous system, and this level of control enables heart rate to accommodate the increased body oxygen need characteristic of exertion or stress. Regulation of heart rate by the autonomic nervous system is discussed in detail in objective 17.

11. **Explain the physiological basis of conduction delay in the AV node.** pp. 83–84

Not all fibers within the cardiac conduction system are the same size or absolutely alike in conduction properties. The fibers in the AV junction conduct impulses more slowly than most other conduction fibers, delaying the arrival of the electrical impulse in the AV node. Conduction within the AV node itself is also slower, and the cumulative effect is a delay that allows the ventricles time to fill properly before they contract, pumping blood out of the heart.

12. **Define the functional properties of cardiac muscle.** pp. 77–84

The heart is made up of three groups of cardiac muscle fibers: atrial, ventricular, and specialized excitatory and conductive fibers. Atrial and ventricular cardiac muscle is striated in the same way that skeletal muscle is structured, and contraction is much the same except for one notable difference. Cardiac muscle has unique structures called intercalated discs that physically connect muscle fibers and enable extremely swift conduction of impulses from fiber to fiber (with a speed approximately 400 times that of a normal cell membrane). This uniquely rapid conduction of an impulse among muscle fibers enables cardiac muscle to function effectively as a single contractile unit. This collective functional unit is termed a syncytium. The heart has two syncytia, the atrial syncytium and the ventricular syncytium. The atria contract together in a superior to inferior direction, expelling blood into the ventricles. The ventricles contract together in an inferior to superior direction, pumping blood into the pulmonary arteries and aorta. The syncytia are separated physically and physiologically by the fibrous structure that supports the atrioventricular valves. The only normal route for impulse conduction from the atria to the ventricles is through the AV node.

Thus, the syncytial myocardial cells have the functional properties of excitability (they can respond to an electrical stimulus), conductivity (they can send an impulse to an adjoining cell), and contractility (they respond to an electrical impulse by contracting).

The even more specialized myocardial cells of the conduction system have the same properties plus an additional one, automaticity. The conductive fibers show excitability and contractility similar to those of other myocardial cells. They have an even higher degree of conductivity, which enables them to transmit an impulse so quickly that it triggers syncytial myocardium to contract in a unified manner. Their unique property is automaticity: They have the ability to depolarize without any external stimulation. This property, which is also called self-excitability, is the basis for electrical initiation of each heartbeat. The conductive cells with the highest degree of automaticity (normally those in the SA node) act as the pacemaker for the whole cardiac unit.

13. **Define the events comprising electrical potential.** pp. 77–84

Impulse conduction and subsequent muscle fiber contraction are based functionally on depolarization of cells that maintain an electrical resting potential in the unstimulated state. Cardiac muscle cells (atrial, ventricular, and excitatory/conductive) expend energy to maintain a difference between the ion concentrations in the cell and those in the extracellular fluid. Pumps in the cell membrane expel sodium ions (Na^+) from the inside of the cell, making the inside of the cell more negatively charged than the surrounding extracellular fluid. This negative resting potential can be measured, and it is typically about –90 mV for a myocardial cell.

14. **List the most important ions involved in myocardial action potential and their primary function in this process.** p. 82

The three most important ions in cardiac function are potassium, sodium, and calcium. Proper amounts of potassium in the extracellular fluid and sodium in the internal cellular environment are vital to establish and maintain the resting potential. Extracellular concentration of calcium ions is vital for excitation of the cardiac contractile process.

15. **Describe the events involved in the steps from excitation to contraction of cardiac muscle fibers.** pp. 77–84

Impulse conduction and subsequent muscle fiber contraction are based functionally on depolarization of cells that maintain an electrical resting potential in the unstimulated state and are described in objective 13 above.

When a myocardial cell is stimulated by an electrical impulse, the membrane opens to ions. As Na^+ ions rush into the cell, the internal charge actually becomes positive relative to the outside environment—with a potential of roughly +20 mV—a change of 110 mV. The rapid influx of Na^+ ions and resultant change of membrane polarity is termed the action potential. During this same period when the membrane is permeable to ions, there is also a slower influx of Ca^{++} ions, which further increases the positive charge within the myocardial cell. After depolarization (the switch from a negative to a positive internal electrical potential) is complete, the syncytial muscle contracts as a unit. Just as rapidly (in a fraction of a second), the membrane pumps become active again, expel the excess ions, and re-establish the resting potential through repolarization of the membrane (re-establishment of the resting, negative potential).

16. Describe the clinical significance of Starling's law.   p. 78

Starling's law states that as the stretch on cardiac muscle increases (that is, as preload increases), the greater will be the force of the subsequent contraction. When preload increases, contraction pressure increases. Because the major factor determining preload is venous return from the body (or the lungs), the greater the venous return, the greater the preload and the greater the ventricular contraction pressure. If an excessive volume flows into the atrium, the atrium will become overly stretched and eventually weaken. For the left ventricle, which pumps blood to the body (including the vital brain, myocardium, and kidneys), preload is determined by venous return from the lungs.

17. Identify the structures of the autonomic nervous system and their effect on heart rate, rhythm, and contractility.   pp. 78-80

The sympathetic and parasympathetic components of the autonomic nervous system act in opposition to each other, and the balance of their effects regulates heart function. The sympathetic nervous system innervates the heart through the cardiac plexus of nerves, which is located at the base of the heart. Its neurotransmitter, norepinephrine, acts to increase heart rate and cardiac contractility. There are two types of receptors in the sympathetic nervous system. Alpha receptors are found mostly in the peripheral blood vessels, where they modulate vasoconstriction. The $beta_1$ receptors are mostly found within the heart; they are responsible for the increase in heart rate and contractility with sympathetic stimulation. ($Beta_2$ receptors are chiefly in the lungs and peripheral blood vessels, and their stimulation results in bronchodilation and vasodilation.) Parasympathetic innervation of the heart is through the vagus nerve (cranial nerve X). Its neurotransmitter is acetylcholine, and parasympathetic stimulation of the heart (most of the nerve fibers of the vagus end in the atria, although some innervate the upper ventricles) results in slowed heart rate and slowed atrioventricular conduction.

18. Define and give examples of positive and negative inotropism, chronotropism, and dromotropism.   p. 80

Inotropy refers to the strength of myocardial contraction. Sympathetic nervous stimulation acts as a positive inotropic agent, one that increases cardiac contractility. Parasympathetic stimulation, by acting as an opposite to sympathetic activity, acts as a negative inotropic agent. Chronotropy refers to heart rate (*chronos* = time). A positive chronotropic agent increases heart rate, whereas a negative chronotropic agent decreases heart rate. Sympathetic nervous stimulation acts as a positive chronotropic agent, whereas parasympathetic stimulation acts as a negative chronotropic agent. Dromotropy refers to the rate of impulse conduction. A positive dromotropic agent increases conduction speed, whereas a negative dromotropic agent slows impulse conduction.

19. Discuss the pathophysiology of cardiac disease and injury.   pp. 97–157

Adequate heart function depends on adequate venous return and other vascular factors, as well as the intrinsic factors of myocardial health and function and adequacy of the electrical conduction system. Hypertension, atherosclerosis, and diabetes are risk factors for cardiac disease because they damage blood vessels, including the coronary arteries. Impaired perfusion of the myocardium (particularly the left ventricle responsible for cardiac output to the body) can lead to ischemia or MI. If infarction occurs, the amount of functional myocardium decreases, and this can ultimately lead to a decrease in cardiac output dependent on the area involved and the amount of myocardium lost.

There are innate disorders of the electrical conduction system, including developmental variants such as the accessory pathways that can make dysrhythmias more likely (such as Wolff-Parkinson-White syndrome). In addition, ischemia or infarction of the fibers of the conduction system can also make development of dysrhythmias more likely, including some (such as the tachycardias and the ventricular dysrhythmias) that can impair cardiac output to some degree or be directly life-threatening by precluding any adequacy of cardiac output (namely, ventricular fibrillation).

External agents that can harm cardiac function and possibly damage cardiac tissue include drugs. In some cases, drugs used to treat cardiac dysfunction can cause different cardiac problems.

20. Explain the purpose of ECG monitoring and its limitations.   **p. 84**

The electrocardiogram (*electro* = electrical, *cardio* = heart, *gram* = record) visualizes the heart's electrical activity as recorded from skin-surface electrodes. The heart is the largest generator of electrical energy in the body, and this is conducted through the body to the skin. An ECG machine records changes in current as a positive impulse (shown on the machine or on a paper printout as an upward deflection), a negative impulse (shown as a downward deflection), or no change (a flat, isoelectric line). The pattern shown over time is a chronological record of the heart's electrical activity, and it is called a rhythm strip.

The ECG in no way assesses the contractility of the myocardium or the pumping ability of the left ventricle, only the electrical activity in the different regions of the heart. There are other limitations of ECG monitoring. Artifacts may occur on the tracing, deflections that do NOT reflect the electrical activity of the heart. Artifacts may be due to a variety of causes, including muscle tremor, shivering, movements by the patient, loose electrodes, interference at the 60-hertz range, and machine malfunction. It is important that you be able to recognize artifacts and try to eliminate them from the tracing.

21. Correlate the electrophysiological and hemodynamic events occurring throughout the entire cardiac cycle with the various ECG wave forms, segments, and intervals.   **pp. 88–95**

The components of an ECG tracing reflect the electrical changes in the heart with each impulse conducted through the heart (Figure 2-16):

- *P wave.* This first component of the ECG reflects atrial depolarization. On Lead II, it appears as a positive, rounded wave that comes before the QRS complex. Normally, this correlates hemodynamically with the opening of the AV valves and atrial contraction, which completes the filling of the ventricles with blood.
- *QRS complex.* This second component of the ECG reflects ventricular depolarization. The Q wave is the initial negative deflection after the P wave; the R wave is the first positive deflection after the P wave; and the S wave is the first negative deflection after the R wave. You should note that not all three waves need be present, and the shape of the QRS complex can vary among individuals. Normally, this correlates hemodynamically with the opening of the semilunar valves and ventricular contraction, pumping blood into the pulmonary arteries and aorta.
- *T wave.* The T wave, which follows the QRS complex, reflects repolarization of the ventricles. It is normally positive in Lead II, rounded, and moves in the same direction as the QRS complex. This is the correlate of ventricular relaxation after contraction.
- *U wave.* A U wave is an occasional finding; when it occurs, it follows the T wave and is usually positive in deflection. U waves are normal in some individuals. You should note that it reflects electrolyte abnormalities in other patients.

In addition, three time intervals and a segment of the ECG reading also have clinical significance:

- *P-R interval (called PRI or P-Q interval, PQI).* The P-R interval is the distance from the beginning of the P wave (the beginning of atrial depolarization) to the beginning of the QRS complex (the beginning of ventricular depolarization). It represents the time taken to send the impulse from the atria to the ventricles (the delay at the AV junction and node). The R wave is absent in some individuals, and in these patients you will see a P-Q interval instead. The terms PRI and PQI are used interchangeably.

- *QRS interval.* The QRS interval is the distance from the first deflection of the QRS complex to the last, and it represents the time necessary for ventricular depolarization and onset of ventricular contraction.
- *Q-T interval.* This is the distance from the beginning of the Q wave to the beginning of the T wave, and it represents the total duration of ventricular depolarization. The duration of the Q-T interval normally has an inverse relationship with heart rate. At increased heart rates (tachycardia), the Q-T interval is generally shortened. With bradycardia, Q-T interval is generally lengthened.
- *S-T segment.* This is the distance from the S wave to the beginning of the T wave, and generally it is isoelectric. In some states such as myocardial ischemia, this segment may be either elevated or depressed.

22. Identify how heart rates, durations, and amplitudes may be determined from ECG recordings. pp. 88–95

ECG graph paper is standardized such that paper always moves across the recording stylus at 22 mm/sec. (Each small box represents 0.04 second, and each large box is equivalent to five small boxes, or 0.20 second.) ECG paper also has time interval markings at the top of the paper, with marks placed at 3-second intervals (or 15 large boxes, 15 × 0.20 = 3.0 seconds).

Three methods exist for quickly establishing heart rate. First, if a patient has a regular rhythm, you can take the number of heartbeats in 6 seconds, multiply by 10, and get rate in beats per minute (bpm). Second, you can measure the R-R interval (also in a patient with a regular rhythm) in seconds, divide into 60, and you have heart rate per minute. If the R-R interval is 0.65 second, 60 ÷ 0.65 = 92 bpm. (Other methods using the R-R interval are described on text page 96) The triplicate method, also useful only in the case of a regular rhythm, requires you to find an R wave that falls on a dark line bordering a large box. You can then assign numbers corresponding to heart rate to the next six dark lines to the right: This equates to 300, 150, 100, 75, 60, and 50 bpm. The number corresponding to the dark line closest to the peak of the next R wave is a rough estimate of heart rate. Last, you can use a commercial heart rate calculator ruler. If you prefer this method, make sure you are comfortable with at least one alternative method that does not require a physical aid!

The same standardization of time allows you to calculate the durations of the physiologically important intervals in the ECG tracing: Normal P-R interval duration is 0.12–0.20 sec; QRS interval duration is 0.08–0.12 sec; and Q-T interval is 0.33–0.42 sec. A prolonged P-R interval is one that lasts longer than 0.20 second and represents an extended delay in the AV node. A prolonged Q-T interval is one longer than 0.42 second and is thought to be related to an increased risk of certain ventricular dysrhythmias and sudden death.

The amplitude of deflections is also standardized: When a machine is properly calibrated, an amplitude of two large boxes represents 1.0 mV.

23. Relate the cardiac surfaces or areas represented by the ECG leads. p. 85

A pair of electrodes constitutes a lead. In hospital settings, a specific 12-lead configuration is standard for ECGs. In the field, a 3-lead system is often used, although one lead is adequate for detection of life-threatening dysrhythmias. The chapter presents placement for a 3-lead ECG, as well as placement information for a 12-lead ECG.

A 3-lead configuration uses Leads I, II, and III, and it shows three axes of the heart (Figure 2-13):

- Lead I (bipolar placed on a limb: positive = left arm, negative = right arm), axis 0° (parallel to collarbones)
- Lead II (bipolar placed on a limb: positive = left leg, negative = right arm), axis 60° (right atrium downward toward apex)

- Lead III (bipolar placed on a limb: positive = left leg, negative = left arm), axis 120° (left atrium downward toward apex)

Addition of three unipolar (also termed augmented) leads adds additional axes of view:

- aVR (augmented/unipolar on right arm), axis 210°
- aVL (augmented/unipolar on left arm), axis –30°
- aVF (augmented/unipolar on left foot), axis 90°

Normal recordings from the augmented leads are similar to those for Leads I, II, and III except that the deflections for aVR are inverted. The inversion is because the axis is negative, that is, it points upward toward the base of the heart instead of downward toward the apex.

The six precordial (chest) leads permit a view of the horizontal plane of the heart, which makes it possible to distinguish activity in different parts of the left ventricle and in the septum. They are designated V_1–V_6; the letter V identifies them as unipolar leads.

The deflections are primarily downward for Leads V_1 and V_2 because the leads are nearer the base of the heart than the apex, and thus they reflect the direction of electronegativity during depolarization. Deflections are primarily upward for Leads V_4, V_5, and V_6 because they are nearer the apex, and thus they are in the direction of electropositivity during depolarization.

Table 2-2 (text page 95) summarizes the portions of the heart examined by each set of leads:

- Leads I and aVL evaluate activity in the left side of the heart in a vertical plane.
- Leads II, III, and aVF evaluate activity in the inferior (diaphragmatic) side of the heart.
- Lead aVR evaluates activity in the right side of the heart in a vertical plane.
- Leads V_1 and V_2 evaluate activity in the right ventricle.
- Leads V_3 and V_4 evaluate activity in the interventricular septum and the anterior wall of the left ventricle.
- Leads V_5 and V_6 evaluate activity in the anterior and lateral walls of the left ventricle.

Overall, Leads V_1–V_4 view the anterior surface of the heart, and Leads I and aVL view the lateral surface of the heart. Leads II, III, and aVF view the inferior surface of the heart. Abnormal activity in a given set of leads, particularly in combination with a clinical picture consistent with acute myocardial infarction, can allow earlier identification and intervention in the ischemia-infarction process.

Lead II gives the best view of the ECG waves, and it best depicts the conduction system's activity. In single-lead systems, the lead used is generally Lead II or a lead called modified chest lead 1 (MCL_1). The chapter, as well as the remainder of the text, uses Lead II as its monitor lead. A monitor lead can provide (1) the rate of heartbeat, (2) the regularity of heartbeat, and (3) the time for conduction of impulse throughout various parts of the heart.

A monitor lead CANNOT provide (1) the presence or location of infarct, (2) the axis deviation or chamber enlargement, (3) the right-to-left differences in conduction or impulse formation, and (4) the quality or presence of pumping action.

24. Differentiate among the primary mechanisms responsible for producing cardiac dysrhythmias. pp. 94–95, 97–157

Major causes of cardiac dysrhythmias include the following: (1) myocardial ischemia, (2) necrosis or infarction, (3) autonomic nervous system imbalance, (4) distention of the heart chambers (especially the atria, secondary to congestive heart failure), (5) blood gas abnormalities, including hypoxia and abnormal pH, (6) electrolyte imbalances (primarily calcium, potassium, and magnesium), (7) trauma to the myocardium (namely, cardiac contusion), (8) drug effects and drug toxicity, (9) electrocution, (10) hypothermia, (11) CNS damage, (12) idiopathic events, (13) normal occurrences.

Note that dysrhythmias in a healthy heart are of little significance.

25. Describe a systematic approach to the analysis and interpretation of cardiac dysrhythmias. pp. 95–97

The following characterize normal sinus rhythm: (1) heart rate between 60 and 100 bpm; (2) regular rhythm, with constant P-P and R-R intervals; (3) P waves that are normal in shape, upright, and appear only before each QRS complex; (4) P-R interval that is constant and lasting 0.12–0.20 second; and (5) QRS complex with normal shape and duration less than 0.12 second. Any deviation from the normal electrical rhythm constitutes a dysrhythmia. The term arrhythmia is properly reserved for states in which there is no cardiac electrical activity.

Dysrhythmias can be approached in a number of ways, including nature of origin (namely, changes in automaticity versus disturbances in conduction), magnitude (major versus minor), severity (life-threatening versus non-life-threatening), and site (or location) of origin. This book classifies dysrhythmias into six categories by origin: (1) dysrhythmias originating in the SA node; (2) dysrhythmias originating in the atria; (3) dysrhythmias originating within the AV junction; (4) dysrhythmias sustained or originating in the AV junction; (5) dysrhythmias originating in the ventricles; (6) dysrhythmias resulting from disorders of conduction.

26. Describe the dysrhythmias originating in the sinus node, the AV junction, the atria, and the ventricles. pp. 99–157

Sinus bradycardia results from slowing of impulse generation in the SA node and may be due to increased parasympathetic (vagal) tone, intrinsic disease of the SA node, drug effects (typically digitalis, propranolol [a beta blocker], or quinidine), or it may be found as a normal finding in a healthy, well-conditioned person.

Sinus bradycardia on the ECG: rate less than 60 bpm, rhythm regular, pacemaker site SA node, P waves upright and normal in shape, P-R interval normal in duration and constant, QRS complex normal in duration.

Clinical significance occurs when decreased heart rate causes decreased cardiac output, hypotension, angina, or CNS symptoms; this is especially likely when rate is less than 50 bpm. Slow heart rate may also lead to atrial ectopic or ventricular ectopic rhythms. However, in a healthy athlete, sinus bradycardia may have no clinical significance.

Sinus tachycardia results from an increased rate of SA node discharge, and it may result from any of the following: exercise, fever, anxiety, hypovolemia, anemia, pump failure, increased sympathetic tone, hypoxia, or hyperthyroidism.

Sinus tachycardia on the ECG: rate greater than 100 bpm, rhythm regular, pacemaker site SA node, P waves upright and normal in shape, P-R interval normal, and QRS complex normal in duration.

Clinical significance occurs when sinus tachycardia is a compensatory mechanism for decreased stroke volume. If the rate is greater than 140 bpm, cardiac output may fall because ventricular filling time is inadequate. Very rapid rates increase myocardial oxygen demand and may precipitate ischemia or even infarct in diseased hearts. Prolonged sinus tachycardia accompanying acute myocardial infarction (AMI) is often an ominous finding suggesting cardiogenic shock.

Sinus dysrhythmia often results from a variation of the R-R interval. It may be a normal finding sometimes related to the respiratory cycle and changes in intrathoracic pressure. Pathologically, sinus dysrhythmia can be caused by increased parasympathetic (vagal) tone.

Sinus dysrhythmia on the ECG: rate 60–100 bpm and varying with respiration, rhythm irregular, pacemaker site SA node, P waves upright and normal in shape, P-R interval normal, and QRS complex normal.

Clinical significance is minimal. Sinus dysrhythmia is a normal variant, particularly in the young and the aged.

Sinus arrest occurs when the SA node fails to discharge an impulse, resulting in short periods of cardiac standstill. This standstill can persist until pacemaker cells lower in the conductive system discharge (generating escape beats) or until the sinus node resumes discharge. Sinus arrest can result from ischemia of the SA node, digitalis toxicity, excessive parasympathetic (vagal) tone, or degenerative fibrotic disease.

Sinus arrest on the ECG: rate is normal to slow, depending on the frequency and duration of the arrest, rhythm is irregular, pacemaker site is the SA node, P waves are upright and normal in shape, P-R interval and QRS complex are normal.

Clinical significance is that frequent or prolonged episodes may compromise cardiac output, resulting in syncope or other problems. There is always the danger of complete loss of SA node activity. Usually, an escape rhythm develops; cardiac standstill, however, may result.

Dysrhythmias originating in the atrioventricular (AV) junction may be due to malfunction in the junctional cells themselves or due to a slowing or blockage in conduction of an impulse from the atria to the ventricles through the AV junction. The group of dysrhythmias termed atrioventricular (AV) blocks originate within the AV junction, and they can be due to either pathology within the AV junctional tissue or to a physiological block such as atrial fibrillation.

First-degree AV block actually involves a delay in conduction at the level of the AV node rather than a complete blockage. Thus, first-degree AV block is not a rhythm itself but a condition imposed on an underlying rhythm; you must be able to establish the underlying rhythm. Although first-degree AV block can occur in a healthy heart, it is most commonly due to ischemia at the AV junction.

First-degree AV block on the ECG: rate dependent upon underlying rhythm, rhythm usually regular although it can be slightly irregular, pacemaker site either SA node or atrial, P waves normal, P-R interval longer than 0.20 sec (this is diagnostic), and QRS complex usually less than 0.12 second, but may be bizarre in shape if conductive system disease exists in the ventricles.

Clinical significance lies not in first-degree block, which is usually no danger itself, but rather in the possibility that the observed AV block may precede development of a more advanced block.

Type I second-degree AV block (also termed *second-degree Mobitz I or Wenckebach*) represents an intermittent block at the AV node. The characteristic cyclic pattern features progressively longer P-R intervals followed by a completely blocked impulse. The cycle is repetitive, and the P-P interval remains constant. The ratio of conducted to nonconducted impulses (seen as P waves to QRS complexes) is commonly 5:4, 4:3, 3:2, or 2:1. The pattern may be either constant or variable. Although this type of AV block occurs in healthy hearts, it is most common with ischemia at the AV junction. Additional causes include increased parasympathetic (vagal) tone and drug effect.

Type I second-degree AV block on the ECG: atrial rate is unaffected, whereas ventricular rate may be either normal or slowed. Atrial rhythm is typically regular, whereas ventricular rhythm is irregular because of the nonconducted beats, pacemaker site may be either in SA node or atria, P waves are normal, but the P waves for nonconducted impulses are not followed by QRS complexes. P-R interval becomes progressively longer until QRS complex is dropped, then the cycle repeats. QRS complex is usually shorter than 0.12 second but may be bizarre in shape if conductive system disease exists in the ventricles.

Clinical significance lies in decreased cardiac output if beats are frequently dropped; symptoms include syncope and angina. Note that this block may occur as a transient phenomenon immediately after an inferior wall MI.

Type II second-degree AV block is also called *second-degree Mobitz II* or *infranodal block.* This is also an intermittent block, but it is characterized by P waves that are not conducted to the ventricles without any change in length of the P-R interval before a beat is dropped. The ratio of conduction (P waves to QRS complexes) is commonly 4:1, 3:1, or 2:1, and the ratio may either be constant or vary. A 2:1 Mobitz II block is often indistinguishable from a 2:1 Mobitz I block. Type II second-degree block is usually associated with acute MI and septal necrosis.

Type II second-degree AV block presentation on the ECG: atrial rate is unaffected, whereas ventricular rate is usually bradycardic. Rhythm may be regular or irregular, dependent on whether conduction ratio is constant or variable. Pacemaker site is in the SA node or atria. P waves are normal, although some P waves are not followed by QRS complexes. The P-R interval is constant for conducted beats, but may be longer than 0.21 second. QRS complex may be normal, although it is often longer than 0.12 second because of the abnormal depolarization sequence.

Clinical significance is in the possibility of decreased cardiac output. Because this block is often associated with cell necrosis secondary to MI, it is considered more serious than Mobitz I. Many Mobitz II blocks develop into full AV blocks.

Third-degree AV block, or *complete block,* is characterized by the absence of conduction between the atria and ventricles due to complete electrical block at or below the AV node. In this case, the atria and ventricles pace independently of each other. The sinus node frequently functions normally, depolarizing the atrial syncytium, whereas an escape pacemaker below the atria paces the ventricular syncytium. Third-degree block can occur with acute MI, digitalis toxicity, or degeneration of the conductive system as can occur in the elderly.

Third-degree AV block on the ECG: Atrial rate is unaffected. Ventricular rate is 40–60 bpm if escape pacemaker is junctional, less than 40 bpm if pacemaker is lower in the ventricles. Both the atrial and ventricular rhythms are usually regular. Pacemaker site is typically SA node for atria, AV junction or ventricular for ventricles. P waves are normal but show no relationship to QRS complexes, often falling within the T wave and QRS complex. There is no relationship between the P-R interval and either P waves or R waves. The QRS complex is longer than 0.12 second if the pacemaker is ventricular and less than 0.12 second if pacemaker is junctional.

Clinical significance lies in severe compromise of cardiac output due to decreased ventricular contraction rate and loss of coordinated atrial kick.

A third group of dysrhythmias can originate in the AV junction or AV node, and these include premature junctional contractions, junctional escape complexes and rhythms, accelerated junctional rhythm, and paroxysmal junctional tachycardia. All four of these dysrhythmias share some ECG features: (1) There are inverted P waves on Lead II resulting from the retrograde depolarization of the atria. The P wave's relation to QRS depolarization depends on the relative timing of atrial and ventricular depolarization. The P wave can appear first if the atria depolarize first, or the QRS can come first if the ventricles depolarize first. If all chambers depolarize at the same time, the P wave and QRS complex can be superimposed, which effectively masks the P wave. P-R interval is less than 0.12 second, and there is normal duration of the QRS complex.

Premature junctional contractions (PJCs) result from a single impulse originating in the AV node that occurs before the next expected sinus beat; thus the beat is considered "premature." A PJC causes a compensatory pause when the SA node discharges before the premature impulse reaches it. A PJC is associated with a noncompensatory pause if the premature impulse depolarizes the sinus node and interrupts the heart's normal cadence. PJCs can result from a number of conditions, including use of alcohol, tobacco, or caffeine, sympathomimetic drugs, ischemic heart disease, hypoxia, digitalis toxicity, or from no apparent cause (idiopathic).

PJC presentation on the ECG: Rate and rhythm depend on underlying rhythm, and rhythm is usually regular except for the PJC. Pacemaker site is an ectopic focus in the AV junction. P waves are inverted and may appear before or after the QRS complex. P-R interval is less than 0.12 second if P wave occurs before QRS and is actually an R-P interval if P wave follows QRS complex. QRS complex itself is usually normal, although it may be longer than 0.12 second if the PJC is through the partially refractory ventricles.

Clinical significance of isolated PJCs is minimal. Frequent PJCs suggest organic heart disease and may be precursors of other junctional dysrhythmias.

A *junctional escape beat,* or a *junctional escape rhythm,* is a dysrhythmia that results when the primary pacemaker, usually the SA node, is slower than that of the AV node. The AV node becomes the pacemaker, generally discharging at its typical 40–60 bpm. This is a compensatory mechanism that prevents cardiac standstill. Junctional escape has several etiologies, including increased vagal tone, which can result in SA node slowing, pathological SA node discharge, or heart block.

Junctional escape rhythm presentation on the ECG: Rate typically 40–60 bpm, rhythm irregular in single junctional escape complex or regular in junctional escape rhythm. Pacemaker site is the AV node. P waves are inverted and may have any relationship to the QRS complex. P-R interval is less than 0.12 second if P wave occurs before QRS and is actually an R-P interval if P wave follows QRS complex. QRS complex is generally normal, although it may be greater than 0.12 second.

Clinical significance is decreased cardiac output due to slowed heart rate, with associated risk for precipitation of angina, syncope, or other problems. If rate is fairly rapid, rhythm may be well tolerated.

Accelerated junctional rhythms result from increased automaticity in the AV junction, causing the AV junction to discharge faster than its intrinsic rate. If the rate is fast enough, it will override the SA node. Accelerated junctional rhythm is not fast enough to qualify as tachycardia; however, it is considered accelerated because it is much faster than the typical junctional rate. A common cause is ischemia of the AV junction.

Accelerated junctional rhythm on ECG: Rate is 60–100 bpm, rhythm is regular, and pacemaker site is AV junction. P waves are inverted and may have any relationship with the QRS complex. P-R interval is less than 0.12 second if P wave occurs before QRS and is actually an R-P interval if P wave follows QRS complex. QRS complex is normal.

Clinical significance lies in the possible cause of ischemia, which can precipitate other, much less well-tolerated dysrhythmias.

Paroxysmal junctional tachycardia (PJT) develops when rapid AV junctional depolarization overrides the SA node. It often occurs in paroxysms (sudden episodes), which may last minutes or hours before terminating abruptly. It may be due to increased automaticity of a single AV nodal focus or by a reentry phenomenon at the AV node. PJT is often more appropriately called paroxysmal supraventricular tachycardia (PSVT) because the rapid rate may make it indistinguishable from paroxysmal atrial tachycardia. PJT may occur at any age and may or may not be related to underlying heart disease. Stress, overexertion, tobacco, and caffeine may precipitate it. However, it is frequently associated with underlying atherosclerotic heart disease (ASHD) and rheumatic heart disease. PJT rarely occurs with MI. It can occur with accessory pathway conduction such as Wolff-Parkinson-White syndrome.

PJT on the ECG: Rate 100–180 bpm, with characteristically regular rhythm except at onset and termination of paroxysm. Pacemaker site is AV junction. If present, P waves are inverted and may have any relationship with the QRS complex. Turning up the speed of the ECG recording to 55 mm/sec spreads out the complex and may aid in identifying P waves. P-R interval is less than 0.12 second if P wave occurs before QRS complex and is actually an R-P interval if P wave follows QRS complex. QRS complex is normal.

Clinical significance in younger patients with good cardiac reserve is minimal for a short time, and the patient usually perceives the PJT as palpitations. However, rapid rate decreases ventricular filling time and thus markedly decreases cardiac output. The reduced diastolic phase of the cardiac cycle can also compromise coronary artery perfusion. PJT can precipitate angina, hypotension, or congestive heart failure.

Dysrhythmias can also originate in atrial tissue outside the SA node or in the internodal pathways.

Atrial tachycardia, also called *ectopic tachycardia* or *wandering pacemaker,* is the passive transfer of pacemaker sites from the SA node to other latent sites in the atria or AV junction. Often more than one pacemaker site is present, causing variation in the R-R interval and P wave morphology. Atrial tachycardia can arise as a variant of sinus dysrhythmia, as a normal phenomenon in the very young or aged, or as part of ischemic heart disease or atrial dilation.

Atrial tachycardia on the ECG: Rate is usually normal, and rhythm is slightly irregular. Pacemaker site varies among SA node, atrial tissue, and AV junction. P wave morphology changes from beat to beat (as pacemaker site changes), or there may be no P waves present. P-R interval varies. It may be less than 0.12 second, normal, or longer than 0.20 second. QRS complex is normal.

Clinical significance is minimal because there are usually no detrimental effects. Occasionally, atrial tachycardia may precede other atrial dysrhythmias such as atrial fibrillation, and sometimes it may signal digitalis toxicity.

Multifocal atrial tachycardia (MAT) is usually found in acutely ill patients, and about 60% of them will have significant pulmonary disease. Certain medications used for pulmonary indications (such as theophylline) may worsen the dysrhythmia. At least three different P waves are noted, indicating the various ectopic foci. MAT can result from pulmonary disease, metabolic disorders (namely, hypokalemia), ischemic heart disease, or occur after recent surgery.

Multifocal atrial tachycardia on the ECG: Rate greater than 100 bpm, rhythm irregular. Pacemaker sites are ectopic sites in the atria. There are organized, discrete nonsinus P waves with at least three different forms. P-R interval varies, and the duration of the QRS complex may be less than 0.12 second, normal, or longer than 0.20 second, dependent on the AV node's refractory status when the ectopic impulse reaches it.

Clinical significance lies in the fact most affected patients are acutely ill; this dysrhythmia may indicate a serious underlying medical illness.

Premature atrial contractions (PACs) result from a single electrical impulse originating in the atria outside the SA node, which in turn causes a premature depolarization before the next expected SA impulse. Because the premature impulse depolarizes the atrial syncytium and the SA node, there is a noncompensatory pause in the underlying rhythm. PACs may result from use of caffeine, tobacco, or alcohol, use of sympathomimetic drugs, ischemic heart disease, hypoxia, digitalis toxicity, or no apparent cause (idiopathic).

PACs on the ECG: Rate and rhythm depend on underlying rhythm, with rhythm generally regular except for PAC. Pacemaker site is an ectopic focus in the atria. The P wave of the PAC is different than the P waves of the underlying rhythm. It occurs earlier than the next expected P wave and may be masked by the preceding T wave. The P-R interval is usually normal, although it may vary with the location of the ectopic focus. Foci near the SA node have a P-R interval of 0.12 second or longer, whereas ectopic foci near the AV node have an interval of 0.12 second or less. The QRS complex is usually normal, although duration may exceed 0.12 second if the PAC is abnormally conducted through the partially refractory ventricles. If the ventricles are refractory and do not depolarize, there will not be a QRS complex.

Clinical significance is slight for isolated PACs. However, frequent PACs may indicate organic heart disease and may precede other atrial dysrhythmias.

Paroxysmal supraventricular tachycardia (PSVT) occurs when rapid atrial depolarization overrides the SA node; this often occurs in a sudden onset paroxysm that may last minutes to hours before terminating abruptly. It may be caused by increased automaticity of a single atrial focus or by reentry at the AV node. PSVT may occur at any age and often is not associated with underlying heart disease. It may be precipitated by stress, overexertion, tobacco, or caffeine. It frequently is associated with underlying atherosclerotic cardiovascular disease and rheumatic heart disease. PSVT is rare in patients with MI; it can occur in patients with Wolff-Parkinson-White syndrome.

PSVT on the ECG: Rate 150–250 bpm, rhythm usually regular except at onset and termination of paroxysm. Pacemaker site is in the atria outside the SA node. The atrial P waves vary slightly from the sinus P waves. The atrial P wave may be impossible to see, especially when rate is rapid. Turning up the speed of the machine to 50 mm/sec spreads out the complex and may help in identifying P waves. The P-R interval is usually normal, although it may vary with location of the ectopic focus. Ectopic pacemakers near the SA node have intervals close to 0.12 second, whereas foci near the AV node have intervals of 0.12 second or less. The QRS complex is normal.

Clinical significance is less in younger patients with good cardiac reserve, who may tolerate PSVT well for short periods. Patients often perceive PSVT as palpitations. Rapid rates are associated with decreased cardiac output due to inadequate ventricular filling time. The shortened diastolic phase of the cardiac cycle can compromise coronary artery perfusion. PSVT may precipitate angina, hypotension, or congestive heart failure.

Atrial flutter results from a rapid atrial reentry circuit and an AV node that physiologically cannot conduct all impulses through to the ventricles. The AV junction may allow impulses in a 1:1, 2:1, 3:1, or 4:1 ratio or greater, resulting in a discrepancy between atrial and ventricular rates. AV block may be consistent or variable. Atrial flutter may occur in normal hearts but is usually associated with organic disease. Atrial dilation with congestive heart failure is a cause of atrial flutter. MI is only rarely a cause.

Atrial flutter on the ECG: Atrial rate 250–350 bpm, with ventricular rate dependent on ratio of AV conduction. Atrial rhythm is regular; ventricular rhythm may be regular or irregular if block is variable. Pacemaker sites are in the atria outside the SA node. Rather than a P wave, F (flutter) waves are present, which resemble sawteeth or a picket-fence pattern. This pattern may be difficult to identify in a 2:1 flutter. However, if the ventricular rate is 150 bpm, suspect 2:1 flutter. The P-R interval is usually constant but may vary, and the QRS complex is normal.

Clinical significance depends on ventricular rate. Flutter with normal ventricular rates is generally well tolerated. Rapid ventricular rates may compromise cardiac output and result in symptoms. Atrial flutter often occurs in conjunction with atrial fibrillation and is then termed atrial fib-flutter.

Atrial fibrillation results from multiple areas of reentry within the atria or from multiple ectopic foci bombarding an AV node that physiologically cannot handle all the incoming impulses. AV conduction is random and highly variable. Atrial fibrillation may be chronic and is often associated with underlying heart disease, such as rheumatic or atherosclerotic heart disease or congestive heart failure. Atrial dilation occurs with congestive heart failure and often causes atrial fibrillation.

Atrial fibrillation on the ECG: Atrial rate approximately 350–750 bpm, ventricular rate highly variable depending on conduction through AV node. Rhythm is slightly irregular.

Pacemaker sites are numerous ectopic foci in the atria. P waves are not discernible. Fibrillation (f) waves are present, indicating chaotic atrial activity. There is no P-R interval, but the QRS complex is normal.

Clinical significance is in loss of atrial contraction with atrial kick, thus reducing cardiac output 20–25%. There is frequently a pulse deficit between the apical and peripheral pulse rates. If rate of ventricular response is normal, as often occurs in patients on digitalis, the rhythm may be well tolerated. If the ventricular rate is less than 60 bpm, cardiac output may fall. Suspect digitalis toxicity in patients with atrial fibrillation and a ventricular rate less than 60 bpm. If ventricular response is rapid and coupled with loss of atrial kick, cardiovascular decompensation may occur with hypotension, angina, infarct, congestive heart failure, or shock.

Patients with accessory pathways such as those with Wolff-Parkinson-White who develop atrial flutter or atrial fibrillation present special concerns. Verapamil, which decreases conduction through the AV node and may shorten the refractory period of the accessory path, may precipitate either ventricular tachycardia or ventricular fibrillation.

Dysrhythmias originating in the ventricles are associated with many causes, including ischemia, hypoxia, and certain medications. The location of the pacemaker site dictates the shape of the QRS complex.

A *ventricular escape beat (ventricular escape rhythm* or *idioventricular rhythm)* results when impulses from higher pacemakers fail to reach the ventricles or when the discharge rate of higher pacemakers falls to less than that of the ventricles (normally 15–40 bpm). Ventricular escape rhythms are compensatory mechanisms that prevent cardiac standstill. There are several etiologies, including slowing of supraventricular pacemaker sites or high-degree AV block. They are frequently the first organized rhythms seen following successful defibrillation.

Ventricular escape rhythms on ECG: Rate generally 15–40 bpm or less, with irregular rhythm in a single ventricular escape complex. Escape rhythm is usually regular unless the pacemaker site is low in the ventricular conduction system. The pacemaker site is the ventricles, and there are no P waves and no P-R intervals. The QRS complex is longer than 0.12 second and bizarre in shape.

Clinical significance lies in decreased cardiac output secondary to slow heart rate. Ventricular escape rhythms are a safety mechanism that you should NOT suppress. Escape rhythms may be either perfusing or nonperfusing.

Accelerated idioventricular rhythm, a subtype of ventricular escape rhythm, is an abnormally wide ventricular dysrhythmia typically associated with an acute MI. The rate is usually 60–110 bpm, and the patient does not require treatment unless hemodynamic instability is present, in which case the ventricular focus should be treated with atropine or overdrive pacing. The principal goal is treatment of the underlying MI.

Premature ventricular contraction (PVC) is a single ectopic impulse arising in a focus in either ventricle that occurs before the next expected beat in the underlying rhythm. PVCs may result from increased automaticity in the ectopic cell or by a reentry mechanism. The alteration in ventricular depolarization results in a wide and bizarre QRS complex and may, in addition, cause the T wave to deflect in the direction opposite to the QRS complex. Because PVCs normally do not depolarize the SA node and interrupt its rhythm, these ectopic beats lead to a fully compensatory pause. Occasionally, a PVC is interpolated between two sinus beats without causing any disturbance in the underlying rhythm. If more than one PVC is observed, it may be possible to distinguish whether there is one (unifocal) or multiple (multifocal) ectopic foci. PVCs with the same morphology imply the same focus. If the coupling interval (the distance between the preceding beat and the PVC) is constant for multiple PVCs, then the PVCs are probably unifocal. PVCs often occur in cluster patterns, including bigeminy (where every other beat is a PVC), trigeminy (where every third beat is a PVC), and quadrigeminy (where every fourth beat is a PVC). Repetitive PVCs are a pattern of two or more PVCs without a normal (sinus) beat between them, and they typically occur as couplets or triplets. More than three consecutive PVCs are often considered ventricular tachycardia. Causes of PVCs include myocardial ischemia, increased sympathetic tone, hypoxia, acid-base disturbances, electrolyte imbalances, normal variation, and idiopathic cases.

PVCs on the ECG: Rate depends on underlying rhythm and rate of PVCs, rhythm of PVCs interrupts regularity of underlying rhythm and is occasionally irregular, and pacemaker site is within a ventricle. P waves are absent; however, a normal sinus P wave may appear before a PVC. There is thus no P-R interval. The QRS complex of the PVC is longer than 0.12 second and bizarre in morphology.

Clinical significance may be slight in patients without heart disease, who sense the PVC as a skipped beat. In patients with myocardial ischemia, PVCs may suggest ventricular irritability and may precede lethal ventricular dysrhythmias. PVCs are often classified as benign or malignant. Malignant PVCs show at least one of five traits: (1) more than six PVCs/minute; (2) R on T phenomenon; (3) couplets or runs of ventricular tachycardia; (4) multifocal in nature; and (5) associated chest pain. Because the ventricles do not fill properly with most PVCs, you will usually not feel a pulse during the PVCs themselves. Grades 0–5 on the Lown system equate the combination of malignant PVC traits to a numerical score. Grade 0 has no PVCs, whereas Grade 4 has repetitive PVCs (couplets or triplets) and Grade 5 shows R on T phenomenon.

Treatment is indicated for patients with a prior history of heart disease or symptoms or if the PVCs are malignant.

Ventricular tachycardia (VT) consists of three or more consecutive ventricular complexes at a rate of 100 bpm or higher. This rhythm overrides the heart's normal pacemaker, and thus the atria and ventricles are asynchronous. In monomorphic VT all complexes appear the same, whereas in polymorphic VT the complexes appear in difference sizes and shapes. The causes for VT are the same as for PVCs.

VT on the ECG: Rate roughly 100–250, with regular or slightly irregular rhythm, and pacemaker site in a ventricle. If P waves are present, they are not associated with the QRS complexes. There is no P-R interval, and the QRS complex is longer than 0.12 second and bizarre in morphology.

Clinical significance lies in the poor stroke volume and rapid rate associated with VT, which may cause severe compromise in cardiac output and coronary artery perfusion. Always remember that VT may deteriorate into ventricular fibrillation. Treatment type depends on whether VT is perfusing or nonperfusing.

Ventricular fibrillation is a chaotic ventricular rhythm that usually results from many reentry circuits within the ventricles. There is no ventricular depolarization or contraction. Although many causes have been identified, it is notable that most result from advanced coronary artery disease.

Ventricular fibrillation on ECG: There is no organized rate or rhythm, and P waves are usually absent. P-R interval is absent, as are QRS complexes. The pacemaker sites are numerous ectopic foci within the ventricles.

Clinical significance is the lethal nature of this dysrhythmia due to lack of cardiac output or organized electrical pattern within the heart.

Asystole is cardiac standstill marked by absence of all cardiac electrical activity. Asystole may be the primary event in cardiac arrest; it is usually associated with massive MI, ischemia, and necrosis. It may result from heart block when no escape pacemaker takes over, and asystole is often the final outcome of ventricular fibrillation.

Asystole on the ECG: No electrical activity with complete absence of P waves, QRS complexes, and T waves.

The likelihood of successful resuscitation is very low.

Artificial pacemaker rhythm results from regular cardiac stimulation by an electrode implanted in the heart and connected to a power source. Demand pacemakers represent an escape rhythm. Ventricular pacemakers stimulate only the right ventricle, resulting in an idioventricular-type rhythm. Dual-chambered pacemakers (also called AV sequential pacemakers) stimulate the atria and then the ventricles. Pacemakers are typically implanted in patients who have chronic high-grade heart block or sick sinus syndrome or who have had episodes of severe symptomatic bradycardia.

Pacemakers on the ECG: Rate varies with the preset rate of the pacemaker. Rhythm is regular if the heart is paced constantly, whereas rhythm is irregular if pacing is on demand. Pacemaker site depends on electrode placement. Ventricular pacemakers will not produce a P wave. Any sinus P waves seen are unrelated to the paced QRS complexes. Dual-chambered pacemakers produce a P wave behind each atrial spike. The spike is an artifact caused by each firing of the pacemaker, and it may be an upward or downward deflection. QRS complexes are usually longer than

0.12 second and bizarre in morphology, and they often resemble those of ventricular escape rhythms. A QRS complex should follow each pacemaker spike. When this occurs, the pacemaker is said to be "capturing" the ventricles. With demand pacemakers, some natural QRS complexes may appear, and these will not be associated with any spike.

27. Describe the process and pitfalls of differentiating wide QRS complex tachycardias. pp. 144–145

Ventricular tachycardia (VT) is the paradigm of a tachycardia with a wide, frequently bizarre QRS complex. In the discussion under objective 26, you learned that nonperfusing VT requires immediate treatment in order to restore tissue oxygenation. Drugs that may be useful include lidocaine, procainamide, or amiodarone. Synchronized cardioversion is generally the next alternative treatment. In cases with chest pain, dyspnea, or systolic BP less than 90 mmHg, synchronized cardioversion is indicated as the immediate treatment. *Torsade de pointes*, a subtype of VT, is commonly caused by certain antidysrhythmic drugs, including procainamide and amiodarone. Thus, prompt recognition of *torsade de pointes*—before initiating any treatment—is vital because you do NOT want to use the antidysrhythmics normally used for VT.

When you look at your initial rhythm strip, the QRS complexes of VT are relatively uniform in appearance and amplitude (check Figure 2-49). In contrast, the QRS complexes of *torsade de pointes* characteristically are not uniform in appearance and amplitude. Instead (as shown in Figure 2-50), the QRS complexes are wide and change in amplitude over the span of several complexes. The span of complexes also tends to vary roughly around a central point. Look at Figure 2-50, and draw a line joining the peaks of the upward deflections and another line connecting the lowest points of the downward deflections. You will see that the two lines almost form a "fish" shape that has its ends at a central point and that the strip shows one such large shape after another. This is the twisting about a point that is implicit in the French *torsade de pointes*. Another characteristic on ECG is a Q-T interval lengthened to 600 milliseconds or more during the breaks between the twisting spans of widened QRS complexes.

28. Describe the conditions of pulseless electrical activity. pp. 154–155

Pulseless electrical activity (PEA, also called electrical mechanical dissociation) means that electrical complexes are present on ECG, but there are no accompanying cardiac contractions. This is the paradigm of the situation in which you should treat the patient rather than the monitor. The ECG may show normal sinus rhythm, but your patient will be pulseless. Underlying conditions that can result in PEA and their general treatment (dependent on local protocol) include (1) hypovolemia/fluid resuscitation; (2) cardiac tamponade/pericardiocentesis; (3) tension pneumothorax/needle thoracostomy; (4) hypoxemia/intubation and oxygen; and (5) acidosis/sodium bicarbonate, as well as massive pulmonary embolism and rupture of the ventricular wall.

29. Describe the phenomena of reentry, aberration, and accessory pathways. pp. 98, 115, 157

Reentry (of an impulse) occurs when two branches of a conduction pathway are altered by a pathologic process such that conduction is slowed in one branch and a unidirectional block is caused in the other. In this case, a normal, anterograde depolarizing impulse travels slowly through the branch with slowed conduction and is blocked in the other. After the impulse travels through the branch with slowed conduction, it enters the branch with the block and is then conducted in the opposite, retrograde direction back toward the source of the impulse. Because this tissue is no longer refractory, it is depolarized by the returning impulse (the one with retrograde directionality). This reentry of an impulse back into the pathway of origin can result in rapid rhythms such as paroxysmal supraventricular tachycardia or atrial fibrillation.

Aberration, or aberrant conduction, reflects conduction of an impulse through the heart's conductive system in abnormal fashion. Aberrant conduction reflects a single supraventricular beat that is conducted through the ventricles in a delayed manner. In bundle branch block (either the right or left bundle can be affected), all supraventricular impulses traveling through the affected branch are delayed. If both branches are affected, third-degree heart block exists. Note that the impulses in these cases arise above the level of the ventricles, unlike the pure ventricular rhythms. In incomplete bundle branch block, the QRS complex will be normal. In complete bundle branch block, there will be a widened QRS complex on the ECG, and this may cause confusion as to whether the rhythm is supraventricular or ventricular in origin. Although there are exceptions, you can use the following guidelines to try to distinguish bundle branch block from a pure ventricular rhythm: (1) a changing bundle branch block suggests SVT with aberrancy; (2) a trial of carotid sinus massage may slow conduction through the AV node and terminate a reentrant SVT or slow conduction of other supraventricular dysrhythmias, whereas it will have no effect on ventricular dysrhythmias; (3) AV block (AV dissociation) indicates ventricular origin; (4) a full compensatory pause, usually seen after a ventricular beat, indicates ventricular tachycardia (VT); (5) fusion beats suggest VT as well; and (6) a QRS duration of longer than 0.14 second usually indicates VT.

An accessory pathway is an extra conduction pathway within the conduction system. In Wolff-Parkinson-White syndrome (WPW), the extra conduction pathway is the bundle of Kent, a pathway that is between the atria and ventricles. The presence of this extra (or accessory) pathway means that the depolarizing impulse effectively bypasses the AV node, shortening the P-R interval and prolonging the QRS complex. Although most patients with the syndrome are asymptomatic, WPW is associated with a high incidence of tachydysrhythmias, usually through a reentry phenomenon. WPW is also referred to as a pre-excitation syndrome because the ventricles are electrically excited before the impulse can arrive via the AV node. Although it is not always present on ECG monitoring, a delta wave (a slur on the upstroke of the QRS complex) is indicative of WPW.

30. Identify the ECG changes characteristically produced by electrolyte imbalances and specify their clinical implications. p. 157

You should always suspect hyperkalemia in patients with a history of renal failure who are on dialysis because potassium tends to be retained in the body. On an ECG, an early sign of hyperkalemia is tall, peaked T waves in the precordial leads. As the blood level rises higher, conduction decreases and the P-R and Q-T intervals increase in length. At very high potassium levels, an idioventricular rhythm may develop and eventually become a classic sine wave. In hypokalemia, the opposite ion disturbance, prominent U waves occur. Very low blood potassium levels can cause a widened QRS complex.

Clinically, hyperkalemia causes the heart to dilate and become flaccid and heart rate slows. Elevation of blood potassium to 2–3 times the normal value can cause so much heart weakness and abnormalities in rhythm that death may ensue.

31. Identify patient situations where ECG rhythm analysis is indicated. pp. 97–157

You will have specific guidelines for ECG monitoring. They will include direct medical cardiac causes such as history of heart disease, MI, or dysrhythmia, as well as any current evidence of dysrhythmia or hemodynamic instability or patient complaints suggestive of angina or acute MI. They will also cover traumatic causes (chest injury that may involve the heart or lungs) and evidence suggesting inadequate oxygenation in the body (such as altered level of consciousness) that may reflect cardiovascular compromise. Last, you may have guidelines recommending monitoring in some metabolic situations (such as hypothermia). Remember that you always treat the patient, not the ECG.

32. Recognize the ECG changes that may reflect evidence of myocardial ischemia and injury and their limitations. pp. 94–95

Changes in the S-T segment are usually looked for as evidence of myocardial ischemia or acute MI. Ischemic tissue produces abnormalities such as S-T segment depression (the norm is an isoelectric line) or an inverted T wave, with inversion usually symmetrical. Tissue injury, which occurs next in the early phase of an MI, may elevate the S-T segment. Finally, as tissue dies a significant Q wave develops. (Such a Q wave is at least one small square wide, lasting 0.04 second or more, or is more than one-third the height of the QRS complex.) Q waves may also indicate extensive transient ischemia. It is often difficult to interpret an ECG without knowledge of the patient's baseline ECG, and this is particularly true in patients with history of cardiac disease such as prior MI.

33. Correlate abnormal ECG findings with clinical interpretation.   pp. 97–157

See objectives 26–28, 30, 32, and 35. You may also find a J wave (or Osborn wave) on ECG monitoring. This wave is a slow, positive, rounded deflection at the end of the QRS complex that accompanies hypothermia. Other ECG changes seen with hypothermia include T wave inversion, P-R, QRS, or Q-T prolongation, sinus bradycardia, atrial flutter or fibrillation, AV block, PVCs, ventricular fibrillation, or asystole.

34. Identify the major mechanical, pharmacological, and electrical therapeutic objectives in the treatment of the patient with any dysrhythmia.   pp. 97–157

The descriptions of dysrhythmias, their clinical significance, and ECG findings associated with them are given in objective 26 above. Treatments for the conditions are discussed below.

- *Sinus bradycardia.* The overall goal of treatment is satisfactory heart rate, with subsequently adequate cardiac output and blood pressure and decreased risk of more dangerous dysrhythmias. Thus, treatment is based on symptoms, and no treatment may be needed unless hypotension or ventricular irritability is present. If treatment is needed, give a 0.5 mg bolus atropine sulfate, and repeat every 3–5 minutes until rate is satisfactory or you have given 0.04 mg/kg atropine. If atropine fails, consider transcutaneous cardiac pacing (TCP), if available.
- *Sinus tachycardia.* Treatment is directed at the underlying cause. Hypovolemia, fever, anemia, or other cause should be corrected. The overall goal is to reduce heart rate to a level compatible with adequate ventricular filling time, with supports in place to maintain an adequate stroke volume.
- *Sinus dysrhythmia.* Sinus dysrhythmia is a normal variant, particularly in the young and aged. Treatment is thus typically not required.
- *Sinus arrest.* If the patient is extremely bradycardic or symptomatic, give a 0.5 mg bolus atropine sulfate. The goal of pharmacologic therapy is to bring rate up to a level where symptoms are eliminated because cardiac output is adequate.
- *First-degree AV block.* Treatment is generally restricted to observation unless heart rate drops significantly. If possible, avoid administration of any drug that will further slow AV conduction, such as lidocaine and procainamide. The goal of treatment, if needed, is to preserve or improve AV conduction, eliminating the risk of development of a higher degree of heart block. When necessary, treatment may be needed to increase heart rate to a level compatible with adequate cardiac output.
- *Type I second-degree AV block* (also termed *second-degree Mobitz I* or *Wenckebach*). Treatment is generally restricted to observation. If possible, you want to avoid administration of any drug that will further slow AV conduction, such as lidocaine and procainamide. If heart rate falls and the patient becomes symptomatic, give 0.5 mg atropine IV. Repeat every 3–5 minutes until rate is satisfactory or you have given 0.04 mg/kg of atropine. If atropine fails, consider TCP if available. Overall goal is preservation or improvement of AV conduction and maintenance of a heart rate associated with adequate cardiac output.
- *Type II second-degree AV block* (also called *second-degree Mobitz II* or *infranodal block*). Definitive treatment is pacemaker insertion to preserve a normal rhythm and adequate cardiac output. In the prehospital setting, give medications if needed to stabilize the patient. Use caution in giving atropine to patients with second-degree Mobitz II blocks because the atropine may increase atrial rate but also worsen the AV nodal block. Consider TCP if available. If the patient remains symptomatic, do not delay application of TCP while waiting for IV access or time for atropine to take affect.
- *Third-degree AV block.* Definitive treatment is pacemaker insertion to preserve adequate cardiac output. In the prehospital setting, give medications if needed to stabilize patient. Use caution in giving atropine to patients with third-degree blocks because the atropine may increase atrial rate but also worsen the AV nodal block. Consider TCP if available. If the patient remains symptomatic, do not delay application of TCP while waiting for IV access or time for atropine to take affect. NEVER use lidocaine to treat third-degree block with ventricular escape beats.
- *Premature junctional contractions (PJCs).* Treatment is restricted to observation if the patient is asymptomatic.

- *Junctional escape rhythm.* Treatment in the field is generally restricted to observation (as patients are asymptomatic); however, care is needed if hypotension or ventricular irritability is present. If needed, give 0.5 mg bolus atropine, and repeat every 3–5 minutes until rate is satisfactory or you've given 0.04 mg/kg atropine. If atropine fails, consider TCP if available. Overall goal is preservation of cardiac output and blood pressure and prevention of more dangerous ventricular dysrhythmias.
- *Accelerated junctional rhythm.* Treatment goal is to correct ischemia.
- *Paroxysmal junctional tachycardia (PJT).* Treatment in the patient who is not tolerating PJT, as evidenced by hemodynamic instability, consists of the following sequence of steps. (1) Vagal maneuvers. (2) Therapy with adenosine (Adenocard), followed by verapamil if rate does not respond and there are no contraindications to verapamil. Verapamil should not be used with beta blockers. Verapamil-induced hypotension can often be reversed with 0.5–1.0 gm calcium chloride IV. (3) Electrical therapy with synchronized cardioversion if ventricular rate is higher than 150 bpm or patient is hemodynamically unstable. If time allows, use presedation. Apply synchronized DC countershock of 100 joules. Remember that DC countershock is contraindicated if digitalis toxicity is suspected. The overall goal is to reach a heart rate compatible with adequate ventricular filling time and good cardiac output, as well as to ensure adequate coronary artery perfusion.
- *Atrial tachycardia.* Treatment options for symptomatic patients include consideration of adenosine or verapamil to lower heart rate and prevent other dysrhythmias, including atrial fibrillation.
- *Multifocal atrial tachycardia.* Treatment of the underlying medical condition usually resolves the dysrhythmia. Specific antidysrhythmic therapy is usually not needed.
- *Premature atrial contractions (PACs).* Treatment for the symptomatic patient is oxygen via nonrebreather mask and establishment of IV access, along with consultation with medical direction. Field goal is to maintain tissue oxygenation and prepare for possible development of other, more clinically significant dysrhythmias.
- *Paroxysmal supraventricular tachycardia (PSVT).* Treatment for patients who are not tolerating the rapid heart rate, as evidenced by hemodynamic instability, should consist of the following series of techniques: (1) Vagal maneuvers. Note that carotid sinus massage should not be done in patients with carotid bruits or known cerebrovascular or carotid artery disease. (2) Pharmacological therapy with adenosine IV. If this fails and patient has normal blood pressure and a narrow QRS complex, consider use of verapamil if no contraindications exist. (3) Electrical therapy with synchronized cardioversion. DC countershock is contraindicated when digitalis toxicity is suspected. The overall goal is attainment of heart rate compatible with adequate cardiac output and coronary perfusion.
- *Atrial flutter.* Treatment is indicated for cases with rapid ventricular rates and hemodynamic compromise. Immediate cardioversion is indicated in unstable patients. Occasionally, you may use pharmacological therapy with stable patients, especially if the rapid ventricular rate is causing congestive heart failure. Several medications slow ventricular rate, including diltiazem (Cardizem), verapamil, digitalis, beta blockers, procainamide, and quinidine. Procainamide and quinidine are often used to convert back to sinus rhythm. Consult local medical direction for protocol specifics.
- *Atrial fibrillation.* Prehospital treatment is necessary when rapid ventricular rates with hemodynamic instability occur. Electrical therapy with immediate cardioversion is required in unstable patients—persons with heart rates greater than 150 bpm and associated chest pain, dyspnea, decreased level of consciousness, or hypotension. Pharmacological therapy may be useful, especially when rapid heart rate is causing congestive heart failure. Drugs that may be used include diltiazem, verapamil, digitalis, beta blockers, procainamide, and quinidine. Atrial fibrillation is a documented risk factor for stroke because atrial dilation allows for stagnation of blood and development of clots. You may wish to consider administration of an anticoagulant. Consult medical direction for specifics of possible pharmacological options. Immediate treatment goal is improvement of cardiac output. (Ultimate goal is adjustment of digitalis level, if toxicity is cause.)

  Patients with accessory pathways such as those with Wolff-Parkinson-White who develop atrial flutter or atrial fibrillation present special concerns. Verapamil, which decreases conduction through the AV node and may shorten the refractory period of the accessory path, may precipitate either ventricular tachycardia or ventricular fibrillation.

- *Ventricular escape rhythms.* Treatment depends on whether the rhythm is perfusing or not. If perfusing, the goal is to increase heart rate with atropine or, if it fails, TCP if available. With a nonperfusing rhythm, follow your pulseless electrical activity (PEA) protocol, including airway stabilization and CPR and IV epinephrine. Direct treatment is aimed at the primary problem, such as hypovolemia, hypoxia, cardiac tamponade, acidosis, or other. Consider a fluid challenge.
- *Accelerated idioventricular rhythm.* This is a subtype of ventricular escape rhythm and is an abnormally wide ventricular dysrhythmia typically associated with an acute MI. The rate is usually 60–110 bpm, and the patient does not require treatment unless hemodynamic instability is present, in which case the ventricular focus should be treated with atropine or overdrive pacing. The principal goal is treatment of the underlying MI.
- *Premature ventricular contractions (PVCs).* Treatment is indicated for patients with a prior history of heart disease or symptoms or if the PVCs are malignant. Administer oxygen and establish IV access. If the patient is symptomatic, give lidocaine at a dose of 1.0–1.5 mg/kg body weight. Give an additional bolus of 0.5–0.75 mg/kg every 5–10 minutes as needed until a total of 3.0 mg/kg has been reached. If PVCs are effectively suppressed, start a lidocaine drip at a rate of 2–4 mg/minute. Reduce dose in appropriate patients, and consider procainamide or bretylium if the ceiling dose of lidocaine has been reached or the patient is allergic to lidocaine. Overall goal is adequate ventricular filling and cardiac output and prevention of ventricular tachycardia or ventricular fibrillation.
- *Ventricular tachycardia (VT).* Treatment type depends on whether VT is perfusing or nonperfusing. If there is a pulse (perfusing VT), give oxygen and place an IV line. Give lidocaine IV at 1.0–1.5 mg/kg and additional doses of 0.5–0.75 mg/kg up to a total of 3.0 mg/kg. If unsuccessful, try procainamide or amiodarone as a second-line agent. Instability (namely, chest pain, dyspnea, or systolic BP less than 90 mmHg) calls for synchronized cardioversion. If you note instability at the outset of treatment, such as falling blood pressure or altered level of consciousness, initiate cardioversion immediately after starting oxygen and an IV. If there is no pulse (nonperfusing VT), treat as for ventricular fibrillation. Treatment goals are to maintain adequacy of cardiac output and coronary artery perfusion and to prevent ventricular fibrillation.
- *Ventricular fibrillation.* Treatment of ventricular fibrillation and nonperfusing VT is the same: Initiate CPR and follow with DC countershock at 200 joules. If unsuccessful, repeat at 200–300 joules; if still unsuccessful, try at 360 joules. Subsequent to countershock, control airway and establish IV access. Epinephrine 1:10,000 is the drug of first choice; give every 3–5 minutes as needed. If unsuccessful, consider second-line agents such as lidocaine, bretylium, amiodarone, procainamide, or even magnesium sulfate.
- *Asystole* (or *cardiac standstill*). Treatment is CPR, airway management, oxygenation, and medication. If there is any doubt of an underlying rhythm, attempt defibrillation.

35. Describe artifacts that may cause confusion when evaluating the ECG of a patient with a pacemaker. pp. 84–85, 152–153

ECG findings for patients with pacemakers are given in objective 26 above.

Note that any patient who has a demand pacemaker may have normal ECG sequences when the pacemaker has not been activated. There will not be any spikes during this time period, only when the pacemaker has been activated. In contrast, patients with a fixed-rate pacemaker will always have spike artifacts because the pacemaker is continually firing at its preset rate.

36. List the possible complications of pacing. p. 153

Possible problems with pacemakers include the following: (1) The battery fails. If batteries fail before they are replaced, pacing stops and the patient's underlying rhythm returns. (2) The pacemaker runs away. In this case (rarely seen with newer pacemakers), the pacemaker discharges at a rapid rate rather than the preset rate. In the older pacemakers, this is most likely to be seen when the battery runs low. Newer models avoid this possible problem by gradually increasing rate as the battery runs low. (3) Failure of a demand pacemaker to shut down when the innate rate exceeds the preset rate. When this happens, the heart's pacemaker and the artificial pacemaker compete, with both pacing the myocardium. If a paced beat falls during the absolute or relative refractory period, it can precipitate ventricular fibrillation. (4) Failure to capture. In this instance, battery failure or displacement of the pacemaker lead results in pacemaker discharge (with resultant ECG spike) that does not lead to depolarization of the myocardium (thus there is no QRS complex following the spike). Bradycardia often is seen.

37. List the causes and implications of pacemaker failure.   p. 153

As seen in objective 36, battery failure, although unlikely, is probably the most common cause of pacemaker dysfunction or failure. Displacement of the discharge lead can also lead to pacemaker failure. In these cases, the patient's underlying rhythm is usually seen, and it is often bradycardic and sufficiently low in cardiac output to cause symptoms (or the pacemaker would not have been implanted). In other patients, asystole can occur when a fixed-rate pacemaker fails.

    The failure of a demand pacemaker to shut down (a different way in which pacemaker function is lost) may lead to ventricular fibrillation if a paced beat occurs while the myocardium is in absolute or relative refractory state.

38. Identify additional hazards that interfere with artificial pacemaker function.   p. 153

You should always examine unconscious patients for evidence of a pacemaker: Batteries, for instance, are often palpable under the skin (commonly in the axillary or shoulder region). You can treat bradydysrhythmias, asystole, and ventricular fibrillation in patients with failed pacemakers as you would in other patients, but you must be careful not to discharge defibrillation paddles directly over the battery pack.

39. Recognize the complications of artificial pacemakers as evidenced on an ECG.   pp. 152–153

See objective 35 above.

CASE STUDY REVIEW

The Case Study Review for this chapter is found in Part 2.

CONTENT SELF-EVALUATION

MULTIPLE CHOICE

_____ 1. From innermost to outermost, the three tissue layers of the heart are:
   A. the endocardium, the pericardium, and the myocardium.
   B. the endocardium, the myocardium, and the syncytium.
   C. the endocardium, the myocardium, and the pericardium.
   D. the myocardium, the epicardium, and the pericardium.
   E. the epicardium, the myocardium, and the endocardium.

_____ 2. The blood supply to the left ventricle, interventricular septum, part of the right ventricle, and the heart's conduction system comes from the two branches of the left coronary artery, which are the:
   A. anterior descending artery and the circumflex artery.
   B. anterior descending artery and the posterior descending artery.
   C. circumflex artery and the posterior descending artery.
   D. circumflex artery and the marginal artery.
   E. marginal artery and the posterior descending artery.

_____ 3. Stimulation of the heart by the sympathetic nervous system results in:
  A. negative inotropic and chronotropic effects.
  B. negative chronotropic and dromotropic effects.
  C. positive chronotropic and dromotropic effects.
  D. positive inotropic and chronotropic effects.
  E. positive inotropic and dromotropic effects.

_____ 4. Specialized myocardial structures called intercalated discs enable the atria to act as an electrophysiologic syncytium and the ventricles to act as another one.
  A. True
  B. False

_____ 5. All of the following can cause an artifact on ECG EXCEPT:
  A. an artificial pacemaker.   D. shivering by the patient.
  B. an enlarged heart.   E. loose electrodes.
  C. movement by the patient.

_____ 6. A prolonged QT interval is longer than 0.38 second.
  A. True
  B. False

_____ 7. Common causes of dysrhythmias include all of the following EXCEPT:
  A. myocardial ischemia or infarction.
  B. electrolyte and pH disturbances.
  C. CNS or autonomic nervous system damage.
  D. drug effects.
  E. hyperthermia.

_____ 8. In the bradycardia algorithm, the first drug in the intervention sequence is:
  A. procainamide.   D. isoproterenol.
  B. epinephrine.   E. dopamine.
  C. atropine.

_____ 9. Of the atrial dysrhythmias listed below, which is often an indication of serious underlying medical disease?
  A. atrial tachycardia
  B. atrial flutter
  C. premature atrial contractions (PACs)
  D. multifocal atrial tachycardia (MAT)
  E. paroxysmal supraventricular tachycardia (PSVT)

_____ 10. The diagnostic finding for first-degree AV block on ECG is:
  A. the presence of some QRS complexes not preceded by a P wave.
  B. a P-R interval longer than 0.20 second.
  C. a QRS complex widened to longer than 0.12 second.
  D. an R-T interval widened for those beats with an initial P wave.
  E. the presence of some P waves without following QRS complexes.

_____ 11. The chief difference between Type I and Type II second-degree AV block is the pattern of lengthening P-R interval before the blocked impulse in Type I second-degree AV block.
  A. True
  B. False

_____ 12. All of the following statements about third-degree AV block are true EXCEPT:
  A. the atrial rate is unaffected, and ventricular rate depends on site of ventricular pacemaker.
  B. P waves are normal but show no relationship to the QRS complex.
  C. there is an absence of conduction between the atria and the ventricles.
  D. both atrial and ventricular rhythms are usually regular.
  E. QRS complexes are normal in length.

_____ 13. Never use lidocaine to treat third-degree heart block in patients with ventricular escape beats.
   A. True
   B. False

_____ 14. All of the following statements about ECG findings for dysrhythmias originating in the AV junction are true EXCEPT:
   A. P-R interval is less than 0.12 second.
   B. P waves are inverted in Lead II.
   C. T waves are blunted and widened.
   D. QRS complexes are normal in duration.
   E. P waves are masked if atrial depolarization occurs during ventricular depolarization.

_____ 15. Caffeine, tobacco, alcohol, and sympathomimetic drugs are common causes of:
   A. junctional escape rhythms.   D. premature junctional contractions.
   B. accelerated junctional rhythm.   E. junctional bradycardia.
   C. paroxysmal junctional tachycardia.

_____ 16. All of the following statements about dysrhythmias originating in the ventricles are true EXCEPT:
   A. ischemia, hypoxia, and drug effects are common causes.
   B. T waves are blunted and widened.
   C. P waves are absent.
   D. the pacemaker site determines QRS morphology.
   E. QRS complexes are 0.12 second or longer in duration.

_____ 17. _Torsades de pointes_ varies in both cause and ECG appearance from other forms of:
   A. ventricular escape rhythm.   D. premature ventricular contraction.
   B. accelerated idioventricular rhythm. E. ventricular tachycardia.
   C. ventricular fibrillation.

_____ 18. Possible characteristics of malignant PVCs include all EXCEPT:
   A. R on T phenomenon.
   B. couplets or longer runs of ventricular tachycardia.
   C. more than eight PVCs per minute.
   D. multifocal origin within the ventricles.
   E. accompanying chest pain.

_____ 19. Nonperfusing ventricular tachycardia and ventricular fibrillation are treated identically, including initiation of CPR followed by:
   A. epinephrine 1:10,000 IV bolus.   D. DC countershock at 200 joules.
   B. adenosine IV bolus.   E. atropine IV bolus.
   C. transcutaneous cardiac pacing (TCP).

_____ 20. Causes of asystole include all of the following EXCEPT:
   A. pre-existing alkalosis (respiratory or metabolic).
   B. hyperkalemia.
   C. hypokalemia.
   D. drug overdose.
   E. hypothermia.

MATCHING

Write the letter of the definition or description regarding cardiac function in the space provided next to the term to which it applies. The same description or definition may be used more than once or not at all.

_____ 21. cardiac cycle

_____ 22. diastole

_____ 23. systole

_____ 24. ejection fraction

_____ 25. preload

_____ 26. afterload

_____ 27. cardiac output

_____ 28. stroke volume

A. the ratio of blood pumped from the ventricle compared with the amount contained at the end of diastole
B. the series of events between the end of a cardiac contraction to the end of the next
C. the resistance against which the heart must pump
D. the phase of the cardiac cycle during which the heart contracts
E. the amount of blood pumped by the ventricle during one cardiac contraction
F. the amount of blood pumped by the ventricle during one minute
G. the phase of the cardiac cycle during which the heart muscle is relaxed
H. the end-diastolic volume in the ventricle
I. the phase of the cardiac cycle during which blood enters the coronary arteries

Write the letter of the clinical effect in the space provided next to the electrolyte or condition that produces that effect.

_____ 29. sodium

_____ 30. calcium

_____ 31. potassium

_____ 32. hypercalcemia

_____ 33. hypocalcemia

_____ 34. hyperkalemia

_____ 35. hypokalemia

A. rapid movement strongly influences repolarization
B. increased myocardial contractility
C. rapid movement strongly influences depolarization
D. influences myocardial depolarization and contraction
E. decreased automaticity and conduction
F. decreased myocardial contractility and increased electrical irritability
G. increased electrical irritability

Write the letter of innate rate of impulse discharge in beats per minute (bpm) in the space provided next to the part of the cardiac conduction system to which it applies.

_____ 36. Purkinje system

_____ 37. AV node

_____ 38. SA node

A. 60–100 bpm
B. 15–40 bpm
C. 40–60 bpm

Write the letter of the portion of the heart in the space provided next to the ECG leads that give a picture of its activity.

_____ 39. Leads II, III, and aVF

_____ 40. Leads V_1 and V_2

_____ 41. Leads V_3 and V_4

_____ 42. Leads V_5 and V_6

A. the right ventricle
B. the anterior and lateral walls of the left ventricle
C. the inferior (diaphragmatic) wall of the heart
D. the interventricular septum and the anterior wall of the left ventricle

LABEL THE DIAGRAMS

Supply the missing labels for the drawing showing the chambers of the heart by writing the appropriate letters in the spaces provided for Figure 1.

A. right ventricle
B. interatrial septum
C. left atrium
D. right atrium
E. interventricular septum
F. left ventricle

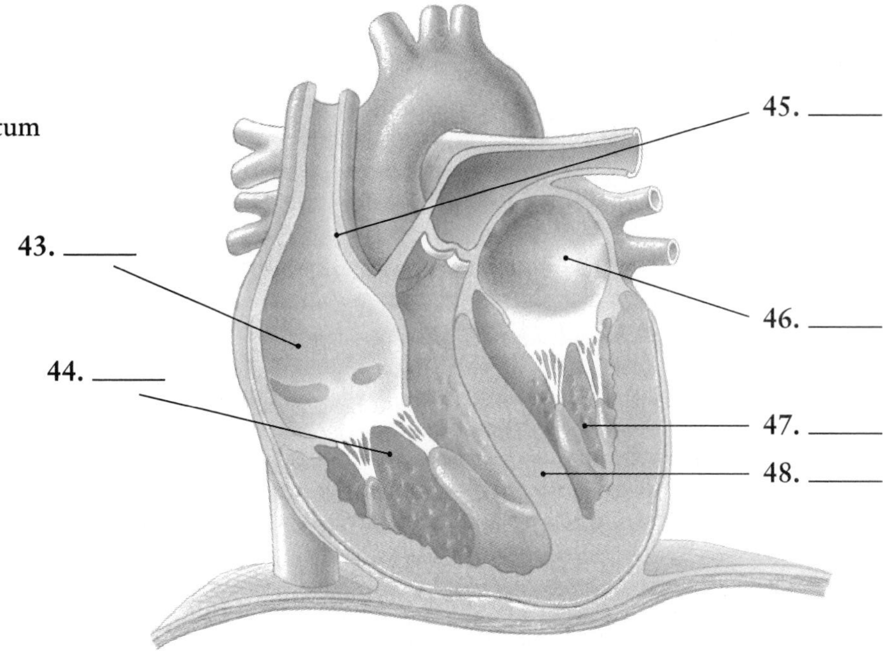

43. _____

44. _____

45. _____

46. _____

47. _____

48. _____

Figure 1

Supply the missing labels for the drawing showing the cardiac conductive system by writing the appropriate letters in the spaces provided for Figure 2.

A. Purkinje fibers
B. left bundle branch
C. SA node
D. AV node
E. bundle of His
F. Internodal atrial pathway
G. AV junction

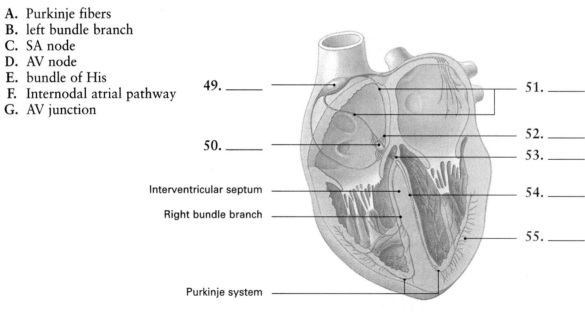

49. _____

50. _____

Interventricular septum

Right bundle branch

Purkinje system

51. _____

52. _____

53. _____

54. _____

55. _____

Figure 2

Use the terms below to fill in the missing labels for Figure 3 in the spaces provided.

A. QRS complex
B. Ventricular depolarization
C. Atrial depolarization
D. T wave
E. Ventricular repolarization
F. P wave

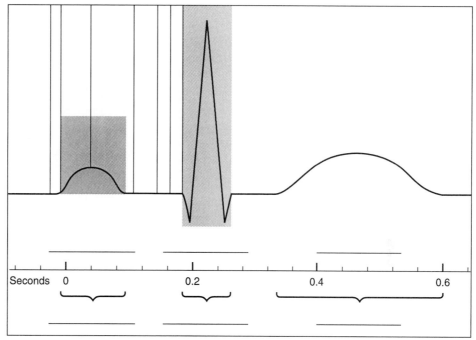

Figure 3

FILL-IN-THE-BLANKS

56. The _____ valves lie between the atria and ventricles, whereas the _____ valves lie between the ventricles and the arteries into which they open.

57. The four properties of cells in the cardiac conductive system are _____ , _____ , _____ , and _____ .

58. If only one ECG lead can be applied, the one most likely to be used as a monitoring lead is _____ , because it gives the best view of ECG waves and depicts the conduction system's activity.

59. ECG machines are standardized such that the paper moves across the stylus at the rate of _____ .

60. When properly calibrated, a deflection of _____ large box(es) is equivalent to 1 mV.

61. One small horizontal box on an ECG is equivalent to _____ , and one large box is equivalent to _____ .

62. The time-interval markings placed at the top of ECG paper are located at intervals of _____ .

63. Prominent U waves and a widened QRS complex are both ECG evidence of this electrolyte imbalance: _____ .

SPECIAL PROJECT

ECG Interpretation

The chapter introduces a five-step procedure for analyzing ECG strips: (1) analysis of rate; (2) analysis of rhythm; (3) analysis of P waves; (4) analysis of P-R interval; and (5) analysis of QRS complexes.
Look at each of the five ECG tracings shown and complete the information grid asked for below each tracing.

ECG #1

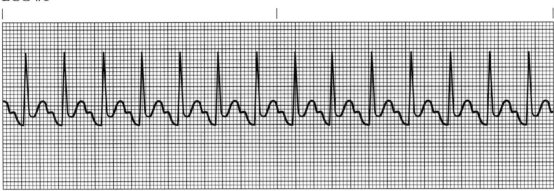

Rate: _____

Rhythm: _____

P waves: _____

P-R interval: _____

QRS complexes: _____

Overall rhythm (or Dysrhythmia): _____

ECG #2

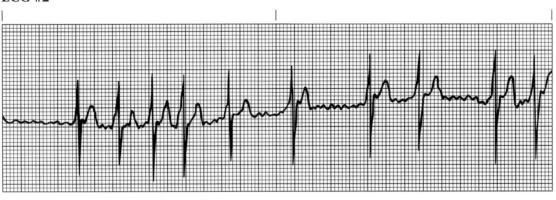

Rate: _____

Rhythm: _____

P waves: _____

P-R interval: _____

QRS complexes: _____

Overall rhythm (or Dysrhythmia): _____

ECG #3

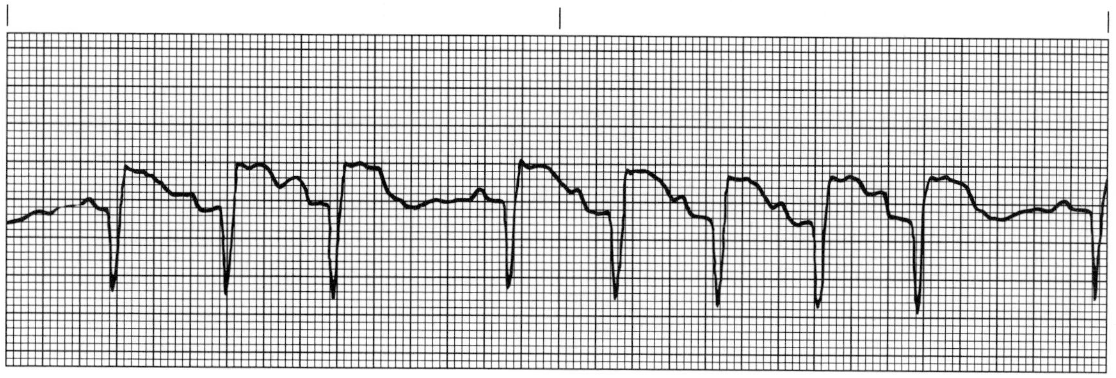

Rate: _____

Rhythm: _____

P waves: _____

P-R interval: _____

QRS complexes: _____

Overall rhythm (or Dysrhythmia): _____

ECG #4

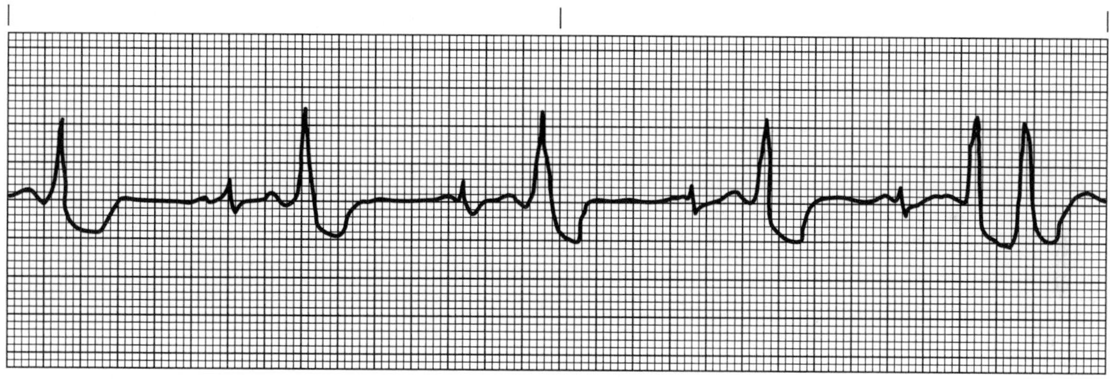

Rate: _____

Rhythm: _____

P waves: _____

P-R interval: _____

QRS complexes: _____

_____

Overall rhythm (or Dysrhythmia): _____

_____

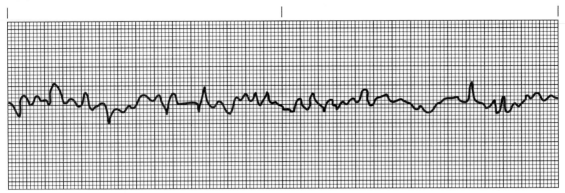

Rate: _____

Rhythm: _____

P waves: _____

P-R interval: _____

QRS complexes: _____

Overall rhythm (or Dysrhythmia): _____

CHAPTER 2
Cardiology

Review of Chapter Objectives

After reading this part of the chapter, you should be able to:

40. Identify and describe the components of the focused history as it relates to the patient with cardiovascular compromise.   **pp. 162–166**

The focused history for cardiac situations uses the same format you learned for pulmonology, the SAMPLE format: Signs/Symptoms, Allergies, Medications, Past medical history, Last oral intake, and Events preceding the incident.

- *Signs/Symptoms.* The most common symptoms of cardiac disease/compromise include chest pain or discomfort, dyspnea, cough, syncope, and palpitations.

  Use the OPQRST format (also something you encountered with pulmonology) to assess chest pain or discomfort: Onset of pain, Provocation/Palliation of pain, Quality of pain, Region where felt/Radiation, Severity, and Timing (duration). (See also objective 54 for full detail.) Questions concerning dyspnea are similar: You want to know how long it has lasted and whether it is continuous or intermittent. Was onset rapid or gradual? Does anything specific either worsen or palliate the dyspnea, and is it exertional or not? Last, be sure to see if orthopnea exists: Does sitting upright give any relief? Questions about cough center on whether it is chronic or acute and whether it suggests congestive heart failure (dry or productive, presence of any wheezing with cough, etc.).

  In addition, observe and question for these possible signs/symptoms: level of consciousness, diaphoresis, restlessness/anxiety, feeling of impending doom, nausea/vomiting, fatigue, palpitations, edema of extremities or positional (sacral), headache, syncope, behavioral change, facial expression, limitation of activity, signs of recent trauma. Many signs/symptoms of cardiovascular disease and compromise can be subtle or change (either rapidly or gradually) over time.
- *Allergies.* Check for allergies to medication (prescription and over-the-counter) or X-ray contrast dyes. Try to distinguish between details suggestive of side effect (such as GI upset) and those of allergy (rash, hives, anaphylactic shock).
- *Medications.* Check both for current medications (again, prescription and over-the-counter) and recent medication changes. If there has been a recent change, ask why. Look for use of cardiovascular drugs such as nitroglycerin, propranolol or other beta blockers, digitalis (digoxin, Lanoxin), diuretics (Lasix, Dyazide), antihypertensives (Capoten, Prinivil, Vasotec), antidysrhythmics (Quinaglute, Mexitil, Tambocor), and lipid-lowering agents (Mevacor, Lopid). If possible, check directly (by inspecting med tray, if there is one) or indirectly (by history) about drug compliance and bring containers to the hospital with you.
- *Past medical history.* Ask directed questions about history of heart disease, MI, stroke, high blood pressure, as well as why suggestive drugs are taken. Specific problems you should inquire about include history of rheumatic heart disease (valvular problems), previous cardiac surgery,

congenital cardiac anomalies, pericarditis or other inflammatory cardiac disease, or congestive heart failure (CHF). Relevant problems of other organ systems include pulmonary disease/COPD, diabetes mellitus, renal disease, hypertension, atherosclerosis. Also ask whether there is any family history of illness/death (particularly early deaths before age 50) from cardiovascular disease or other relevant disorders. Last, be sure to ask whether patient smokes or smoked tobacco and whether he/she knows his/her cholesterol level.

- *Last oral intake.* Valuable as a screening question for anyone with a possible surgical condition, this also gives you the chance to ask about most recent caffeine or tobacco use, as well as whether there was a recent fatty meal. (For some patients, this may help steer you to gallbladder disorders.)
- *Events preceding incident.* Ask what the patient was doing just before onset of symptoms. Was there emotional stress or physical exertion? Was there sexual activity? If the patient is male, does he take Viagra? It is often uncomfortable to take a sexual history, but sometimes the information gained is life saving, and you can explain to the patient the possible importance of the answer.

41. **Identify and describe the details of inspection, auscultation, and palpation specific to the cardiovascular system.**   **pp. 166–170**

Always do visual inspection first. (1) Look for tracheal position. If isn't in its normal midline position but is toward one side, there may be a pneumothorax. (2) Check neck veins for signs of jugular distention (have the patient elevated about 45° and with head turned to the side). Jugular venous distention (JVD) is evidence of back pressure from causes such as heart (pump) failure or cardiac tamponade. (3) Thorax and chest movement while breathing should be observed with proper exposure so you can see chest shape (barrel chests may indicate COPD) and effort during respiration, such as retractions of the soft tissues between the ribs. Accessory muscles used when breathing is difficult may include those of the neck, back, and abdomen. Always look for surgical scars; a scar over the sternum may indicate prior cardiac surgery. (4) Evaluate the epigastrium while the chest wall is exposed, looking for distention and visible pulsations. Pulsations may signal an aortic aneurysm dissection or rupture. (5) Position-dependent edema may be found in the ankles or sacral area, depending on whether the patient has been sitting or lying in bed. Pitting edema (a depression that persists after you stop applying firm pressure) is significant. (6) Skin changes associated with cardiovascular disease include pallor and diaphoresis (indicating increased sympathetic tone and peripheral vasoconstriction) or a mottled appearance (often an indicator of chronic cardiac failure). (7) Subtle changes associated with cardiovascular disease include not only surgical scars but subcutaneous batteries for a pacemaker or nitroglycerin skin patches.

Auscultation includes listening to the lungs, to the heart, and over the carotid arteries. (1) Assess the lung fields for equality and for sounds such as rales (crackles), rhonchi (whistling or snoring-like sounds), or wheezes, which may signal pulmonary edema or primary pulmonary disease. Note that patients with pulmonary edema may have foamy, blood-tinged sputum evident at the mouth and nose. In advanced cases, you may even hear a gurgling-like sound as the patient breathes. (2) It is difficult to auscultate the heart well in the field because of the number and intensity of background noises. Ideally, you want to listen for heart sounds at four classic sites: aortic, pulmonic, mitral (left AV valve), and tricuspid (right AV valve). The point on the chest wall where heartbeat is loudest or is best felt is called the point of maximum impulse (PMI). (3) Auscultation over the carotid arteries may reveal bruits, murmur sounds due to turbulent flow. A bruit over any artery indicates partial obstruction due to atherosclerosis. Never attempt carotid sinus massage in a patient with a bruit because you might dislodge atherosclerotic material that could lodge in a cerebral artery causing a stroke or other mishap.

Palpation should cover three areas: peripheral pulse, thorax, and epigastrium. (1) Determine rate and regularity of the pulse as well as equality. A pulse deficit (intensity less than expected) may indicate underlying peripheral vascular disease and should be reported to medical direction. (2) Thoracic palpation is extremely important and may reveal crepitus, akin to "bubble wrap" crackling under your fingers, which suggests subcutaneous emphysema. Check for tenderness or possible rib fracture. Remember that at least 15% of MI patients have some associated chest wall tenderness. (3) Abdominal exam may reveal distention or pulsations.

42. Identify and define the heart sounds and relate them to hemodynamic events in the cardiac cycle. pp. 168–169

Everyone is familiar with the lub-dub of normal heart sounds. The first component, called S_1, is produced by the closing of the AV valves during ventricular systole (at the beginning of the ventricular contraction that expels blood into the aorta and pulmonary artery). The second heart sound (S_2) is produced by the closure of the aortic and pulmonary valves as the ventricles begin to relax and the heart fills with blood again (at early diastole).

43. Describe the differences between normal and abnormal heart sounds. pp. 168–169

Any extra heart sounds (beyond S_1 and S_2) are abnormal. The sound termed S_3 is associated with congestive heart failure, and it has a cadence like that of the word Kentucky; when it is present, it follows S_2. The fourth heart sound, S_4, appears just before S_1 when it is present, and it is associated with increased effort of atrial contraction. Its cadence resembles that of Tennessee.

44. Define pulse deficit, pulsus paradoxus, and pulsus alternans. pp. 169, 205

A pulse deficit is the less intense of two peripheral pulses that you would expect to be equal, for instance, the right and left carotid or right or left radial pulses. The pulse with the deficit often reflects an artery that is partially blocked by atherosclerosis. Pulsus paradoxus is related to a change in blood pressure with respiration. Specifically, pulsus paradoxus exists when systolic blood pressure decreases by more than 10 mmHg with inspiration, and it is due to compression of either the great vessels or the ventricles. Pulsus alternans exists when the pulse alternates between weak and strong intensity over time. In such cases, pulses may be felt as thready or weak on examination.

45. Identify the normal characteristics of the point of maximal impulse (PMI). p. 169

The point on the chest wall where heartbeat is loudest on auscultation is usually the point where palpation finds the strongest impulse of the beating heart. This location is called the point of maximum impulse (PMI). You can find additional information about the PMI and cardiac examination in Volume 2, Chapter 2, "Physical Examination," of this series.

46. Based on field impressions, identify the need for rapid intervention for the patient in cardiovascular compromise. pp. 160–170

As with any other patient, your first responsibilities are to check airway, breathing, circulation, and the possibility of shock. Only after you have managed life-threatening problems (and if new, life-threatening problems don't develop) can you communicate with and support the patient and family. Note that interventions in the field beyond the absolutely essential are generally limited to administration of analgesia or nitrates for chest pain, treatment of pulmonary edema, and administration of appropriate analgesia for peripheral vascular emergencies. Do be sure, however, to look for the obvious and subtle signs of cardiovascular disease during the focused history and physical. The discovery of an abdominal pulsation that might signal aortic aneurysm dissection or rupture in a patient with some signs of early shock changes the dynamic for intervention and transportation greatly.

47. Describe the incidence, morbidity, and mortality associated with myocardial conduction defects. pp. 186, 198, 240–254

Remember that dysrhythmias arising from coronary heart disease, or CHD (often part of myocardial ischemia or infarction), cause many of the sudden deaths associated with CHD, and these deaths are too numerous. About 225,000 Americans have CHD-induced deaths before they can reach a hospital; this amounts to roughly one death per minute. Dysrhythmias are the most common complication of MI and the most common cause of death from an MI. Life-threatening dysrhythmias can develop very early in the course of myocardial ischemia and can cause sudden death (immediate or within one hour of onset of symptoms).

Conduction abnormalities also arise directly from disease or from drug effects or electrolyte abnormalities. Among the forms of AV block, third-degree block is the most serious: In this type, none of the impulses originating in the atria reach the ventricles. Ventricular rate and rhythm are dependent on development of a ventricular escape rhythm. This can lead to morbidity through symptomatic bradycardia and heart failure. In some situations, cardiac arrest and death may result. Bundle branch block can result from age-related deterioration, MI, or transient causes such as drugs and electrolyte abnormalities. Part of your concern with cases of left bundle branch block should lie in the fact that nothing else can be determined from the ECG regarding possible ischemic change. Thus, a patient with left bundle branch block can have a significant MI and ECG changes will not be seen; this can increase the morbidity or mortality from the MI.

48. Identify the clinical indications, components, and the function of transcutaneous and permanent artificial cardiac pacing. pp. 152–153, 186, 188–189

Permanent artificial pacemakers are generally inserted into patients who have chronic high-grade AV block or sick sinus syndrome or who have had episodes of severe symptomatic bradycardia in the past. The pacemaker (the pulse generator) is implanted near the heart, and its discharge lead is inserted into either the right ventricle or right atrium and ventricle, depending on whether it is a ventricular-type pacemaker or a dual-chambered pacemaker (see Figure 2-54). The battery packs are usually palpable in their subcutaneous position (often in the shoulder or axillary region). Permanent pacemakers are of two functional types: either they can pace continuously or they can pace when the heart's natural rate falls below a preset number of beats per minute. (The two types are called fixed-rate and demand pacemakers.) In all cases, the pacemaker should enable the patient to have a heart rate and rhythm that supports adequate cardiac output.

Transcutaneous cardiac pacing (TCP) allows electrical pacing of the heart through the skin via specially designed thoracic electrodes. You will need to have one of the newer cardiac monitor/defibrillators with an appropriate built-in pacing device. TCP may be highly beneficial for patients with symptomatic bradycardia such as high-degree AV block, atrial fibrillation with slow ventricular response, or other significant bradycardias and asystole. You can use TCP if pharmacological intervention fails and if the patient is hypotensive or hypoperfusing to try to establish a rate and rhythm compatible with adequate cardiac output. You can also use TCP to provide overdrive pacing to suppress recurrent tachycardia or in *torsade de pointes*, a specific form of ventricular tachycardia.

49. Explain what each setting and indicator on a transcutaneous pacing system represents and how the settings may be adjusted. pp. 188–189

One system setting is for heart rate: The range available is typically 60 to 80 bpm, and medical direction will consult with you about setting the appropriate rate. The output setting (in amps) should initially be set to 0 and then gradually increased until you see the pacemaker spike on ECG that shows ventricular capture. Maintenance rate and output are arranged with medical direction. With a patient in asystole, output is generally begun at the maximum setting, with output gradually lowered if ventricular capture occurs.

50. Describe the techniques of applying a transcutaneous pacing system. pp. 188–189

There are eleven steps involved in applying and monitoring TCP. (1) Establish IV access and ECG monitoring and administer oxygen. (2) Place the patient in a supine position. (3) Confirm symptomatic bradycardia (the usual indication) and medical direction's order for TCP. (4) Apply the pacing electrodes according to the manufacturer's directions. Be sure they adhere well to the skin. (5) Connect the electrodes. (6) Set desired heart rate on the pacemaker. (7) Turn output setting to 0. (8) Turn on pacer. (9) Slowly increase output until you see ECG spikes indicating ventricular capture. (10) Check the patient's pulse and blood pressure and adjust rate and amperage (output) per instructions from medical direction. (11) Monitor patient response to treatment.

51. Describe the characteristics of an implanted pacemaking system. pp. 152–153

See the first part of objective 48 on permanent pacemakers.

52. Describe the epidemiology, morbidity, mortality, and pathophysiology of angina pectoris.
pp. 191, 194

Angina pectoris, or pain in the chest, occurs when the myocardial demand for oxygen exceeds the available supply through the coronary arteries. Myocardial ischemia causes the chest pain. Usually, reduced blood flow through the coronary arteries is correlated with permanent partial obstruction by atherosclerotic lesions. Angina can also result from spasm of the coronary arteries (arterial vasospasm), temporarily reducing the diameter of the lumen and blood flow. About two-thirds of patients with vasospastic angina (commonly called Prinzmetal's angina) have atherosclerosis involving the coronaries. Epidemiologically, though, this still means roughly one-third of patients with Prinzmetal's angina do not have significant coronary atherosclerosis and thus may not fit the risk factor profile for atherosclerosis.

The epidemiology, morbidity, and mortality of cardiovascular disease, including coronary heart disease (CHD, disease of the coronary arteries) are covered in depth in objectives 1 and 3 of Part 1 of this chapter.

53. Describe the assessment and management of a patient with angina pectoris.
pp. 194–196

During assessment, remember that weak or absent peripheral pulses (especially when symmetric or global) may signal pending shock, which requires immediate intervention. Pallor and cyanosis of the skin or cold extremities also suggest shock. Because angina is a progressive disorder, a history of angina does not mean that the current episode is "safe." If it is important enough to activate EMS, it is important enough for your full attention and the suspicion of serious underlying problems such as acute MI. Listen to the history of the current event: The chief complaint is usually sudden onset chest pain. Pain may radiate or be localized to the chest. Angina usually lasts 3–5 minutes, although it may last as long as 15 minutes, and it is generally relieved by rest and/or nitroglycerin. Prinzmetal angina is often accompanied by S-T segment elevation on ECG, which may indicate myocardial tissue ischemia. Breathing may or may not be labored, but you should check for lung sounds after ensuring the airway is patent. Listen for congestion, especially at the bases. Although the anginal patient's rate and rhythm may be altered, they may be normal, and peripheral pulses should be equal and normal. Typically, blood pressure rises during the anginal episode and normalizes afterward. Ask the patient for his/her baseline BP, as hypertension may be present. If it is possible without prolonging the time on-scene, get an ECG tracing. A 12-lead ECG provides more information and should be done if possible.

Management includes placing the patient at physical and emotional rest to decrease myocardial oxygen demand: Give oxygen, generally at high-flow rate. Establish IV access on scene or en route to the hospital. Conduct the ECG; do not, however, delay transport to perform it. You can give nitroglycerin sublingually as a tablet or spray. If symptoms persist after 1–2 doses, raise your suspicion for a more serious condition such as acute MI. Nifedipine and other calcium channel blockers can also be used for relief of anginal pain: Morphine may be used for nonresponsive chest pain.

Patients with an initial episode of angina or an episode that does not respond to medication are usually admitted for observation. Immediate transport is indicated if relief does not come after oxygen and nitrates. The absence of relief may signal the beginning of infarction, and in this case reperfusion is crucial. Hypotension may occur, especially if nitroglycerin has been given. It indicates transport as well because it can lead to or worsen hypoperfusion of myocardial tissue. S-T segment changes, particularly elevation, also indicate the need for rapid, efficient transport: Transport should be WITHOUT lights or siren, if possible, in order to minimize patient anxiety.

If the patient refuses transport, be sure you clearly explain that immediate evaluation is vital because of the potential for problems such as MI. If you can't reverse the patient's decision, be sure the patient reads and signs the refusal and understands the potential risks. Ask that they contact their cardiologist or other physician for follow-up as soon as possible.

54. Identify what is meant by the OPQRST of chest pain assessment.
pp. 162–163

Use the OPQRST format (also something you encountered with pulmonology) to assess chest pain or discomfort: Onset of pain, Provocation/Palliation of pain, Quality of pain, Region where felt/Radiation, Severity, and Timing (duration). Questions about onset include when pain began and what was happening at the time. Ask a patient who has had prior episodes of chest pain to compare this one with prior episodes. If it is described as similar to pain that signaled a prior heart attack, you can strongly assume the pain is cardiac in origin. Questions on provocation and palliation of pain also may point to angina or toward another cause. In particular, ask about any relationship to exertion of any type or palliation with rest. If there have been multiple episodes, ask whether it takes less to trigger an episode now than in the past. Ask a general question about the quality of the pain and let the patient describe it. Common words include sharp, tearing, pressured, or heavy. Radiation of chest pain may occur to arm(s), neck, jaw, and/or back. Again, ask if this pattern fits earlier episodes. Ask the patient to evaluate the severity of the pain on a scale of 1–10 (be sure you use the same scale that will be used at the hospital in order to standardize response significance): You can ask the same question later to assess efficacy of therapy. Timing questions get information on how long the pain has lasted (write down the time the patient first noted pain as this may affect decisions later regarding possible thrombolytic therapy) as well as whether pain has been constant or intermittent or has changed with time (Better? Worse?).

55. List other clinical conditions that may mimic signs and symptoms of coronary artery disease and angina pectoris. pp. 191, 194

Causes of chest pain fall into four categories: cardiovascular, respiratory, gastrointestinal, and musculoskeletal. You'll note that the causes range from the troublesome but benign (dyspepsia, or heartburn) to the life threatening (aortic dissection). Cardiovascular causes include coronary artery disease and angina, but also pericarditis and dissection of the thoracic aorta. Respiratory causes include pulmonary embolism, pneumothorax, pneumonia, and pleurisy (pleural inflammation). GI causes are diverse: cholecystitis (gallbladder origin), pancreatitis, hiatal hernia, esophageal disease, gastroesophageal reflux (GERD), peptic ulcer disease, and dyspepsia. Musculoskeletal causes include chest wall syndrome, costochondritis, acromioclavicular disease, herpes zoster (shingles), chest wall trauma, and chest wall tumors. You should always be prepared to treat patients with chest pain as if they may have cardiac ischemia or another major disease process. Only after you have excluded these possibilities should you consider the less critical causes.

56. Identify the ECG findings in patients with angina pectoris. pp. 194–195

An ECG should be done on-scene; if that would delay transport, it may be done en route. If possible, get a 12-lead ECG because it provides more information. Typical findings in patients with angina include S-T depression and/or T wave inversion. After relief of pain, ECG usually returns to baseline. The most common finding in angina is S-T depression, although Prinzmetal patients typically show S-T elevation. Note that S-T segment changes are not specific, and dysrhythmias and ectopy may not be seen either. Be sure to transmit the ECG to medical direction and discuss as necessary.

57. Based on the pathophysiology and clinical evaluation of the patient with chest pain, list the anticipated clinical problems according to their life-threatening potential. pp. 191, 194

Because angina, whether typical (obstructive) or vasospastic (namely, Prinzmetal's angina), reflects myocardial ischemia, progression to myocardial infarction is always possible. ECG monitoring may pick up signs of ischemia or infarction, as well as related cardiac problems such as dysrhythmia and ectopy, all of which can rapidly develop into life-threatening conditions. Aortic dissection is a life-threatening emergency, as can be pericarditis if pressure on the heart decreases cardiac output to the point of hypoperfusion of the heart (causing angina) or other vital organs such as the brain. Pulmonary embolism may also present as a life-threatening emergency if the embolus is very large or affects flow into both lungs. Pneumothorax and pneumonia are always serious, but they may also be life threatening in a patient with previously compromised cardiopulmonary function. Pleurisy, suspected cholecystitis or pancreatitis, and esophageal disease and peptic ulcer disease are also serious. If any of the GI conditions involve hemorrhage, the patient's condition may become unstable, especially if cardiopulmonary compromise exists. Always carry a degree of suspicion of impending or possible shock. Other causes, including the musculoskeletal causes as well as GI problems such as hiatal hernia, merit medical workup, but these patients are unlikely to be unstable on-scene or during transport. In some cases, such as known GERD, dyspepsia, or costochondritis, a patient with no other signs of a serious condition and no change in condition while you are on-scene may refuse transport. You should always advocate follow-up as quickly as possible with the personal physician because the complaint was severe enough to warrant the call to EMS.

58. Describe the epidemiology, morbidity, mortality, and pathophysiology of myocardial infarction. pp. 196–197

Each year about 466,000 Americans die from coronary heart disease (CHD), and myocardial infarction (MI) is the usual direct cause of death. In addition, an American suffers a nonfatal MI every 29 seconds. Myocardial infarction, the death of myocardial tissue, is the result of prolonged oxygen deprivation or when myocardial oxygen demand exceeds oxygen supply for an extended period. MI is most often associated with atherosclerotic heart disease (ASHD, which is the same as atherosclerotic coronary heart disease). The precipitating event is often development of a thrombus in a partially occluded artery, with the thrombus completely occluding the vessel. Other pathophysiologic bases for MI include coronary artery spasm, microemboli as can be seen with cocaine use, acute volume overload, hypotension (causing myocardial hypoperfusion), or acute respiratory failure (leading to acute hypoxia). Trauma can also cause MI, often by loosening atherosclerotic plaque in the coronary artery, blocking it.

The region of the heart affected and the size of the eventual infarcted area depend on the coronary artery involved and the specific site of the obstruction. Most infarctions involve the left ventricle. Obstruction of the left coronary artery or its branches may result in infarction of the anterior or lateral ventricle or the interventricular septum. Right coronary artery occlusions tend to result in infarction of the inferior or posterior wall of the left ventricle or infarction of the right ventricle.

The pathophysiologic progression of events starts with ischemia, followed by cell death. The infarcted tissue becomes necrotic and eventually forms scar tissue, if the affected individual survives. Ischemic tissue at the periphery of the infarct will survive but may become the origin of dysrhythmias. Dysrhythmias are the most common complication of MI and the most common cause of death from an MI.

Infarction of myocardium can cause congestive heart failure. Heart failure implies that the heart is working poorly but adequately. If the heart cannot meet body oxygen demand, cardiogenic shock results. Last, if the damaged portion of the ventricular wall is too weakened, it may form a ventricular aneurysm and rupture, causing death.

Based on pathophysiology, the basic strategies of intervention are pain relief and reperfusion. For reperfusion to be effective, rapid, safe transport is essential.

59. List the mechanisms by which a myocardial infarction may be produced from traumatic and nontraumatic events. p. 196

See objective 58 above.

60. Identify the primary hemodynamic changes produced in myocardial infarction. pp. 196–197

In order for myocardial tissue to become ischemic, there is either hypoperfusion or low blood oxygen. Hypoperfusion is the typical cause of ischemia and eventual infarction. If the affected myocardium includes conductive tissue, dysrhythmias such as ventricular tachycardia or ventricular fibrillation may result. Even if rhythm is preserved, it is possible that infarction can cause pump failure of either the right or left ventricle or both, resulting in heart failure. If the pump failure is severe, cardiogenic shock develops.

61. List and describe the assessment parameters to be evaluated in a patient with a suspected myocardial infarction. pp. 196–197

Initial size-up, inspection, and vital signs may reveal a lot. Is breathing labored? Is the patient diaphoretic and pale? Are there other signs of shock? Remember that blood pressure usually elevates during an episode of ischemia and then returns to normal. Hypotension more likely suggests cardiac compromise and possible shock. Peripheral pulses should be regular and equal. Irregularities may suggest dysrhythmia.

As you move through the OPQRST mnemonic, look for these signs of MI: sudden onset chest pain that proves to be severe, constant, and unrelenting over a period longer than 30 minutes. Pain may radiate to the arms (usually the left), neck, back, or into the epigastrium. Myocardial ischemia can easily produce pain in the 8–10 range and the pain may be associated with nausea and vomiting. Unlike the situation with angina, neither rest nor nitroglycerin will palliate MI pain. Remember that patients with diabetes mellitus may NOT have this picture even when an MI is in evolution. These patients may minimize the severity of their discomfort or simply complain of feeling unwell. Typically, these patients do not have nausea and vomiting. MIs typically evolve over 48–72 hours, and so the pain seen at 24–48 hours may be very different than if you had seen the patient in the first 12–24 hours after onset of discomfort.

Emotion may suggest MI. Patients with severe chest pain often are very frightened and complain of a sense of doom or fear of death. Denial of emotional upset or severity of pain does not mean a benign episode. Denial may hide severe fear or pain.

Auscultation of the lung fields may show clear fields or congestion in the bases. Other physical findings typical of MI include pallor and diaphoresis, coldness in the extremities, and possible change in body temperature. Heart rate and rhythm may be irregular or not. Blood pressure may be baseline, high, or low.

The ECG should be checked first for underlying rhythm and any sign of dysrhythmia. If you have a 12-lead ECG, look at the S-T segment and QRS complex. Check S-T segment for height, depth, and overall contour. Note any depression or elevation. A pathological Q wave (one deeper than 5 mm and wider than 0.04 sec) can indicate infarcted tissue or extensive transient ischemia. Anticipate dysrhythmias.

Next, assess whether the patient is a likely candidate for rapid transport and reperfusion therapy with thrombolytic agents. The time window for thrombolytic therapy to be effective is generally considered to be the first 6 hours from onset of symptoms. Consult medical direction. Note that some patients will have contraindications to thrombolytic therapy, including bleeding or clotting disorders, possible blood in the stool, uncontrolled hypertension, recent trauma, recent hemorrhagic stroke, or recent surgery. Generally, signs of acute injury or pathological Q waves indicate transport for reperfusion if you are within the 6-hour window. If you are uncertain whether the patient meets criteria for reperfusion therapy, assume that he/she does. Be sure to relay information to medical direction including time of pain onset, any S-T segment change (particularly elevation), and location of ischemia or infarct according to a 12-lead ECG.

62. **Identify the anticipated clinical presentation of a patient with a suspected acute myocardial infarction.** pp. 197–199

See objective 61.

63. **Differentiate the characteristics of the pain/discomfort occurring in angina pectoris and acute myocardial infarction.** pp. 197–198

Typical picture of angina: The chief complaint is usually sudden onset chest pain. Pain may radiate or be localized to the chest. Angina usually lasts 3–5 minutes, although it may last as long as 15 minutes, and it is generally relieved by rest and/or nitroglycerin. Breathing may or may not be labored, but you should check for lung sounds after ensuring airway is patent.

Typical picture of MI: There is a sudden onset chest pain that proves to be severe, constant, and unrelenting over a period longer than 30 minutes. Pain may radiate to the arms (usually the left), neck, back, or into the epigastrium. An MI can produce pain in the 8–10 range and the pain may be associated with nausea and vomiting. Unlike the situation with angina, neither rest nor nitroglycerin will palliate MI pain. Blood pressure may be high, low, or baseline, but it is unlikely to change solely with decrease in pain.

64. **Identify the ECG changes characteristically seen during evolution of an acute myocardial infarction.** p. 198

See objective 61.

65. Identify the most common complications of an acute myocardial infarction. pp. 196–199

Dysrhythmias are the most common complication and one of the most common causes of death associated with MI. Congestive heart failure, or even overt cardiogenic shock, can also occur with an MI, especially when the infarcted area is very large or represents tissue loss on top of previous losses from prior MIs. Rupture of ventricular aneurysms, weakened areas of a ventricular wall due to MI, is another complication and cause of sudden death.

66. List the characteristics of a patient eligible for thrombolytic therapy. pp. 198–201

The most essential element of eligibility is time from onset of symptoms, as a duration beyond 6 hours from onset is generally correlated with poor success of thrombolytic therapy. In addition, patients who have contraindications to thrombolytic therapy include persons with bleeding or clotting disorders, possible blood in the stool (GI bleeding), uncontrolled hypertension, recent trauma, recent surgery, or recent hemorrhagic stroke.

67. Describe the "window of opportunity" as it pertains to reperfusion of a myocardial injury or infarction. pp. 198–199

Reperfusion therapy with a thrombolytic agent is most likely to be successful from the onset of symptoms to 6 hours later. Sometimes the window is expanded slightly for a younger patient or one with serious complications.

68. Based on the pathophysiology and clinical evaluation of the patient with a suspected acute myocardial infarction, list the anticipated clinical problems according to their life-threatening potential. pp. 197–201

Dysrhythmias are the most common complication and one of the most common causes of death associated with myocardial infarction. Cardiogenic shock results from loss of cardiac function such that the minimal oxygen needs of the body are not met. A lesser loss of cardiac function can result in congestive heart failure. An uncommon complication that can result in death is rupture of a ventricular aneurysm.

69. Specify the measures that may be taken to prevent or minimize complications in the patient suspected of myocardial infarction. pp. 199–201

Act expediently and calmly and keep the patient in as much physical and emotional rest as possible. Provide supplemental oxygen to decrease myocardial oxygen demand and increase available oxygen. Always have good IV access (possibly more than one IV line). Be sure to ask about medication allergies (especially to any that may have been used previously in a cardiac setting) before the patient or family may become unable to give you this information. Transport as rapidly as possible with no lights or sirens if possible. Delay in transport, however, is preferable to a patient's refusal to leave the scene.

70. Describe the most commonly used cardiac drugs in terms of therapeutic effect and dosages, routes of administration, side effects, and toxic effects. pp. 175–180

The classes of drugs you are most likely to use in the setting of an MI are antidysrhythmics, sympathomimetics, and drugs specific for use in the setting of ischemia (including the thrombolytics), along with less frequently used prehospital medications.

Antidysrhythmics
Antidysrhythmics control or suppress dysrhythmias. Among the most commonly used are atropine, lidocaine, procainamide, bretylium, adenosine, amiodarone, and verapamil.

- Atropine sulfate is a parasympatholytic agent (one that decreases parasympathetic effect by acting as an anticholinergic) used to treat symptomatic bradycardias, especially those arising in the atria, and is sometimes used as part of a treatment regimen for asystole. Dose is 0.5–1.0 mg IV for bradycardia and 1.0 mg for asystole, repeated every 3–5 minutes as needed until a total dose of 0.04 mg/kg is reached. Endotracheal (ET) doses are 2.0–2.5 times the IV doses.

Side effects include blurred vision, dilated pupils, dry mouth, tachycardia, and drowsiness. It has no contraindications in the EMS setting.

- Lidocaine is a first-line antidysrhythmic used to treat and prevent life-threatening ventricular dysrhythmias such as ventricular tachycardia. It suppresses abnormal irritability in the ventricles while having little effect on normal myocardial tissue. Dose is 1.0–1.5 mg/kg slow IV push (50 mg/min) for ectopy, or normal IV push in cardiac arrest. An IV drip is prepared by mixing 1 gram into 250 cc D_5W or saline. Typical maintenance dose is 2–4 mg/minute. Maximum bolus dose is 300 mg. The drug can be given IV bolus, IV drip, or through an ET tube. Side effects include drowsiness, seizures, confusion, bradycardia, heart blocks, and nausea and vomiting. Lidocaine is contraindicated by the presence of second- or third-degree AV block.

- Procainamide is a second-line antidysrhythmic to lidocaine, and it is used for ventricular dysrhythmias refractory to lidocaine or for patients who are allergic to lidocaine. It is administered by slow IV bolus or IV drip. IV bolus is 100 mg given over 5 minutes, with a maximum dose of 17 mg/kg. Discontinue when the dysrhythmia is suppressed, hypotension ensues, the QRS complex widens 50%, or the maximum dose is given. Drip rate is the same as for lidocaine. Side effects and contraindications are the same as for lidocaine.

- Bretylium is a second-line antidysrhythmic used to treat life-threatening ventricular dysrhythmias, especially ventricular fibrillation. Although its mechanism of action is poorly understood, bretylium apparently raises the ventricular fibrillation threshold. Bretylium is administered by IV bolus and IV drip. Dose is 5 mg/kg IV push with drip rate of 1–2 mg/min. A subsequent dose of 10 mg/kg is repeated if the dysrhythmia persists. Maximum dose is 30 mg/kg. Side effects include hypo- or hypertension, dizziness, syncope, seizures, and nausea and vomiting. Bretylium is now being used less frequently because of development of other agents.

- Adenosine is used to manage supraventricular tachydysrhythmias. It is a naturally occurring nucleoside that acts on the AV node to slow conduction and inhibit reentry pathways. It is given by IV rapid bolus through a venous site as close to the heart as possible. Flush the line with saline immediately after giving adenosine to ensure drug delivery. Initial dose is 6 mg (rapid push) followed by a 15–30 cc saline flush. If the tachydysrhythmia is not eliminated, a second dose of 12 mg and, if needed, a third dose of 12 mg may be given. Maximum dose is 30 mg. Side effects include apprehension, burning sensation, heavy sensation in the arms, hypotension, chest pressure, diaphoresis, numbness or tingling, dyspnea, tightness in the throat and/or groin pressure, headache, and nausea and vomiting. Adenosine is contraindicated in the presence of second- or third-degree AV block or in sick sinus syndrome unless a pacemaker is present.

- Amiodarone (Cordarone) is an antidysrhythmic used in management of recurring ventricular fibrillation and hemodynamically unstable ventricular tachycardia (nonperfusing tachycardia). Amiodarone is also being used more frequently in the prehospital setting of cardiac arrest. Although it is a second-line drug in the United States, it is a first-line agent in several Commonwealth countries. Dosage is 150–300 mg by slow IV infusion. Side effects include hypotension (the most common), bradycardia, and AV blocks. It is contraindicated in cardiogenic shock, marked sinus bradycardia, and second- or third-degree AV block.

- Verapamil is a calcium channel blocker that slows heart rate in symptomatic atrial tachycardias. It is used to terminate paroxysmal supraventricular tachycardia as well as to control the rapid ventricular response often seen with atrial flutter or fibrillation. It is administered by slow IV bolus with a maximum dose of 30 mg.

Sympathomimetic agents

Sympathomimetic agents are similar to the naturally occurring hormones epinephrine and norepinephrine, and they mimic sympathetic nervous system stimulation on either alpha or beta adrenergic receptors. Alpha receptor stimulation causes peripheral vasoconstriction and beta receptor stimulation increases heart rate and cardiac contractility, causes bronchodilation, and peripheral vasodilation. Stimulation of dopaminergic receptors in the renal and mesenteric vascular beds causes dilation. Commonly used sympathomimetic agents include epinephrine, norepinephrine, isoproterenol, dopamine, and dobutamine.

- Epinephrine, which acts on alpha and beta receptors, is the mainstay of cardiac arrest resuscitation. It is used with ventricular fibrillation, asystole, and pulseless electrical activity. It is also sometimes used for bradycardia refractory to atropine. It is given as IV bolus, subcutaneously, and via ET tube. Dose is 1 mg of 1:10,000 solution given every 3–5 minutes.

- Norepinephrine has alpha agonist properties greater than those of epinephrine. It acts on beta receptors to a lesser degree. It is used occasionally in hemodynamically significant hypotension and cardiogenic shock, although dopamine is the first-line agent for these conditions. Norepinephrine may be effective if total peripheral resistance is low, such as in neurogenic shock. It is administered by IV infusion via drip by placing 4 mg into 1000 cc of D_5W (ONLY) to give a concentration of 4 mcg/cc. Initial loading dose is 8–12 mcg/min to give blood pressure of 80–100 mmHg systolic. Maintenance dose is 2–4 mcg/min. Side effects include anxiety, trembling, headache, dizziness, and nausea and vomiting. It can also cause bradycardia. DO NOT use norepinephrine in patients with hypotension from hypovolemia.

- Isoproterenol is rarely used with the advent of TCP, but it is a potent beta agonist that increases heart rate and cardiac contractility. It is used in bradycardia refractory to atropine and to manage asystole. Isoproterenol is given via IV infusion. Add 1 mg to 250 cc D_5W or saline to give 4 mcg/cc. The drip rate is 2–20 mcg/min. Common procedure is to start with a low dose and titrate upward until a satisfactory rate is achieved. TCP is preferred to use of isoproterenol.

- Dopamine (Intropin) is a vasopressor that increases cardiac output. It stimulates both alpha and beta receptors. It has the advantage over other drugs of preserving renal perfusion at recommended doses. Dose is given via IV drip by mixing 800 mg into 500 cc D_5W or saline to give a concentration of 1600 mcg/cc (400 mg into 250 cc also works). Dopamine's effects are dose-related: At 1–2 mcg/kg/min, renal artery dilation occurs; at 2–10 mcg/kg/min, beta receptors are primarily stimulated; at 10–15 mcg/kg/min, both beta and alpha receptors are stimulated; and at 15–20 mcg/kg/min, alpha receptors are primarily stimulated. Side effects include nervousness, headache, dysrhythmias, palpitations, chest pain, dyspnea, and nausea and vomiting. Note: Dopamine is contraindicated for hypovolemic shock until fluid resuscitation has been completed.

- Dobutamine (Dobutrex), like dopamine, increases cardiac output and increases stroke volume. It has little effect on heart rate and is occasionally used in isolated left heart failure until medications such as digitalis can take effect. Dobutamine is given by IV infusion by mixing 250 mg into 250 cc D_5W or saline to give a concentration of 1000 mcg/cc. Dose is 2–10 mcg/kg/min titrated to effect. Its side effects are the same as dopamine's. Do not use dobutamine as the sole agent in hypovolemic shock unless fluid resuscitation is complete. Dopamine is preferred over dobutamine to increase cardiac output in cardiogenic shock.

Drugs used for myocardial ischemia

Drugs used to treat myocardial ischemia and relieve its pain include oxygen, nitrous oxide, nitroglycerin, morphine, and nalbuphine.

- Oxygen is important because it increases the blood's oxygen content and aids oxygenation of peripheral and cardiac tissues. It is indicated in any situation where hypoxia or ischemia is possible.

- Nitrous oxide (Nitronox) is purely an analgesic with no significant hemodynamic effects. However, delivery in fixed combination with 50% oxygen can increase myocardial oxygen supply. Nitrous oxide is self-administered by inhalation via a modified demand valve to the desired effect. Its effects subside within 2–5 minutes. Side effects include CNS depression and potential respiratory depression. Do not give nitrous oxide to patients who cannot comprehend verbal instructions or who are intoxicated with alcohol or other drugs.

- Nitroglycerin is an organic nitrate that dilates peripheral arteries and veins, reducing preload and afterload and myocardial oxygen demand. It may cause some coronary artery dilation, thus increasing blood flow through the collateral circulation. Nitroglycerin use often helps to distinguish the pain of angina from that of an MI. Nitroglycerin does not relieve the pain of an MI, but it should be given before morphine because it works in conjunction with morphine in an MI. Dosage is one tablet sublingually repeated every 5 minutes up to a total of three tablets. Monitor blood pressure before each dose. Its side effects include headache, dizziness, weakness, hypotension, and tachycardia. Note that nitroglycerin loses potency as soon as the bottle is opened to the air. Always use the nitroglycerin provided on the medical intensive care unit and check the date before administration.

- Morphine sulfate is a narcotic drug that is important in managing MI. It reduces myocardial oxygen demand by reducing both preload and afterload. It also acts directly on the CNS to relieve pain, and it reduces sympathetic discharge, which can further decrease myocardial oxygen demand. Dosage is in 1–2 mg increments via slow IV push, titrated to pain relief. Monitor blood pressure before each dose. Side effects include nausea and vomiting, abdominal cramping, respiratory depression, hypotension, and potential altered mental status. Toxic effects are apnea and severe hypotension. Check for drug allergy before administration.
- Nalbuphine (Nubain) is used in some EMS systems instead of morphine. Nalbuphine is an analgesic, but it lacks the desirable hemodynamic effects of morphine. Dose is 10–20 mg IV, IM, or subcutaneously. Side effects include sedation, clammy skin, dizziness, dry mouth, hypotension, hypertension, and nausea and vomiting. It is contraindicated in patients who have taken depressants or alcohol.

Thrombolytic agents

The use of thrombolytic agents as a definitive treatment for myocardial ischemia is one of the most important recent advances in medicine. In some instances, thrombolytic therapy may even have benefit in the field, and this is especially true in areas with a long transit time to a definitive care facility. Thrombolytic agents are generally very expensive, and their use requires a 12-lead ECG. Alteplase (tPA, Activase) and reteplase (Retavase) are thrombolytic agents. Although aspirin is not a thrombolytic agent, it merits discussion in this section.

- Aspirin is important in treatment of cardiac ischemia because it inhibits platelet aggregation and thus is effective in treating coronary ischemia and stroke secondary to thrombus development. The standard dosage is 325 mg by mouth, although some physicians prefer smaller doses. Baby aspirin may be useful because it can be chewed, thus more quickly reaching a therapeutic blood level. Its most common side effect is GI upset, although bleeding can be a problem in certain patients.
- Alteplase (Activase, tPA). Alteplase, or tPA (tissue plasminogen activator) is a potent thrombolytic agent that is manufactured through recombinant technology, which means it is the same as the biological compound. This minimizes chances of allergic reaction. TPA is effective if given within 6 hours of onset of coronary ischemia. It is given as a bolus dose followed by infusion. The typical dose is 100 mg given over 1.5–2 hours. Complications of tPA include hemorrhage, which can be fatal. Also, when reperfusion occurs, potentially life-threatening dysrhythmias can develop.
- Reteplase (Retavase) is another human plasminogen activator. It functions in a manner similar to tPA and has the same basic side effects and complications. It is administered as a single 10-unit bolus by IV push over 2 minutes. A second 10-unit bolus is given 30 minutes afterward. This dosing regimen makes reteplase attractive for prehospital care.

Other prehospital drugs

Less frequently used agents you may administer in the prehospital setting include furosemide, diazepam, promethazine, and sodium nitroprusside.

- Furosemide (Lasix) is a potent loop diuretic that also relaxes the venous system with effects seen within 5 minutes. Its diuretic effect decreases intravascular fluid volume. Dose is 40 mg slow IV push (40 mg/min). If the patient takes furosemide or another diuretic, you may need to double the dosage. Side effects include hypotension, ECG changes, chest pain, dry mouth, hypokalemia, hypochloremia, hyponatremia, and hyperglycemia. Furosemide should only be used in life-threatening emergencies during pregnancy because it can cause fetal abnormalities.
- Diazepam (Valium) is not an analgesic but rather an anti-anxiety drug, and it may be given to patients who are extremely apprehensive or agitated. Dose is 2–5 mg IV or deep IM.
- Promethazine (Phenergan) has sedative, antihistamine, antiemetic, and anticholinergic properties. It also potentiates narcotics, making it useful in the MI setting by reducing the nausea associated with morphine while enhancing its effects. Dosage is 12.5–25.0 mg given slow IV push or deep IM (25.0 mg/min). Its side effects are drowsiness, sedation, blurred vision, tachycardia, bradycardia, and dizziness. Promethazine is contraindicated in unresponsive patients or those taking large doses of depressants. Extrapyramidal symptoms (namely, dystonia) have been reported with promethazine.

- Sodium nitroprusside (Nipride) is a potent arterial and venous vasodilator, making it popular for use in hypertensive crisis. It is given as an IV infusion, which makes administration more controlled and the patient's response more predictable.

Drugs infrequently used in the prehospital setting

Lastly, certain medications commonly associated with in-hospital use or long-term patient use are included in this discussion. You are most likely to use these often if you work in an emergency department. Drugs in this group include digitalis, beta blockers, calcium channel blockers, and alkalinizing agents.

- Digitalis (digoxin, Lanoxin) is a cardiac glycoside that increases cardiac contractility and cardiac output. It slows impulse conduction through the AV node and decreases the ventricular response to certain supraventricular dysrhythmias such as atrial flutter or fibrillation and paroxysmal supraventricular tachycardia. It is also used long term to treat heart failure. The dose is 8–12 mcg/kg slow IV push over 15–20 minutes. If possible, obtain the patient's digitalis level beforehand (if the patient is on digoxin) before administering any cardiac glycoside. Most patients taking digitalis will remain therapeutic at 10–15 mcg/kg over a 24-hour period. Giving digitalis to patients who already take a cardiac glycoside involves complicated calculations, which makes it impractical for prehospital use in most settings. Its side effects include fatigue, muscle weakness, agitation, hallucinations, headache, malaise, dizziness, vertigo, stupor, blurred vision and yellow-green halo vision, photophobia, diplopia, and nausea and vomiting. Digitalis toxicity, which is not uncommon in some patients, can cause almost any dysrhythmia, including some of the same dysrhythmias it is used to treat, and these will often be refractory to traditional antidysrhythmic drugs. Digitalis is contraindicated in any digitalis-induced toxicity, ventricular fibrillation, or ventricular tachycardia not caused by CHF.
- Beta blockers are frequently used to control dysrhythmias, hypertension, and angina. Many beta blockers such as propranolol (Inderal) are non-selective; other beta blockers such as metoprolol are selective for either B_1 or B_2 receptors. Beta blockers may precipitate CHF, heart block, or asthma in patients predisposed to them. The beta-blocker labetalol (Trandate, Normodyne) effectively decreases blood pressure. It is given by IV bolus and infusion. The IV bolus is 20 mg over 20 minutes and may be repeated at 40–80 mg over 10 minutes. Maximum bolus is 300 mg. Drip is established by mixing 200 mg into 160 cc D_5W, and the drip dose is 2 cc/min.
- Calcium channel blockers are a relatively new class of antihypertensive medication that include verapamil (Isoptin, Calan), diltiazem (Cardizem), and nifedipine (Procardia). Nifedipine is now being used in addition to nitroglycerin to treat angina. Like nitroglycerin, it is a vasodilator but with a different mechanism. It is given orally. Calcium channel blockers are being used increasingly for angina, dysrhythmias, and other cardiovascular problems.
- Alkalinizing agents such as sodium bicarbonate are used late in the management of cardiac arrest, if at all. Occasionally, metabolic acidosis from another disorder may cause pulseless electrical activity, asystole, ventricular tachycardia, or ventricular fibrillation. In these cases, sodium bicarbonate may aid in converting to a perfusing rhythm. Adequate CPR, prompt defibrillation, and appropriate drug administration should always precede the use of bicarbonate. Sodium bicarbonate has few side effects and no contraindications in the emergency setting. Dose is initially 1 mEq/kg followed by 0.5 mEq/kg every 10 minutes. When possible, doses should be based on arterial blood gas (ABG) results.

71. **Describe the epidemiology, morbidity, mortality, and physiology associated with heart failure.** pp. 202–204

Heart failure is the clinical syndrome in which the heart's pumping capacity is compromised so that cardiac output cannot meet the body's needs. Heart failure can be typed as right ventricle or left ventricle failure or bilateral heart failure. Left ventricular failure occurs when the left ventricle's ability to pump fails, causing back pressure of blood into the pulmonary circulation, which results in pulmonary edema. Right ventricular failure is due to loss of pumping ability in the right ventricle, resulting in back pressure of blood into the systemic venous circulation causing venous congestion. The most common cause of right heart failure is pre-existent left heart failure. Other causes of right ventricular failure include systemic hypertension, pulmonary hypertension due to COPD, or *cor pulmonale*. All of these causes relate to an initial increase in the pressure in the pulmonary arteries, which then results in right ventricular enlargement, and, if untreated, right ventricular failure. Pulmonary embolism causes right ventricular failure if the clot is large enough to block a major pulmonary vessel.

72. Identify the factors that may precipitate or aggravate heart failure. pp. 202–204

There are many causes of heart failure, including valve disorders and coronary or myocardial disease. Dysrhythmias may aggravate heart failure by further decreasing cardiac output, decreasing myocardial perfusion, or both. Other factors that can contribute to heart failure include excess fluid or salt intake, fever (sepsis), hypertension, pulmonary embolism, or excessive alcohol or drug use. Failure can manifest with exertion in a patient who has an underlying disease or who has progressive cardiac disease. Specific causes of left heart failure include MI, valvular disease, chronic hypertension, and dysrhythmias. Because MI is a common cause of left ventricular failure, suspect that all patients with pulmonary edema may have had an MI. Causes of right ventricular failure include initial MI of the left ventricle, systemic hypertension, pulmonary hypertension due to COPD, and *cor pulmonale*. Another major cause of right ventricular failure is pulmonary embolism.

73. Define acute pulmonary edema and describe its relationship to left ventricular failure. p. 202

As the left ventricle's pumping ability falls, it cannot pump out all of the blood delivered to it from the lungs. Consequently, left atrial pressure rises and is transmitted to the pulmonary veins and the pulmonary capillary beds. When pulmonary capillary pressure increases sufficiently, blood plasma is forced into the alveoli and interstitial spaces; this is pulmonary edema (swelling of the lungs). Progressive fluid accumulation in the alveoli decreases the lungs' oxygenation capacity and can cause hypoxia that can be fatal.

74. Differentiate between early and late signs and symptoms of left ventricular failure and those of right ventricular failure. pp. 203–204

For left ventricular failure, the cardinal symptom is dyspnea due to pulmonary edema. Signs include cyanosis, tachycardia, noisy, labored breathing, rales, cough, blood-tinged, frothy sputum, and a gallop rhythm of the heart. The major signs of right ventricular failure: neck veins engorged and pulsating, edema of body and extremities, engorged liver and spleen, abdominal distention with ascites (fluid), as well as tachycardia.

Congestive heart failure (CHF) is a general term for ventricular failure (left, right, or both) that causes excess fluid to accumulate in body tissues (hence, congestion). The excess fluid is manifest as edema, which may be pulmonary, peripheral, sacral, or within the abdomen as ascites. You may find it in the acute setting of MI, pulmonary edema, or pulmonary hypertension. In the chronic setting, it can reflect cardiac enlargement.

75. Define and explain the clinical significance of paroxysmal nocturnal dyspnea, pulmonary edema, and dependent edema. pp. 204–205

Paroxysmal nocturnal dyspnea (PND) is an episode of waking during the night due to shortness of breath, and it reflects the presence of pulmonary edema. If these episodes become more frequent (more nights or more times/night), it suggests worsening of the underlying pathophysiologic process. Pulmonary edema reflects backup of fluid into the pulmonary alveoli and interstitium, but it does not necessarily imply etiology. Left ventricular failure, however, is probably the best known and most common cause, and you should look for other signs of congestive heart failure in a patient who presents with signs of pulmonary edema. If pulmonary edema seems to be very acute in onset, look for precipitating causes, such as cardiac dysrhythmia or acute MI. Dependent edema represents edema in the gravity-dependent portions of the body. For a bedridden patient, this often manifests as sacral edema. Sometimes edema will be so severe it will eliminate your ability to find a pulse in the affected area (such as a pedal pulse). If edema is severe enough to be pitting edema (a situation in which you press firmly into the affected tissue, lift the finger, and find that the depression caused by your finger persists), you can make a semi-quantitative evaluation by scoring as 0 to 4+.

76. List the interventions prescribed for the patient in acute congestive heart failure.   pp. 205–206

Manage a patient with severe CHF by assessing in an ongoing manner for life-threatening symptoms and intervene promptly while readying the patient for rapid transport. Do not allow the patient to exert in any way, including standing up. Positioning in a seated position with feet dangling promotes venous pooling and, consequently, reduced preload. Administer high-flow oxygen. If necessary, provide positive-pressure ventilations with either a demand valve or a bag-valve-mask device. Establish an IV line at a keep-vein-open rate or place a saline or heparin lock. Place ECG electrodes. If the patient is extremely diaphoretic, apply tincture of Benzoin first so electrodes will be tightly adherent to skin. Record a baseline ECG and continue monitoring.

Medication use will be according to your local protocols or the order of medical direction. Always remember to ask about drug allergies or reactions to any medication.

Transport as a nonemergency unless clinical conditions say otherwise. Indications for emergency transport include hypertension or hypotension, severe respiratory distress or pending respiratory failure, or life-threatening dysrhythmias. If you feel nonemergency transport will compromise the patient's condition, use lights and siren.

77. Describe the most commonly used pharmacological agents in the management of congestive heart failure in terms of therapeutic effect, dosages, routes of administration, side effects, and toxic effects.   pp. 175–180, 206

The drugs most likely to be used in the setting of left ventricular failure and pulmonary edema include morphine sulfate, nitroglycerin, furosemide (Lasix), dopamine (Intropin), dobutamine (Dobutrex), promethazine (Phenergan), and nitrous oxide (Nitronox). Dosages and other information on these medications are given in objective 70 above.

78. Define and describe the incidence, mortality, morbidity, pathophysiology, assessment, and management of the following cardiac related problems: pp. 206–216

Cardiac tamponade
Cardiac tamponade exists when an accumulation of material (air, pus, serum, blood, or a combination) inside the pericardium places pressure on the heart such that diastolic filling is impaired and stroke volume falls. Tamponade may evolve gradually; common progressive causes include pericarditis and benign or malignant neoplasms. Rare medical causes of tamponade include hypothyroidism and renal disease. Acute onset tends to occur when the cause is trauma or MI. Specific traumatic causes include CPR and penetrating and nonpenetrating chest trauma. Regardless of cause and regardless of gradual or acute onset, cardiac tamponade can lead to death.

During the initial patient assessment, you may suspect cardiac tamponade. If so, limit history taking to questions that might reveal a precipitating cause. Use the OPQRST mnemonic to get information about the patient's symptoms: The most frequent chief complaints in tamponade are chest pain or dyspnea, and pain may be either dull or sharp. On physical exam, cardiac tamponade often presents with a characteristic picture: dyspnea and orthopnea, with clear lung sounds. Typically, peripheral pulses are rapid and weak. In the early stage, venous pressure is often elevated and you may see jugular vein distention. Blood pressure often reveals a decrease in systolic pressure, pulsus paradoxus, and narrowing pulse pressures. Heart sounds may be normal early in tamponade, but they are more likely (especially later) to become muffled or faint because of the presence of the tamponade-producing material in the pericardial sac.

Use of the ECG, whether single monitor lead or 12-lead, is not a diagnostic tool, but it may support your clinical suspicions. ECG findings are generally inconclusive; however, ectopy is usually a late sign due to irritation of the heart's epicardial tissue by the pericardial effusion. QRS and T wave voltages are low, and nonspecific T wave changes occur. S-T segments may elevate. Electrical alternans (weak voltage alternating with normal voltage) may appear in the P, QRS, T, or S-T segments.

Management is primarily supportive except when shock or low perfusion is detected. Maintain airway and deliver high-flow oxygen. If clinically indicated, use endotracheal intubation and maintain circulation with IV support, medications, or CPR. Again, before giving any medication ask about allergies. Medications frequently used in the setting of cardiac tamponade include morphine sulfate, nitrous oxide, furosemide, dopamine, and dobutamine. Rapid transport is indicated.

Hypertensive emergency

Hypertensive emergency occurs when there is a life-threatening elevation of blood pressure. This develops in about 1% of patients with hypertension. Clinically, the emergency is usually characterized by a rapid increase in diastolic pressure (generally, to greater than 130 mmHg) accompanied by restlessness and confusion, blurred vision, and nausea and vomiting. It often occurs with hypertensive encephalopathy, a consequence of severe hypertension marked by severe headache, vomiting, visual changes including transient blindness, paralysis, seizures, and stupor or coma. With modern medications, hypertensive encephalopathy has become rare, although it is still seen in the hospital setting. Both ischemic and hemorrhagic strokes are more common results of severe hypertension and can have devastating consequences. Hypertensive emergency can also cause left ventricular failure and pulmonary edema.

The major causes of hypertensive emergency include noncompliance with antihypertensive drugs or other prescribed medications and lack of treatment for hypertension. Risk factors include age (older age) and race (hypertension is more common in blacks, and morbidity and mortality appear to be higher, too). Among pregnant women, one cause of hypertension is preeclampsia (also called toxemia of pregnancy), which can appear at any point after the 20th week of pregnancy.

Assessment findings on physical exam of a patient with hypertensive emergency commonly include a chief complaint of headache accompanied by any of the following: nausea, vomiting, blurred vision, shortness of breath, epistaxis, and dizziness (vertigo). The patient may be semiconscious or unconscious and seizing. In toxemia of pregnancy, the woman usually has edema of hands or face. Photosensitivity and headache are common complaints in this group. Determine whether there is a documented history of hypertension and to what degree prescribed medications have been taken. Find out whether the patient may have borrowed someone else's medications or taken herbal or over-the-counter drugs. Skin may be pale or flushed, normal, cool, or warm. Look for edema. The patient may confirm PND, orthopnea, vertigo, epistaxis, tinnitus, or visual acuities. Look for possible motor or sensory deficits in parts of the body or on one side. ECG findings are generally inconclusive unless there is an underlying cardiac condition such as angina or MI. If left ventricular failure is present, pulmonary edema may be present. Otherwise, lungs are generally clear. The pulse is strong and may feel bounding. Hypertension is present with systolic pressure greater than 160 mmHg and/or diastolic pressure greater than 90 mmHg. Signs or symptoms of hypertensive encephalopathy in the presence of measured hypertension should be considered hypertensive emergency.

Management centers on positioning for comfort and watching for possible airway compromise if vomiting or stroke occurs. Give oxygen and decide upon transport based on clinical presentation. Attempt supportive IV therapy on-scene or en route. Place pregnant patients on their left sides and transport as smoothly and quietly as possible.

Medications that may be used in the prehospital setting have notably changed recently; know your local protocol. Medications often used include morphine, furosemide, nitroglycerin, sodium nitroprusside, and labetalol (Trandate, Normodyne).

Cardiogenic shock

Cardiogenic shock is the extreme state of heart failure: Cardiac output is so low it cannot sustain minimal physiologic activity. Clinically, you will see it after existing dysrhythmias, hypovolemia, or altered vascular tone have been corrected, leaving only the possibility of endogenous pump failure. This failure of the heart and overwhelming of any compensatory mechanisms usually happens after an extensive MI, often involving more than 40% of the left ventricle, or with diffuse ischemia. Note that cardiogenic shock can occur at any age, but it is most often seen as an end-stage event in geriatric patients with underlying disease. Mortality rate is high for elderly patients following massive MI or septic shock because end-organ damage is so severe that life cannot be sustained.

Numerous mechanisms can lead to cardiogenic shock, and onset may be gradual or acute. Among mechanical causes are tension pneumothorax and cardiac tamponade. Interference with ventricular emptying or afterload (such as pulmonary embolism and prosthetic or natural valve dysfunction) can also cause shock. Impairment in cardiac contractility is also a general cause: examples include MI, myocarditis, and recreational drug use. Trauma is another general cause, either primarily through cardiac damage or secondarily through hypovolemia. Finally, shock can develop secondarily to underlying conditions such as neurologic, GI, renal, or metabolic disorders.

Assessment findings depend on whether the patient is in an early phase of shock or a most advanced state. Look for evidence of a possible contributing cause such as hypovolemia, sepsis, or trauma. Among direct cardiac causes, you will most often see cardiogenic shock in the setting of MI if the MI affects the anterior wall or 40% or more of the left ventricle. Information about the patient's medications may give clues about pre-existing pump compromise. Inquire about the degree of compliance with medication regiments and ask about borrowed or over-the-counter drugs, which might have unpredictable interaction effects.

The altered mental status associated with advancing shock may begin as restlessness and progress through confusion to loss of consciousness. Airway findings include dyspnea, productive cough, or labored breathing. Tachypnea is often present due to pulmonary edema. Also common is a history of paroxysmal nocturnal dyspnea. Typical ECG findings include tachycardia and atrial dysrhythmias such as atrial tachycardia. Ectopy is also common.

MI often precedes cardiogenic shock; symptoms will be compatible with those expected with MI. Expect hypotension to develop as shock progresses. Systolic pressure will often fall to less than 80 mmHg. Try to correct any discovered dysrhythmias.

Management of cardiogenic shock begins by placing the patient in a position of comfort. With pulmonary edema, this may be sitting upright. Treatment consists mostly of caring for underlying conditions (such as MI or CHF) and supportive care. Remember to treat heart rate and rhythm and transport rapidly. Medications that may be used in this setting include the vasopressors dopamine, dobutamine, and norepinephrine. Other medications include morphine, promethazine, nitroglycerin, nitrous oxide, furosemide, digitalis, and sodium bicarbonate.

Cardiac arrest

Cardiac arrest and sudden death account for 60% of all deaths from coronary heart disease. Cardiac arrest is defined as the absence of ventricular contractions that immediately results in systemic circulatory failure. Sudden death is any death that occurs within one hour of the onset of symptoms. At autopsy, signs of MI are not present, and authorities generally believe lethal dysrhythmia secondary to severe atherosclerosis is the most common cause of death. The risk factors for sudden death are similar to those for ASHD and CHD. Other causes of sudden death include drowning, acid-base imbalance, electrocution, drug intoxication, electrolyte imbalance, hypoxia, hypothermia, pulmonary embolism, stroke, hyperkalemia, trauma, and end-stage renal disease.

Assessment for cardiac arrest shows an unresponsive, apneic, pulseless individual. After initiating CPR, place ECG leads and initiate monitoring. Dysrhythmias you may find include ventricular tachycardia or fibrillation, asystole, or PEA. If you find asystole, confirm it in two or more leads. Question bystanders with the goal of finding some specific, prognostic information: Did anyone witness the arrest? If CPR was begun before you arrived, try to learn as precisely as possible the length of time between arrest and initiation of effective CPR. Often, the emergency room physician will also want to know total down time from the beginning of the arrest until arrival at the emergency department. Also, try to get a list of the patient's medications as well as a past history.

Management starts with simultaneous efforts on the ABCs. Ventilate with a bag-valve mask using 100% oxygen. Intubate or insert an airway as quickly as possible. If ECG changes indicate defibrillation or synchronized cardioversion, perform it in conjunction with CPR, stopping CPR only long enough to apply the pads or paddles and deliver the shock. If the patient has an internal pacemaker or defibrillator, be sure not to defibrillate over the device.

After starting CPR and advanced airway management, get IV access with a venous site as close to the heart as possible (for instance, the antecubital area in the arm or the external jugular vein). Follow IV medications with a 30–45 second flush to ensure complete delivery. After each flush, set the line to a keep-vein-open rate. Agents used with cardiac arrest include atropine, lidocaine, procainamide, bretylium, epinephrine, norepinephrine, isoproterenol, dopamine, dobutamine, and sodium bicarbonate.

If blood pressure and pulse return, be aware that the blood pressure itself may be low, normal, or high because of the drugs administered. Pulse may return with a bradycardic, normal, or tachycardic rate. Ventricular ectopy is the most serious concern. If the patient presented in ventricular tachycardia or ventricular fibrillation or if ectopy is seen postarrest, use an antidysrhythmic such as lidocaine.

Transport should be done as safely and smoothly as possible and with lights and siren.

79. Identify the limiting factor of pericardial anatomy that determines intrapericardiac pressure. **p. 206**

The limitation is in the volume of material that can be held in the pericardial sac without exerting undue pressure on the heart. The normal volume is about 25 cc in an adult. As this volume is exceeded, pressure is exerted on the heart, and it can eventually reach the point of significantly limiting the extent to which the heart can fill during diastole or contract to expel blood during systole. This is cardiac tamponade.

80. Describe how to determine if pulsus paradoxus, pulsus alternans, or electrical alternans is present. **pp. 205–207**

Pulsus paradoxus is determined by measuring blood pressure during respirations. A systolic pressure that falls more than 10 mmHg during inspiration is pulsus paradoxus. Pulsus alternans is an alternation between weak and strong peripheral pulses; this is determined by palpation of the pulse. Electrical alternans is determined by ECG analysis: It consists of an alternating pattern of normal and very low voltage.

81. Explain the essential pathophysiological defect of hypertension in terms of Starling's law of the heart. **pp. 204, 209–210**

Starling's law states that the greater the stretch on myocardial muscle (the preload), the greater will be the force of contraction. This is true until the muscle is overstretched, at which point contraction becomes weaker. Afterload also affects stroke volume. An increase in afterload (peripheral vascular resistance) is an increase in the pressure against which the ventricle must pump, and thus increased afterload decreases stroke volume. Hypertension, or high blood pressure, is a state in which afterload is chronically increased, and thus this represents a chronic stressor on the ventricular myocardium.

82. Rank the clinical problems of patients in hypertensive emergencies according to their sense of urgency. **p. 208**

Hypertensive emergency in the general sense is a state in which diastolic blood pressure has risen to dangerous levels (greater than 130 mmHg), mandating a lowering of blood pressure within one hour to minimize or avoid risk for end-organ changes such as hypertensive encephalopathy, renal failure, or blindness. Hypertensive encephalopathy is a life-threatening situation in which stroke, coma, left ventricular failure, or pulmonary edema may occur. A hypertensive emergency in a pregnant patient with preeclampsia poses a high risk of the obstetric complication of abruption of the placenta or progression to eclampsia, with its seizures and risk of death for the woman and unborn fetus.

83. Identify the drugs of choice for hypertensive emergencies, cardiogenic shock, and cardiac arrest, including their indications, contraindications, side effects, route of administration, and dosages. **pp. 175–180, 209, 212, 213–214**

- *Hypertensive emergencies:* Drugs include morphine sulfate, furosemide, nitroglycerin, sodium nitroprusside, and labetalol.

- *Cardiogenic shock:* Drugs include dopamine, dobutamine, norepinephrine, morphine sulfate, promethazine, nitroglycerin, nitrous oxide, furosemide, digitalis, and sodium bicarbonate.
- *Cardiac arrest:* Drugs include atropine, lidocaine, procainamide, bretylium, epinephrine, norepinephrine, isoproterenol, dopamine, dobutamine, and sodium bicarbonate.

General descriptions, specific doses, contraindications, and side effects of these medications are given in objective 70 above. Two medications not covered in detail in objective 70 are discussed below.

Labetalol (Trandate, Normodyne). The IV bolus is 20 mg over 20 minutes, and it may be repeated at 40–80 mg over 10 minutes. Maximum bolus is 300 mg. Drip is established by mixing 200 mg into 160 cc D_5W, and the drip dose is 2 cc/min.

Sodium bicarbonate. Sodium bicarbonate is used late in the management of cardiac arrest, if at all. Occasionally, metabolic acidosis from another disorder may cause pulseless electrical activity, asystole, ventricular tachycardia, or ventricular fibrillation. In these cases, sodium bicarbonate may aid in converting to a perfusing rhythm. Adequate CPR, prompt defibrillation, and appropriate drug administration should always precede the use of bicarbonate. Sodium bicarbonate has few side effects and no contraindications in the emergency setting. Dose is initially 1 mEq/kg followed by 0.5 mEq/kg every 10 minutes. When possible, doses should be based on arterial blood gas (ABG) results.

84. Describe the major systemic effects of reduced tissue perfusion caused by cardiogenic shock. pp. 209–210

A chief effect is CNS compromise, which may manifest early as restlessness or agitation and later as confusion or unconsciousness. Impaired renal function due to poor perfusion may be seen as oliguria or anuria. The decrease in blood flow to the extremities as blood is shunted to core organs is seen as cold, clammy, pale skin.

85. Explain the primary mechanisms by which the heart may compensate for a diminished cardiac output and describe their efficiency in cardiogenic shock. pp. 209–210

The three basic mechanisms that increase cardiac output are increase in contractility, increase in preload, or decreasing peripheral resistance. Increased myocardial contractile force will help to increase stroke volume. Increased preload increases the stretch on the myocardium, and, within limits (this is Starling's law), this results in increased contraction force and increased stroke volume. Last, decreasing peripheral resistance (afterload) decreases the force that the ventricles must exert in order to expel blood into the aorta and pulmonary arteries.

86. Identify the clinical criteria and progressive stages of cardiogenic shock. pp. 209–210

See objective 78 above.

87. Describe the dysrhythmias seen in cardiac arrest. p. 213

The dysrhythmias seen most frequently in cardiac arrest are ventricular tachycardia, ventricular fibrillation, asystole, and pulseless electrical activity (PEA). Asystole should always be confirmed in two more ECG leads.

88. Explain how to confirm asystole using the 3-lead ECG. p. 213

An ECG tracing of asystole is shown in Part 1 of this chapter. On each lead, you should see an absence of all cardiac electrical activity: There will be no discernible components of the ECG sequence (no P waves, QRS complexes, or T waves).

89. Define the terms *defibrillation* and *synchronized cardioversion*. pp. 180–181, 183

Defibrillation is the process of passing an electrical current through a fibrillating heart in order to depolarize all cells and allow them to repolarize uniformly, thus restoring an organized cardiac rhythm. Synchronized cardioversion is a controlled form of defibrillation for patients who have some organized cardiac activity with a pulse. A synchronizing circuit interprets the QRS cycle and delivers an electrical discharge during the R wave of the QRS complex, reducing the likelihood of delivering the cardioversion during the vulnerable period of the QRS cycle and reducing the likelihood of triggering ventricular fibrillation. Indications for synchronized cardioversion include perfusing ventricular tachycardia, paroxysmal supraventricular tachycardia, rapid atrial fibrillation, and 2:1 atrial flutter.

90. Specify the methods of supporting the patient with a suspected ineffective implanted defibrillation device. p. 182

When external defibrillation is required, be sure that you do not place paddles over the generator of an implanted automatic defibrillator or pacemaker, because this can damage or disable the implanted device.

91. Describe resuscitation and identify circumstances and situations where resuscitation efforts would not be initiated. pp. 213–216

Objective 78 above covers initial resuscitation procedures as well as care after return of spontaneous pulse. In some situations, the patient will not survive despite resuscitation efforts, and in these cases resuscitation is contraindicated and should not be begun: These settings are rigor mortis, fixed dependent lividity (pooling of blood in gravity-dependent fashion), decapitation, and incineration. Less obvious but equally important settings include those where there is an advance directive to withhold resuscitation.

92. Identify communication and documentation protocols with medical direction and law enforcement used for termination of resuscitation efforts. pp. 214–216

In some settings, resuscitation will begin but criteria for termination of resuscitation may exist. These include (1) age 18 years or older, (2) arrest that is presumed cardiac in origin and not associated with a treatable cause such as hypothermia, overdose, or hypovolemia, (3) successful and maintained endotracheal intubation, (4) ACLS standards having been applied throughout the arrest, (5) on-scene efforts having been sustained for 25 minutes or the patient remaining in asystole through four rounds of ALS drugs, (6) patient rhythm that is asystolic or agonal when the decision to terminate is made and persistence of this rhythm until resuscitation is actually terminated, and (7) victims of blunt trauma who presented in asystole or developed asystole on-scene.

You should be equally familiar with criteria that exclude termination of resuscitation: (1) age under 18 years, (2) cause that might benefit from in-hospital treatment, (3) persistent or recurring ventricular tachycardia or fibrillation, (4) transient return of a pulse, (5) signs of neurologic viability, (6) arrest witnessed by EMS personnel, (7) and family or other responsible party opposed to termination.

Review local protocols and contact medical direction before attempting to terminate resuscitation. The medical director or other physician may use the following information: (1) medical condition of the patient, (2) known etiologic factors, (3) therapy rendered, (4) family's presence and appraisal of the situation, (5) communication of any resistance or uncertainty on the part of the family, and (6) maintenance of continued documentation including ECG.

Law enforcement regulations will require that all local, state, and federal laws pertaining to death be followed. The officer may also be required to assign the patient to the medical examiner if he/she does not have a physician. Check with your local law enforcement agencies to determine their protocols.

93. Describe the incidence, morbidity, mortality, pathophysiology, assessment, and management of vascular disorders including occlusive disease, phlebitis, aortic aneurysm, and peripheral artery occlusion. pp. 217–220

Conditions discussed in the chapter as peripheral vascular emergencies include atherosclerosis (which is an occlusive disease), aneurysm, acute arterial occlusion, and deep venous thrombosis.

- Atherosclerosis is the progressive degenerative disease affecting medium and large arteries that underlies many cardiovascular emergencies. It is the cause of coronary artery disease and can affect the carotid, aortic, and cerebral arteries, among others. In atherosclerosis, fats are deposited under the inner layer of the artery, causing injury that subsequently damages the middle, muscle-containing tissue layer as well. Progression occurs as calcium is deposited in the fatty material, forming plaques. Small hemorrhages typically occur around atherosclerotic plaques, further damaging the artery. As the disease progresses, the luminal diameter narrows and blood flow may be impaired to the distal tissues. Eventually, the artery may become totally blocked. If tearing occurs in the arterial wall, the vessel may become dilated and frail; this constitutes an atherosclerotic aneurysm. Arteriosclerosis is the related process in which disruption of tissue layers destroys the elasticity of the vessel and contributes to hypertension. You are already familiar with some of the clinical states due to atherosclerosis and arteriosclerosis: angina, MI, carotid bruits, and stroke.

- Aneurysms are dilatations of vessels. There are actually several types of aneurysms, including atherosclerotic, dissecting, infectious, congenital, and traumatic. Most aneurysms are due to atherosclerotic damage and occur in the aorta, the largest artery in the body and the one with the highest blood pressure. Infectious aneurysms are usually syphilitic in nature and are now rare. Congenital aneurysms can occur with several disease states including Marfan's syndrome, a genetic disorder of connective tissue. Aortic aneurysms are not uncommon in individuals with Marfan's syndrome because the aortic wall is relatively weak from birth.

   Aneurysms form in the aorta when blood infiltrates the wall through a tear in its innermost layer. An abdominal aortic aneurysm secondary to atherosclerosis is a fairly common finding in persons aged 60 to 70 years and ten times as common in men than in women. Signs and symptoms of an abdominal aneurysm include abdominal, back, or flank pain, hypotension, and an urge to defecate caused by retroperitoneal leakage of blood. Degenerative changes in the smooth muscle and elastic tissue of the aorta cause most dissecting aortic aneurysms. The original tear often results from cystic medial necrosis, a degeneration of connective tissue associated with hypertension and, to some extent, aging. Hypertension is clearly a risk factor; it is present in 75–85% of cases. It occurs most frequently in those older than 40-50 years, although it can occur in younger individuals, especially pregnant women. There can also be a hereditary factor. A dissecting aortic aneurysm is one where a rapid inrushing of blood into the wall causes the layers of the wall to separate and eventually rupture. A dissecting aortic aneurysm is extremely painful, and this is one reason you gently search for pulsating masses during the focused abdominal exam of a patient with back, chest, or abdominal pain.

- Acute arterial occlusion is the sudden blockage of an artery due to trauma, thrombosis, embolus, tumor, or idiopathic means. Emboli are probably most common. They can arise within a chamber of the heart (mural emboli), from a thrombus in the left ventricle, from an atrial thrombus secondary to atrial fibrillation, or from a thrombus caused by abdominal aortic atherosclerosis. Arterial occlusions (from emboli leaving the aorta) most commonly involve vessels in the abdomen or extremities. Emboli leaving the heart via the left ventricle can cause embolic strokes, and emboli leaving the right ventricle (perhaps secondary to atrial fibrillation) can cause pulmonary embolisms.

- Deep venous thrombosis is a blood clot in a vein, usually one in the thigh or calf of the leg. Predisposing factors include recent history of trauma, inactivity, pregnancy, or varicose veins. The patient often complains of gradually increasing pain and tenderness; the affected leg and foot are typically swollen because of occluded venous drainage. Skin may be warm and red. Gentle palpation of the calf and thigh will reveal tenderness, and you may be able to palpate cord-like clotted veins.

   Assessment of peripheral vascular disorders starts with the ABCs. Breathing is usually unaffected except in the case of pulmonary emboli. If you find decompensated shock, the cause is most likely to be aneurysm, arterial occlusion, or pulmonary embolus. Circulation is typically compromised distal to the occlusion. Check circulation for the five Ps: pallor, pain, pulselessness, paralysis, and paresthesias. Also check the skin for mottling distal to the affected area. Use the OPQRST acronym to learn more about the patient's pain or other complaint. Find out if this is a new event or a recurrence.

   On physical exam, alteration in breathing and heart rate and rhythm are most common, with pulmonary embolus and aortic aneurysm the two conditions most likely to be life threatening. Unequal bilateral blood pressures may indicate a high thoracic aortic aneurysm that affects flow to one arm. Peripheral pulses may be normal, diminished, or absent, dependent on the site of obstruction. Bruits may be audible over a carotid artery partially occluded by atherosclerotic material. ECG findings generally do not contribute to diagnosis or treatment. However, if you find ectopy or dysrhythmias, treat them.

Management of the patient with a peripheral vascular emergency is largely supportive. Place the patient in a position of comfort. Give oxygen by nonrebreather mask if you suspect pulmonary embolus, aortic aneurysm, or acute arterial occlusion or if either hypotension or a hypoperfusion state exists. Ask about drug allergies before giving any medication. Agents you may use in this setting include nitrous oxide and morphine. Transport as soon as possible. Indications for rapid transport with lights and siren include any situation in which medications do not relieve symptoms or in which you suspect pulmonary embolism, aortic aneurysm, or arterial occlusion. Also consider hypotension or hypoperfusion to be an emergency meriting rapid transport.

94. Identify the clinical significance of claudication and presence of arterial bruits in a patient with peripheral vascular disorders. pp. 217, 219, 220

Claudication is severe pain in a calf muscle due to inadequate blood supply. It typically occurs with exertion and subsides with rest. It is, in many respects, a peripheral parallel to cardiac angina. Arterial bruits are another sign of partial arterial blockage, usually due to atherosclerosis. Bruits are soft sounds heard over an artery (often the carotids) and represent the turbulent blood flow due to partial obstruction.

95. Describe the clinical significance of unequal arterial blood pressure readings in the arms. p. 220

Unequal bilateral blood pressures may indicate an aneurysm high in the thoracic aorta; this is due to unequal flow to the left and right extremities.

96. Recognize and describe the signs and symptoms of dissecting thoracic or abdominal aneurysm. pp. 218, 220

Pain and evolution of shock (including alterations in heart rate and rhythm) are the most common symptom and sign of a dissecting aortic aneurysm. Abdominal aneurysms often present initially with abdominal, back, or flank pain accompanied by development of hypotension. The patient may complain of an urge to defecate if blood leaks into the retroperitoneal space. Thoracic aneurysms also present with pain; look for unequal bilateral blood pressures in the arms as evidence of the dissecting aneurysm.

97. Differentiate between signs and symptoms of cardiac tamponade, hypertensive emergencies, cardiogenic shock, and cardiac arrest. pp. 206–213

Cardiac tamponade typically presents as dyspnea and chest pain, the latter of which may be either dull or sharp. Onset may be sudden or gradual. Classical physical findings include orthopnea, pulsus paradoxus, and narrowing pulse pressures. (In addition, you may see elevated venous pressures in the early phase represented by jugular venous distention.) The ECG is not a diagnostic tool, but you may well see diminished voltages and electrical alternans.

Hypertensive emergencies often show signs of hypertensive encephalopathy: confusion, headache, vomiting, visual changes, or seizures. The extreme hypertension found on blood pressure measurement (diastolic greater than 130 mmHg) is diagnostic.

Cardiogenic shock presents with the signs typical of shock: tachycardia, hypotension, poor peripheral perfusion. History may reveal evidence of chronic heart disease (medications, surgical scars, PND, or current medication regimen) or an acute event such as an MI as clues to the cardiac origin of shock. The usual heart rhythm is sinus tachycardia, but dysrhythmias are not uncommon. Peripheral edema may be so severe that pulses are not palpable.

Cardiac arrest presents with a completely unresponsive patient with no spontaneous breathing or pulse. ECG may show asystole or PEA or may show a dysrhythmia such as ventricular tachycardia or ventricular fibrillation.

98. Utilize the results of the patient history, assessment findings, and ECG analysis to differentiate between, and provide treatment for, patients with the following conditions: pp. 160–221

- **Cardiovascular disease.** Objectives 93–96 all deal with elements of peripheral vascular disease. Assessment findings are specific to the region of the vascular system affected by occlusion. Central findings such as tachypnea and change in heart rate or rhythm suggest pulmonary embolism or aortic aneurysm. Care is largely supportive unless a life-threatening problem (such as hypotension or dysrhythmia) develops.

- **Chest pain.** Chest pain can have a cardiac (pericarditis, angina, or MI) or vascular (aortic aneurysm) origin, or it can reflect problems of the respiratory system, GI tract, or musculoskeletal system (see objective 55). Look for pain on exertion that is relieved by rest and/or nitroglycerin as a sign of possible angina and pain that is unremitting for an MI. With both you may well see ECG changes including sinus tachycardia, S-T segment depression or elevation, ectopy, or dysrhythmias.

- **In need of a pacemaker.** A patient with a history of high-degree AV block or symptomatic bradycardia or atrial fibrillation has inadequate cardiac output for body needs during the periods of those dysrhythmias. If medications don't convert the dysrhythmia to a rhythm compatible with adequate cardiac output, a pacemaker should be considered. Other patients may have recurrent episodes of life-threatening dysrhythmias such as ventricular tachycardia or ventricular fibrillation, and they may also need a pacemaker.

- **Angina pectoris.** The typical presentation for angina is pain lasting from 3-5 minutes, or perhaps as long as 15 minutes, that is relieved by rest and/or nitroglycerin. Prinzmetal's (vasospastic) angina most often occurs at rest or without a known trigger but has similar duration. Prinzmetal's angina is often accompanied by S-T segment elevation on ECG. A patient with fixed (obstructive) angina may show S-T depression and/or T wave inversion on 12-lead ECG. Relief of pain is generally associated with resolution of ECG disturbances.

- **A suspected myocardial infarction.** The patient with an acute MI has chest pain that is severe, constant, and lasts longer than 30 minutes. Neither rest nor nitroglycerin relieves the pain, and the patient may be fearful or feel a sense of doom. On ECG, check the S-T segment for depression, which suggests ischemia, or elevation, which suggests tissue injury. A pathological Q wave (deeper than 5 mm and longer than 0.04 sec) can indicate either widespread transient ischemia or infarcted tissue. Ectopy and dysrhythmia can appear without warning.

- **Heart failure.** Heart failure, inadequacy of pumping ability to meet the body's oxygen demand, can be left-sided, right-sided, or both. Left-sided ventricular failure typically presents with dyspnea and the following additional signs: cyanosis, tachycardia, noisy, labored breathing, rales, cough, blood-tinged, often frothy sputum, and galloping heart sounds. Decreased lung sounds on exam reflect pulmonary edema. Right-sided ventricular failure typically presents with tachycardia, jugular venous distention, edema of body and extremities, engorged (palpable) liver and spleen, and abdominal distention due to ascites fluid. History will usually reflect past cardiac disease or pulmonary disease (COPD). Paroxysmal nocturnal dyspnea suggests left heart failure.

- **Cardiac tamponade.** Cardiac tamponade may be gradual or acute in onset depending on the origin of the material filling the pericardium and exerting pressure on the heart. Assessment typically finds dyspnea and orthopnea and pulsus paradoxus. ECG is not considered diagnostic, but you may see decreased voltage and electrical alternans in these patients.

- **A hypertensive emergency.** The patient with a hypertensive emergency will have extreme hypertension (diastolic greater than 130 mmHg) and usually will show some signs of hypertensive encephalopathy such as headache, visual change, nausea and vomiting, restlessness, or seizures or coma.

- **Cardiogenic shock.** Cardiogenic shock represents shock of cardiac origin: Exam will show characteristic signs of shock (hyperperfusion to extremities, hypotension, tachycardia) but history and exam will rule out extracardiac causes such as hypovolemia or sepsis. ECG may reveal an underlying acute event such as MI.

- **Cardiac arrest.** Patients in cardiac arrest are unresponsive, apneic, and pulseless. ECG may show asystole, PEA, or ventricular tachycardia or ventricular fibrillation. Confirm arrest in two or more ECG leads before beginning management.

99. **Based on the pathophysiology and clinical evaluation of the patient with chest pain, characterize the clinical problems according to their life-threatening potential.** pp. 191, 194

Among cardiac causes, ischemia and MI are life threatening. Pericarditis becomes immediately life threatening if tamponade develops. Among vascular causes, dissection of the thoracic aorta is also immediately life threatening. Most of the respiratory causes are slightly less urgent (such as pneumonia and pleurisy), although both pulmonary embolism and pneumothorax can be immediately life threatening, especially in an individual with pre-existing respiratory or cardiovascular compromise. The GI causes of chest pain most likely to prove truly urgent are those associated with GI hemorrhage: These may include esophageal disease and peptic ulcer disease. Cholecystitis and pancreatitis are serious medical emergencies, but they are generally slightly less urgent than cases involving active hemorrhage. Hiatal hernia, GERD, and dyspepsia require medical care but are relatively unlikely to require urgent care. Most musculoskeletal causes are not urgent and do not have immediate life-threatening potential, although chest trauma may involve injury to the respiratory and/or cardiovascular systems.

100. **Given several preprogrammed patients with cardiac complaints, provide the appropriate assessment, treatment, and transport.** pp. 160–221

Because cardiovascular disease is so common and so serious, accounting for considerable morbidity and mortality, you will see patients who have the problems or conditions discussed in this chapter. Review objectives 46, 53, 55, 61–65, 68–70, 76–78, 83, 86, and 96–98 in particular to familiarize yourself with care in the setting of chest pain, angina, and MI, as well as care of heart failure and acute cardiovascular emergencies.

CASE STUDY REVIEW

Reread the case study on page 67 in Paramedic Care: Medical Emergencies *before reading the discussion below.*

This case study demonstrates how paramedics react to a typical medical emergency involving chest pain. In addition to observing how the team conducts the patient's initial assessment, note how they respond as the situation quickly changes into a more complex and urgent one.

David and Bart are called to a nursing home to evaluate a man with chest pain. You aren't told if they are given any additional information or if any sense of urgency is conveyed, but a call for chest pain in an adult should always bring differential diagnoses to mind. Cardiac conditions, including angina and acute MI, are at the top of the list.

They find an 80-year-old man who has been in the emotionally stressful situation of a large family gathering and who has developed substernal chest pain that radiates to the left arm. Staff who are present immediately add some useful information: Mr. Henry has a history of this type of pain, but it typically resolves with nitroglycerin. Pain has not subsided today, and so the staff activated EMS. At this point, the possibility of an acute MI becomes quite marked.

The paramedics immediately place Mr. Henry on supplementary oxygen, connect him to a cardiac monitor, and establish IV access. They take the time to do a focused history and begin an exam when Mr. Henry screams and collapses. You don't know if Bart had a chance to take a peripheral pulse or listen to Mr. Henry's heart, so you don't have any information about the patient's heart rate or rhythm when the team came, but the change in condition is unmistakable. After his collapse, Mr. Henry is unresponsive, apneic, and pulseless. The monitor shows coarse ventricular fibrillation. He is in cardiac arrest.

The protocol for cardiac arrest is immediately begun. David charges the defibrillator (note that it was on-scene and ready) and delivers a 200-joule charge. The rhythm does not change, and a second charge of 300 joules is delivered. Because the patient remains in ventricular fibrillation, a third charge of 360 joules is delivered. You aren't told whether CPR is performed between defibrillation attempts, but you can assume this was done because a note is made that CPR is continued when the additional crew arrives within 2 minutes of the time Mr. Henry went down.

At this time, with more people and (probably) more equipment at the ready, management can become more comprehensive, and it does. An endotracheal tube (ET) is placed for airway control, and the patient is ventilated with 100% oxygen. The clear bilateral lung sounds not only confirm ET placement but also indicate pulmonary function is adequate. (There is no evidence of pulmonary edema.) Epinephrine is given IV and a fourth shock is delivered. After this, the patient's heart assumes a slow idioventricular rhythm that improves to sinus tachycardia with a weak but palpable peripheral pulse. As the pulse becomes stronger, chest compressions are stopped. The patient's condition continues to spontaneously improve as systolic blood pressure rises to 110 mmHg.

The complication for which you always need to be ready in the setting of an acute MI or resuscitation from a cardiac arrest is dysrhythmia, and this is seen with Mr. Henry. Even as his clinical condition improves, the ongoing scan of the cardiac monitor shows ectopy: a few premature ventricular contractions (PVCs). This is promptly addressed by administration of a lidocaine bolus followed by IV drip. Mechanical ventilation continues, and the patient is readied for transport.

During transport, the patient's condition continues to improve. Not only does he have an acceptable heart rhythm without PVCs, but he begins to breathe on his own as well. At this point, he has moved from complete loss of airway, breathing, and circulation (the state at the outset of his cardiac arrest) to a controlled airway and spontaneous breathing and circulation. You don't know what report is given to the receiving team, but you do know it will include the following information: the minimal down time between collapse and institution of resuscitation, details about the duration of ventricular fibrillation, and the history of vitals (including cardiac rhythm) from time of cardioconversion to arrival at the emergency department.

You should note one other thing about this case study. The team was able to provide appropriate care in timely fashion and with good result without actually treating the underlying cause, the acute MI. This case study serves as a reminder that you should always treat life-threatening problems as they occur and defer other matters such as field diagnosis until the patient is stable or the emergency department is reached. Familiarity with the algorithms for care of various cardiac emergencies, including cardiac arrest, will help you to reflexively do the correct thing in emergency situations such as the one with Mr. Henry.

CONTENT SELF-EVALUATION

MULTIPLE CHOICE

_____ 1. Chest pain is the most common chief complaint among patients with cardiac disease, but not all patients with cardiac disease will have chest pain.
   A. True
   B. False

_____ 2. Atropine, lidocaine, and adenosine are in which group of drugs?
   A. sympathomimetics
   B. sympatholytics
   C. thrombolytics
   D. antidysrhythmics
   E. drugs used for myocardial ischemia and its pain

_____ 3. Dopamine, dobutamine, and epinephrine are in which group of drugs?
   A. sympatholytics
   B. drugs used for myocardial ischemia and its pain
   C. antidysrhythmics
   D. parasympathomimetics
   E. sympathomimetics

_____ 4. Nitrous oxide, nitroglycerin, and morphine are in which group of drugs?
   A. sympathomimetics
   B. drugs used for myocardial ischemia and its pain
   C. antidysrhythmics
   D. antiatherosclerotics
   E. sympatholytics

_____ 5. A potent loop diuretic used to relax the venous system and decrease intravascular fluid volume is:
  A. promethazine.
  B. alteplase.
  C. furosemide.
  D. sodium nitroprusside.
  E. isoproterenol.

_____ 6. Indications for synchronized cardioversion in an unstable patient include all of the following EXCEPT:
  A. rapid atrial fibrillation.
  B. nonperfusing ventricular tachycardia.
  C. paroxysmal supraventricular tachycardia.
  D. perfusing ventricular tachycardia.
  E. 2:1 atrial flutter.

_____ 7. Potentially urgent noncardiac causes of chest pain include all of the following EXCEPT:
  A. stroke.
  B. peptic ulcer disease.
  C. pneumothorax.
  D. pulmonary embolism.
  E. esophageal disease.

_____ 8. Always consider the possibility of cardiac tamponade when you encounter a patient:
  A. with a chest wall tumor.
  B. with muffled or distant heart and lung sounds.
  C. with a gallop rhythm (S_1, S_2, S_3, S_4 heart sounds).
  D. who has just entered ventricular fibrillation.
  E. who received CPR and later deteriorated.

_____ 9. Causes of cardiogenic shock include all of the following EXCEPT:
  A. subendocardial MI.
  B. tension pneumothorax.
  C. pulmonary embolism.
  D. diffuse myocardial ischemia.
  E. prosthetic valve malfunction.

_____ 10. Return of spontaneous circulation occurs when resuscitation results in resumption of a pulse; spontaneous breathing may or may not return.
  A. True
  B. False

_____ 11. Which of the following is NOT a possible criteria for termination of resuscitation efforts?
  A. successful and maintained endotracheal intubation
  B. patient remains in asystole after four rounds of ALS drugs
  C. on-scene ALS efforts have been sustained for 25 minutes
  D. arrest is associated with blunt trauma, hypothermia, or drug overdose
  E. ACLS standards have been applied throughout the arrest

_____ 12. Digitalis (digoxin) has all of the following effects EXCEPT it:
  A. increases force of cardiac contractions.
  B. suppresses atrial ectopy as an antidysrhythmic.
  C. increases cardiac output.
  D. decreases ventricular response to certain supraventricular dysrhythmias.
  E. decreases conduction through the AV node.

MATCHING

Write the letter of the definition in the space provided next to the term to which it applies.

_____ 13. orthopnea   _____ 17. pulsus alternans

_____ 14. bruit   _____ 18. intermittent claudication

_____ 15. paroxysmal nocturnal dyspnea   _____ 19. thrombophlebitis

_____ 16. pulsus paradoxus

A. inflammation and clots within a vein
B. relief of dyspnea on sitting upright
C. alternation of weak and strong pulse over time
D. pain in the calf muscles secondary to local ischemia
E. episodes of being awakened at night by shortness of breath
F. murmur heard over an artery due to turbulent blood flow
G. drop of more than 10 mmHg in systolic BP with inspiration

Write the letter of the clinical setting in the space provided next to the procedure that should be carried out in that setting.

_____ 20. defibrillation   _____ 23. synchronized cardioversion

_____ 21. transcutaneous cardiac pacing   _____ 24. carotid sinus massage

_____ 22. precordial thump

A. effort made immediately after onset of ventricular fibrillation or pulseless ventricular tachycardia that may cause conversion to organized rhythm
B. passage of electrical current through the heart during a specific part of the cardiac cycle to terminate certain dysrhythmias
C. manipulation of an arterial baroreceptor in an effort to increase parasympathetic tone
D. electrical pacing of the heart with use of special skin electrodes
E. passage of electrical current through a fibrillating heart to depolarize a critical mass of myocardium, resulting in conversion to an organized rhythm

Write the letter of the cardiac condition in the space provided next to the ECG finding that would suggest it.

_____ 25. pathological Q wave

_____ 26. S-T segment elevation

_____ 27. T wave inversion

_____ 28. S-T segment depression

A. infarcted tissue or extensive transient ischemia
B. myocardial ischemia
C. myocardial injury
D. old infarcted tissue that has formed a scar

Write the letter of the probable diagnosis in the space provided next to the appropriate description of the condition. A letter response may be used more than once or not at all.

A. pulmonary edema
B. heart failure
C. acute MI
D. left ventricular failure

E. right ventricular failure
F. cardiac arrest
G. cardiac tamponade
H. hypertensive encephalopathy

_____ 29. Constant chest pain that is not relieved by rest or nitroglycerin and lasts longer than 30 minutes

_____ 30. Dyspnea, tachycardia, noisy, labored breathing, gallop heart rhythm

_____ 31. Syndrome in which the heart's pumping ability does not meet body needs

_____ 32. Unresponsiveness with apnea and pulselessness

_____ 33. Jugular venous distention, engorged liver, edema, tachycardia

_____ 34. Pulsus paradoxus and pulsus alternans

_____ 35. Dyspnea, orthopnea, decreased systolic BP with narrowing pulse pressures

_____ 36. Severe headache, visual disturbance, seizures, stupor, diagnostic vital signs

FILL-IN-THE-BLANKS

37. A(n) _____ infarction affects the full thickness of myocardium and almost always results in pathological Q waves in the leads associated with the region of tissue death.

38. The most common and one of the most life-threatening complications of an acute MI is

   _____ .

39. The typical window for thrombolytic therapy in the setting of acute MI is initiation of therapy within _____ of onset of symptoms.

40. Left ventricular failure causes back pressure of fluid into the pulmonary veins and into the lungs, resulting in _____ _____ , which worsens the patient's overall cardiorespiratory function.

41. _____ _____ is the most common symptom of congestive heart failure (CHF).

42. Sudden death is defined as death within _____ of onset of symptoms.

43. The five Ps of acute arterial occlusion are _____ , _____ , _____ , _____ , and _____ .

44. Starling's law states that the greater the stretch on the myocardium, the _____ the force of the contraction.

45. Because _____ starts to lose strength as soon as it is exposed to the air, it is important to use an unopened bottle and to check expiration date before use.

CHAPTER 2
Cardiology

Review of Chapter Objectives

After reading this part of the chapter, you should be able to:
Note: The asterisked objectives are not included in the DOT Paramedic curriculum.

*101. Explain the placement and view of the heart provided by bipolar, unipolar (augmented), and precordial ECG leads. **pp. 224–228**

Both the bipolar leads and the unipolar leads provide information on the heart's electrical activity as viewed from the frontal plane of the body. The precordial leads are complementary: They provide information as viewed in the horizontal plane. The bipolar leads are I, II, and III. (Recall that Lead II is the usual monitoring lead when looking for dysrhythmias.) The unipolar leads are aVR, aVL, and aVF. (The "a" designation marks them as "augmented" leads.) Finally, the precordial leads are V_1, V_2, V_3, V_4, V_5, and V_6. Figure 2-75 on text page 225 shows the axial view of each of the 12 standard leads (Note: the 12 leads are the 3 bipolar leads [I, II, III], the 3 unipolar/augmented leads [aVR, aVL, and aVF], and the 6 precordial leads [V_1–V_6].

- *Lead I:* The negative electrode is on the right arm and the positive electrode is on the left arm. When electrical current within the heart flows from right to left, it will be recorded as a positive deflection (the current is coming toward the positive electrode).
- *Lead II:* The negative electrode is placed on the right arm and the positive electrode is placed on the left leg. When electrical current flows through the heart in a downward vector from right to left, it will be recorded as a positive deflection. (Look at the position of the heart and you will see that a positive deflection on this lead represents electrical current moving from the base toward the apex of the heart. This is why Lead II is the usual monitoring lead if only one lead is used.)
- *Lead III:* The negative electrode is placed on the left arm and the positive electrode is placed on the left leg. When electrical current flows through the heart in a downward direction parallel to left arm toward the left leg, it will be recorded as a positive deflection.
- *aVR:* The negative electrode is a combination of the left arm and left leg electrodes, whereas the positive electrode is placed on the right arm. (The lead is considered to be augmented because a combination of two electrodes forms the negative electrode.)
- *aVL:* The negative electrode is a combination of the right arm and left leg, whereas the positive electrode is placed on the left arm.
- *aVF:* The negative electrode is a combination of the right arm and left arm. The positive electrode is placed on the left foot.

If you superpose the direction of each of these leads on a single figure of the chest, you can see that the six leads form a complete circle of 360 degrees.

The six precordial leads share the same combined negative electrode: a common ground formed by connecting all limb leads. Placement of the positive electrode for each of the precordial leads is as follows:

- V_1: The positive electrode is placed to the right of the sternum at the fourth intercostal space.
- V_2: The positive electrode is placed to the left of the sternum at the fourth intercostal space.
- V_3: The positive electrode is placed midway between leads V_2 and V_4.
- V_4: The positive electrode is placed at the midclavicular line at the fifth intercostal space.
- V_5: The positive electrode is placed at the anterior axillary line at the same level as V_4 (namely, the fifth intercostal space).
- V_6: The positive electrode is placed at the midaxillary line at the same level as V_4 (namely, the fifth intercostal space).

*102. Discuss QRS axis and axis deviation.   pp. 228–231

The electrical energy recorded by ECG leads is the sum of the energy generated by each individual myocardial cell. The flow of energy over time has magnitude (amount of energy) and direction of flow. Thus, this force with magnitude and direction is considered a vector. If we combine each individual vector of energy flow through the heart at any instant in time, we can get a summed, average vector termed the mean cardiac vector. This summation of the myocardium's electrical forces can be shown as an arrow in a single plane: This is the QRS axis.

The heart's normal electrical axis is +59°; Lead II has the most positive deflection (largest magnitude of QRS) because it lies most closely to the electrical axis. Lead II is at +60°.

Under some circumstances, the axis of an individual's heart is not normal; this phenomenon is called axis deviation. When the axis equals or is greater than +105°, the patient is said to have right axis deviation. Right axis deviation is abnormal and often associated with COPD and pulmonary hypertension. When the axis is equal to or greater than –30°, the patient is said to have left axis deviation. Left axis deviation is abnormal and often associated with hypertension, valvular heart disease, or other diseases.

If is often simpler to break the frontal plane into four quadrants rather than to consider the specific angle of the QRS axis. The quadrant spanning 0° to +90° is considered the norm. (You can also think of the quadrants as part of a clock face; then this same quadrant represents 3:00 to 6:00.) The quadrant from +90° to +180° (or 6:00 to 9:00) is right axis deviation. The quadrant from 0° to –90° (or 3:00 to 12:00) is left axis deviation. Finally, an axis in the fourth quadrant (namely, from –90° to –180°) is generally considered indeterminate or extreme right axis deviation.

You will find that most modern ECG machines calculate QRS axis for you. If the machine does not do so, you can calculate axis based on information from Leads I, II, and III. This method has three steps:

(1) Look at the QRS complex in Leads I, II, and III. If the QRS is NOT negative in any of these leads, then the axis is within normal range.
(2) Look at the QRS complex in Lead I. If it is negative, then look at Leads II and III. If the QRS is variable in Lead II (positive, intermediate, or negative) and is positive in Lead III, then the axis shows right axis deviation.
(3) Look at the QRS complex in Lead III. If it is negative, look at Lead II. If both Leads II and III are negative, then the axis shows left axis deviation.

Conditions that are important for you to recognize clinically, such as bundle branch block, chamber enlargement, and other factors, can affect the QRS axis.

*103. Recognize a normal 12-lead ECG.   pp. 231–232

As you learned in Part 1 of this chapter, a 12-lead ECG gives you information on the same electrical events as viewed from 12 different perspectives and from 2 different planes (frontal and horizontal). Many clinically important abnormalities can be detected on a 12-lead ECG. You should always remember, however, that an ECG only gives you information about the electrical activity in the heart; it does not tell you anything about the pumping efficiency of either ventricle.

The information from the 12 ECG leads can be presented in different graphical ways: Learn the specifics of the ECG machines you will use. One common presentation has information from leads aVR, V_1, and V_4 in the top row; aVL, V_2, and V_5 in the second row; and aVF, V_3, and V_6 in the third row. On the figure tracing, the fourth, or bottom, row has a rhythm strip obtained entirely from lead II.

*104. Explain the evolution and localization of acute myocardial infarction.   **pp. 232–240**

See Part 2, objectives 58–65 for a full discussion of acute myocardial infarction.

Below is a summary of the evolution of an acute MI as seen on an ECG:

(1) An area of myocardium becomes ischemic due to inadequate blood flow (time 0). Impairment of repolarization may show up on ECG as S-T segment depression and/or T wave inversion. The likelihood of ischemia being shown on ECG depends roughly on how much myocardium is involved: The larger the area of ischemia, the more likely it will be shown on ECG.

(2) Prolonged ischemia damages myocardial cells. When a sufficiently large block of myocardium is injured, this is seen as S-T segment elevation and peaked T waves.

(3) As the total period since onset of ischemia approaches 6 hours, some injured cells will die, and the amount of cells infarcted will increase with time. Typically, S-T segment elevation will persist because there are live, injured cells surrounding the area of infarction. Over the next 48 to 72 hours, the infarction becomes complete (that is, all cells die that were too injured to survive). The amount of injured tissue decreases (either because cells die and no longer show any electrical activity or because some injured cells recover), and S-T segment elevation may persist but be lower in amplitude. At the same time, a pathological Q wave may develop as a sign of infarction.

(4) As the infarcted area is replaced by scar tissue over the next few months, the S-T segment usually returns to normal and some R waves may reappear. T wave inversion often persists, and a significant Q wave may persist as a permanent indicator of an old (usually transmural) infarction.

You may be able to localize the area of ischemia, injury, or infarction on ECG by noting which leads have abnormalities and the nature of the abnormal changes.

- The anterior surface of the heart (occlusion in the left anterior descending coronary artery): Leads I, V_2, V_3, and V_4. Lead I and Leads V_2–V_4 lie directly on top of the anterior surface of the heart, and S-T segment elevation, T wave inversion, and development of pathological Q waves in these leads indicates an acute anterior MI. Note that Leads V_2 and V_3 lie directly above the interventricular septum, the wall of tissue through which the ventricular conduction system fibers run.
- The anterolateral surfaces of the heart (occlusion of the circumflex coronary artery, marginal branch of the left circumflex artery, or the diagonal branch of the left anterior descending artery): Leads I, aVL, V_5, and V_6. These leads record current from the anterior and lateral surfaces of the heart. ECG changes representing ischemia, injury, and infarction in these leads indicate an anterolateral infarction.
- The lateral surface of the heart: Leads V_5 and V_6. S-T segment elevation, T wave inversion, and development of pathological Q waves in these leads indicate a lateral MI.
- The high lateral surface of the heart: Leads I and aVL. Changes visualized in these two leads represent ischemia, injury, or infarction of the high lateral surface of the heart. Changes in these leads are often seen in the other lateral leads.
- The inferior surface of the heart (occlusion in the right coronary artery): Leads II, III, and aVF. The inferior, or diaphragmatic, surface of the heart is visualized with leads II, III, and aVF. S-T segment elevation, T wave inversion, and development of pathological Q waves in these leads indicates an inferior MI.
- The inferolateral surface of the heart: Leads II, III, aVF, and V_6. These four leads record current from the inferolateral surfaces of the heart, and ECG changes seen in these leads indicate an MI involving the inferolateral surface of the heart.

- The true posterior wall of the heart (supplied by the distal circumflex artery and the posterior descending or distal right coronary arteries) has no ECG lead directly lying over it. True posterior MIs are rare. However, you may be able to detect them by looking for reciprocal, or mirror, changes in the opposite, anterior leads (V_1 and V_2). Normally, the R wave in Leads V_1 and V_2 is chiefly negative. An unusually large R wave (the reciprocal of the posterior Q wave) and an upright T wave (the reciprocal of a posterior inverted T wave) may indicate a true posterior MI.

*105. **Recognize 12-lead ECG tracings of a variety of conductive abnormalities.** pp. 240–254

Review objective 26 (in Part 1 of this chapter) to refresh yourself about the different types of conduction anomalies: AV blocks (first-degree, Type I second-degree, Type II second-degree, and third-degree) and bundle branch blocks.

Conduction defects in the bundle branches can be described as affecting the right bundle branch, the left bundle branch, or even one fascicle of the thicker left bundle branch. Note that although AV blocks can be diagnosed from a single-lead rhythm strip, you need a 12-lead ECG to diagnose bundle branch blocks. In a bundle branch block, ventricular depolarization will be abnormal. The impulse will be passed properly through the AV node into the bundle of His and then into the right and left bundles, but the block will occur at some distal point. If the right bundle branch is blocked, the impulse will travel properly through the left bundle branch. The impulse will then eventually pass through the interventricular septum to depolarize the right ventricle. Likewise, if a blockage is in the left bundle branch, the impulse will pass properly through the right bundle branch, the interventricular septum, and eventually the left ventricle. Because of the circuitous passage of the depolarizing impulse toward the ventricle whose bundle branch bears the block, depolarization of that ventricle will be delayed. You can see this prolongation of ventricular depolarization as a QRS complex of 0.12 second or longer. In addition, the same delay can result in an abnormal QRS complex shape.

Right bundle branch block

Right bundle branch block results from an electrical obstruction at some point in that bundle branch. The right ventricle is the one affected by the delay in the depolarizing impulse. The right ventricle is also the lower pressure pump, and it has a thinner myocardium than the left ventricle. Thus, under normal circumstances the electrical forces in the right ventricular myocardium are overshadowed by those in the more massive left ventricle. In the case of right bundle branch block, the delayed right ventricular depolarization is anterior and to the right compared with the vector for left ventricular depolarization. A complete right bundle branch block is detected as a prolonged QRS complex (at least 0.12 sec in length) and as an abnormal, later portion of the QRS that is directed toward the right ventricle (and away from the left ventricle).

Look at Lead I and you will see a broad S wave. You will also see a characteristic RSR′ (R-S-R prime) complex in Lead V_1. The RSR′ reflects the abnormal septal depolarization and the subsequent right ventricular depolarization. Lead V_1 overlies the right ventricle and is useful not only for detecting right bundle branch block but also other right ventricular abnormalities.

Clinically, right bundle branch block is a relatively common finding. It is a relatively thin bundle of fibers compared to the left bundle branch and thus it is more vulnerable to injury. Right bundle branch block can result from acute MI, drugs, electrolyte abnormalities, and general age-related deterioration of the cardiac conduction system.

Left bundle branch block

Left bundle branch block is derived from an obstruction at the level of the bundle of His, which divides into the anterior and posterior fascicles of the left bundle branch before terminating in the Purkinje system of the left ventricle. The left ventricle is the one affected by the delay in the depolarizing impulse. The left ventricle is also the higher pressure pump, and it has a thicker myocardium than the right ventricle. Unlike the case of right bundle branch block, the direction of depolarization in left bundle branch block is still right to left, and thus nearly the same as in a normal heart. The QRS complexes in the heart with left bundle branch block are prolonged (at least 0.12 sec in length) and bizarre in appearance. Typically, wide, notched QRS complexes are seen in Leads I, aVL, V$_5$, and V$_6$. The changes are most pronounced in these leads because they visualize the lateral surface of the heart, which is principally the left ventricle. You may also see deep S waves in Lead V$_1$, V$_2$, or V$_3$ or tall R waves in Leads I, aVL, V$_5$, and V$_6$.

Left bundle branch block usually indicates significant and widespread myocardial disease. Like right bundle branch block, it can be caused by MI, drugs, electrolyte abnormalities, and age-related degenerative disease. Most MIs affect the left ventricle, and the presence of a left bundle branch block may mask new-onset ischemic changes associated with an acute MI. Thus, a patient may have a significant acute MI and the "characteristic" ECG changes will not be seen because of the presence of the left bundle branch block. In fact, the presence of left bundle branch block negates any possibility of localizing an MI with use of a 12-lead ECG.

An alternative method to determine whether left or right bundle branch blocks exist (namely, the turn-signal method) is given on text pages 247–248.

Detection of bundle branch blocks, especially left bundle branch blocks, is important in the field for two reasons: (1) The block can mask ischemic changes associated with an acute MI and (2) some S-T segment elevation usually appears in the precordial leads (V$_1$–V$_6$) with left bundle branch blocks, which can make 12-lead tracings useless in the field.

The left bundle branch (which feeds the far thicker left ventricular myocardium) divides into anterior and posterior fascicles. Blocks (termed hemiblocks) can occur in either of these fascicles, and such hemiblocks are a fairly common finding.

Hemiblocks

• Left posterior hemiblock results from blockage of the posterior fascicle and consequent delayed depolarization of the region of the left ventricle that it innervates. Note that a left posterior hemiblock does NOT typically result in a prolonged QRS interval or abnormally shaped QRS complex. Instead, the chief ECG finding is a rightward shift in QRS axis (right QRS deviation). This is often difficult to confirm, especially in the presence of right ventricular or pulmonary disease. Generally, the QRS axis must be equal to or greater than +120° to consider a left posterior hemiblock likely. This form of hemiblock is usually due to degenerative disease of the conductive system or to ischemic heart disease.

• Left anterior hemiblock results from blockage of the anterior fascicle. Anterior hemiblock does NOT result in a delay in ventricular depolarization, and so the QRS complex is of normal duration and is usually of normal shape (without the notching characteristic of bundle branch blocks). Instead, the chief ECG finding is a far leftward shift in QRS axis (typically more negative than −30°), which is manifest as a negative QRS complex in leads II, III, and aVF. A left anterior hemiblock is usually caused by degenerative disease of the conduction system or ischemic heart disease; it is usually a benign finding.

Chamber enlargement

Enlargement of any of the heart's four chambers rarely affects care in the field; however, you should understand the basic pathophysiology because it can causes changes in the ECG that might mislead you into consideration of ischemia. Any disease process that causes prolonged increased in pressure in a chamber can lead to chamber enlargement. Right atrial enlargement (RAE) is often due to pulmonary disease such as emphysema or chronic bronchitis (COPD) or due to pulmonary emboli. In these cases, the problem of origin produces pulmonary hypertension, which causes the increased pressure in the right atrium. Right ventricular hypertrophy (RVH, thickening of the right ventricle due to enlargement by stretching of the individual muscle cells) typically follows. In a similar fashion, left atrial enlargement (LAE), which is often due to long-term systemic hypertension, is a precursor to left ventricular hypertrophy (LVH).

• *Atrial enlargement.* Because the P wave represents atrial depolarization, atrial enlargement affects its formation. The first half of the P wave, which represents right atrial depolarization, is normally rounded like a quarter-circle. The second half of the P wave, which represents left atrial depolarization, has the same quarter-circle shape. RAE appears on a 12-lead tracing as a tall, spiked first half of the P wave (taller than 2 mm, 2 small boxes). LAE appears as a biphasic (two-part), widened P wave of 2.5 mm. Leads II, aVL, V$_1$, and V$_2$ offer the best views of RAE and LAE.

- *Ventricular enlargement.* Because the QRS complex represents ventricular depolarization, ventricular enlargement affects it. Abnormally deep S waves or tall waves in the precordial leads suggest RVH or LVH. RVH generally appears as an R wave taller than 7 mm with a right axis deviation. You need to look at the S wave of V_1 or V_2 and the R wave of V_5 or V_6 to detect LVH. Add the amplitude of the deeper S wave (of V_1 or V_2) to the amplitude of the taller R wave (of V_5 or V_6). A sum equal to or greater than 35 mm indicates LVH. Clinically, it is important for you to be able to detect LVH because its S-T pattern often mimics the S-T segment elevation expected with myocardial injury.

Echocardiography is the usual diagnostic test for chamber enlargement, but 12-lead monitors with programmed interpretative capability may detect the condition. Even if you have one of the most advanced monitors with computerized interpretation, you should remember that they can detect only about 50% of these cases.

*106. Explain prehospital 12-lead ECG monitoring procedures. pp. 255–258

The skills sequence for 12-lead prehospital ECG monitoring is as follows:

(1) Explain what you are going to do to the patient. Reassure the patient that the machine only monitors electrical activity of the heart and will not give a shock.
(2) Prepare all equipment and make sure that the cable is in good shape. Make sure that there are adequate leads and material for skin preparation.
(3) Prep the skin with an appropriate substance to eliminate dirt, oil, sweat, or other materials that may impair adhesion of the electrode to the skin.
(4) Place the four limb leads according to the manufacturer's instructions.
(5) Next, prepare for placement of the precordial leads.
(6) Place Lead V_1 first, putting the positive electrode to the right of the sternum at the fourth intercostal space (see diagram on text page 256 for precordial placements).
(7) Place Lead V_2 next, putting the positive electrode to the left of the sternum at the fourth intercostal space.
(8) Place Lead V_4 by putting the positive electrode at the midclavicular line at the fifth intercostal space.
(9) Place Lead V_3 by putting the positive electrode midway between Leads V_2 and V_4.
(10) Place Lead V_5 by putting the positive electrode at the anterior axillary line at the same level as V_4.
(11) Place Lead V_6 by putting the positive electrode at the midaxillary line at the same level as V_4.
(12) Ensure that all leads are attached.
(13) Turn on the machine.
(14) Check that all leads are properly attached and a good tracing is being received from each of the 12 channels.
(15) Record the tracing.
(16) Examine the tracing. Do not rely completely on the machine's interpretation of the tracing. If necessary, confirm with medical direction.
(17) Give the tracing to the receiving team. If you have a patient with an acute MI and you do not start thrombolytic therapy in the field, you can reduce the door-to-needle time by providing a quality 12-lead tracing to the emergency department staff as soon as the patient arrives.
(18) Perform proper patient pass-off to the hospital personnel.
(19) Be sure you restock all equipment and supplies before the next call.
(20) Compare field interpretation with the emergency department and cardiology interpretations.

CASE STUDY REVIEW

The Case Study Review for this chapter is found in Part 2.

CONTENT SELF-EVALUATION

MULTIPLE CHOICE

_____ 1. A positive deflection on the tracing for a certain lead means that the electrical current is flowing toward the positive electrode for that lead, whereas a negative deflection for the same lead signifies a flow of electrical current away from the positive electrode.
  A. True
  B. False

_____ 2. If current is flowing directly toward the positive lead, the deflection will be less than it would be if the current were flowing obliquely toward the positive lead.
  A. True
  B. False

_____ 3. When the flow of current is exactly perpendicular to the line of the negative and positive electrode for a certain lead, the tracing will show no deflection at all.
  A. True
  B. False

_____ 4. The leads that examine heart activity in the horizontal plane are:
  A. I, II, and III.
  B. aVR, aVL, and aVF.
  C. I, II, III, aVR, aVL, and aVF.
  D. V_1, V_2, V_3, V_4, V_5, and V_6.
  E. all 12 leads.

_____ 5. Right axis deviation exists when the QRS axis lies between:
  A. −29° and +105°.
  B. 0° and +90°.
  C. +90° and +180°.
  D. 0° and −90°.
  E. −90° and −180°.

_____ 6. Left axis deviation exists when the QRS axis lies between:
  A. −29° and +105°.
  B. 0° and +90°.
  C. +90° and +180°.
  D. 0° and −90°.
  E. −90° and −180°.

_____ 7. Myocardial injury is shown on an ECG as:
  A. an isoelectric S-T segment.
  B. S-T segment depression.
  C. S-T segment elevation.
  D. a lengthened QRS complex.
  E. S-T segment prolongation.

_____ 8. On very hot days or with a patient who is diaphoretic, you may wish to apply which substance to the skin in order to achieve a good skin-electrode interface for an ECG?
  A. Betadine
  B. normal saline
  C. rubbing alcohol
  D. soap and water
  E. tincture of Benzoin

MATCHING

Write the letter of the ECG leads in the space provided next to the type of leads they are.

  A. I, II, III
  B. V_1, V_2, V_3, V_4, V_5, V_6
  C. aVR, aVL, aVF

_____ 9. unipolar (augmented)

_____ 10. bipolar

_____ 11. precordial

Localization of myocardial ischemia, injury, or infarction is done by examining the ECG tracings among leads reflecting different regions of the heart. Write the letter of the myocardial region in the space provided next to the leads that examine it.

A. inferior
B. lateral
C. anterolateral
D. high lateral

E. true posterior
F. inferolateral
G. anterior

_____ **12.** II, III, and aVF

_____ **13.** I, V_2, V_3, and V_4

_____ **14.** II, III, aVF, and V_6

_____ **15.** I, aVL, V_5, and V_6

_____ **16.** V_5 and V_6

_____ **17.** I and aVL (sometimes with V_5 and V_6)

_____ **18.** V_1 and V_2 (looking for reciprocal changes)

Write the letter of the description of the conduction disturbance in the space provided next to the name of the disturbance.

_____ **19.** right bundle branch block

_____ **20.** left bundle branch block

_____ **21.** left posterior hemiblock

_____ **22.** left anterior hemiblock

_____ **23.** left atrial enlargement (LAE)

_____ **24.** right ventricular hypertrophy (RVH)

_____ **25.** left ventricular hypertrophy (LVH)

A. prolonged QRS complex with bizarre, notched complexes in Leads I, aVL, V_5, and V_6, along with deep S waves in Lead V_1, V_2, or V_3 or tall R waves in Leads I, aVL, V_5, and V_6
B. R wave > 7 mm tall and presence of right axis deviation
C. prolonged QRS complex with broad S wave in Lead I and RSR′ complex in Lead V_1
D. normal QRS length and appearance; right deviation in QRS axis ($\geq$ +120°)
E. biphasic, widened P wave
F. sum of deeper S wave (in V_1 or V_2) and taller R wave (in V_5 or V_6) $\geq$ 35 mm; possible S-T segment elevation
G. normal QRS length and appearance; left deviation in QRS axis with negative QRS complexes in Leads II, III, and aVF.

SPECIAL PROJECT

Interpreting an ECG

You receive a call to check out the medical status of an elderly man who has been seen wandering along the side of a local highway. As you drive down the road, you pass an empty car and note its license plate in case it belongs to the man you are to check out. About 0.4 mile farther down the road, you spot the man walking unsteadily and slowly along the shoulder and pull in behind him.

The patient is a thin, elderly man who seems out of breath but aware of you and your partner as you approach. When you draw near, you explain that you are paramedics who are there to see if he is all right or needs help. He replies that his name is Adam Benon, that he is 81 years old, and that he has lost his car. You notice that he is tachypneic and breathing with great effort, and you ask him how he feels as you gently take his shoulder and turn him toward the ambulance.

Within a few minutes you learn that Mr. Benon felt dizzy and nauseated while driving and pulled over to the side of the road. The patient cannot remember getting out of the car, but he does remember walking toward the next exit looking for help. He notes that his chest hurts more now than it did a while ago and he feels that he cannot take a deep breath.

Mr. Benon has a regular pulse of 90, and his ECG is shown on the next page.

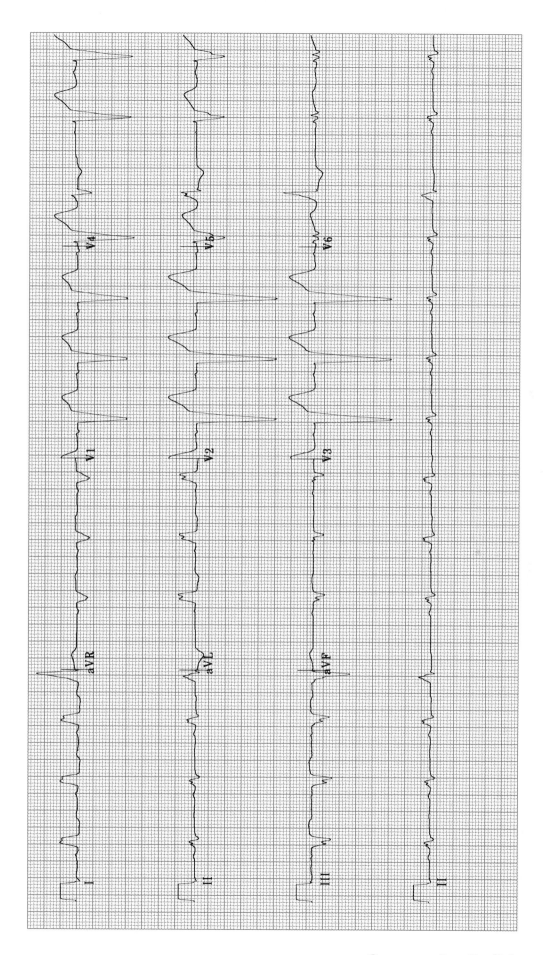

1. What preexisting cardiac problem is strongly suggested by the ECG tracing?

2. What, if any, significance does this hold for your current attempt to determine whether Mr. Benon is having an acute cardiac problem such as ischemia or acute MI?

CHAPTER 3
Neurology

Review of Chapter Objectives

After reading this chapter, you should be able to:

1. **Describe the incidence, morbidity, and mortality of neurological emergencies.**   pp. 262, 289, 299, 300, 302, 304–306, 308

Diseases and conditions of the nervous system affect millions of Americans: You will see neurological emergencies in the field, and you will also see patients who present with another complaint but who have coexisting neurological conditions. Epilepsy affects about 2.5 million persons, who may present with a neurological emergency or have another condition complicated by their seizure disorder. Strokes are medical emergencies, and they affect about 500,000 people annually, of whom about 150,000 die. Strokes are also a frequent source of considerable morbidity. Recent studies have shown that early recognition and intervention in certain strokes due to thromboembolism may decrease their morbidity and mortality. Neoplasms affecting the CNS occur in about 40,000 persons annually; morbidity and mortality depend on variables including tumor type and location. The miscellaneous group termed the degenerative disorders account for considerable morbidity for many Americans, and they often account for premature death, as well. Multiple sclerosis affects about 300,000–400,000 Americans, and typical first presentation is at the age range of 20–40 years. Parkinson's disease affects more than 500,000 Americans, who are typically 60 years or older.

Other neurological conditions are extremely common and of variable cause and morbidity/mortality. For instance, nearly half of all Americans will have a syncopal episode (that is, faint) in their lifetime, and syncope accounts for roughly 3% of all emergency department visits. Headaches of various causes are extremely common, with nearly 45 million persons affected by chronic headaches. Low back pain can be either acute or chronic, and roughly 60 to 90% of Americans will experience some type of lower back pain in their lifetimes.

2. **Identify the risk factors most predisposing to diseases of the nervous system.**   pp. 290, 294–295, 299, 300, 308

Risk factors differ for the various types of neurological conditions. Strokes are vascular in nature (hemorrhagic or occlusive), and the major risk factors for stroke reflect this: atherosclerosis, heart disease, diabetes, abnormal blood lipid levels, hypertension, sickle cell disease, use of oral contraceptives, and the cardiac dysrhythmia atrial fibrillation. Some chronic conditions such as epilepsy reflect different causes and thus have different risk factors: It can develop in patients who have had head trauma, brain tumors, or certain vascular disorders such as stroke. Most cases are considered idiopathic, which means cause is unknown. Syncope is similar in having very different causes: Syncopal episodes can be due to cardiovascular (such as dysrhythmias or mechanical problems) origin or non-cardiovascular (metabolic, neurologic, or psychiatric) origin; indeed, many episodes are considered idiopathic even after workup. Headaches tend to be classified as vascular (such as migraine), tension, or organic (the last including headache due to tumor, infection, or other conditions). Some of the risk factors for low back pain are somewhat gender-related: Symptoms in women over age 60 years often reflect postmenopausal osteoporosis. Occupations involving exposure to vibrations from vehicles or machinery or jobs requiring repetitive lifting also are associated with risk for low back pain. Other causes include compression or trauma to the sciatic nerve or its roots, as can happen with a herniated intervertebral disk. Most cases, though, are also idiopathic.

3. **Discuss the anatomy and physiology of the nervous system.**   pp. 262–275

The nervous system is the body's chief control for virtually every major function. It is divided physically into the central nervous system (CNS) and peripheral nervous system (PNS). The CNS consists of the brain and spinal cord. If the body were visualized as a computer, the CNS would be the central processing unit. Both very basic functions, such as continuance of heartbeat and respiration, and complex functions such as listening to Mozart and anticipating a musical passage you particularly like, are controlled by cells in the brain. Messages within the CNS, as well as those that connect it with the rest of the body, travel as nerve impulses. The complex network of nerves outside the CNS makes up the peripheral nervous system. The messages that carry information regarding critical body functions such as respiration pass through a part of the PNS called the autonomic nervous system; these functions do not require any conscious effort to maintain them. In contrast, messages that involve voluntary, or conscious, actions and thoughts travel through the other part of the PNS, the somatic nervous system. Both the autonomic and somatic nervous systems have two parallel tracks: one of nerves that carry messages to the brain, and a second that carries messages from the brain. In terms of the computer analogy, the PNS carries the various input and output messages that run between the brain and spinal cord and the rest of the body. The autonomic nervous system is also structurally and functionally broken into two parts: the sympathetic and parasympathetic nervous systems. These two parts work together to make sure the net balance of stimulatory and inhibitory messages from the brain keep body functions such as blood pressure within normal limits.

The basic structural and functional unit is the neuron, or nerve cell. As you can see in Figure 3-2 on text page 264, nerve cells have a body that contains the essential cell machinery of nucleus, mitochondria, etc. Nerve processes (usually there are many) that are capable of receiving impulses from other neurons or body cells are called dendrites. An impulse that is picked up by a dendrite travels toward the cell body. Another process, the axon, carries the impulse away from the cell body. Axons may have multiple tips, which means the neuron has the capacity to send the impulse onward to more than one other nerve or other cell. Dendrites associated with neurons of the major senses organs (such as the eye or ear) convert an environmental stimulus into a nerve impulse that can be forwarded via the axon to other nerves, and eventually the brain. Dendrites associated with neurons that monitor internal conditions such as PaO_2 also convert that information into an impulse and send it to the brain. Eventually all such information is analyzed by neurons in the brain and response impulses travel back through the PNS. These impulses eventually affect a motor neuron, causing a muscle cell to contract, or affect another type of cell such as one in a gland. Messages cannot pass directly from an axon to a dendrite because there is a tiny physical gap, called a synapse, between each pair of neurons. As the wave of electrical depolarization (due to ion fluxes of potassium rapidly leaving the neuron and sodium rapidly entering) reaches the axon tip, it causes a chemical called a neurotransmitter to be released into the synapse. (There are multiple neurotransmitters within the body. Either acetylcholine or norepinephrine is found in the neurons of the PNS. Neurotransmitters within the CNS include dopamine and serotonin.) When the neurotransmitter crosses the synapse and is taken up by the dendrite on the other side, a wave of depolarization is started in that dendrite and the nerve impulse is then carried toward the cell body.

Most of the CNS is protected by the bones of the cranium and spine. The spinal column is made up of 33 vertebrae running from the neck to the junction with the pelvis. There is also an inner shock-absorbing, cushioning protection system. The cells of the brain and spinal cord are bathed in cerebrospinal fluid, and there are three layers of protective membranes between the neural surface and the outer, protective bone. These meninges are called the dura mater, arachnoid membrane, and pia mater (in outer-to-inner sequence). (Review Figures 3-4 to 3-6 in the textbook for details of structure.)

As you look at a human brain, it has six obvious structural regions: the cerebrum, the diencephalon, the mesencephalon (or midbrain), the pons, the medulla oblongata, and the cerebellum (see Figure 3-7). Sometimes, this is simplified into the terminology of the forebrain (cerebrum and diencephalon), the midbrain, and the hindbrain (the brainstem—pons, medulla oblongata—and the cerebellum). The largest part of the brain, with its characteristic folded outer surfaces, is the cerebrum. The cerebrum has left and right sides, or hemispheres, which are connected physically and functionally by tissue called the corpus callosum. The cerebrum is responsible for intelligence, learning, memory, and language, as well as analysis and response to sensory and motor activities. The diencephalon is covered by the cerebrum, and it is made up of a number of vital structures: the thalamus, hypothalamus, and the limbic system. This primal part of the brain is responsible for many involuntary functions such as temperature regulation, sleep, water balance, stress response, and emotion. It also has an important role in regulating the autonomic nervous system. The brainstem consists of the mesencephalon, pons, and medulla oblongata. The mesencephalon is located between the diencephalon and the pons, and it plays a role in motor coordination. It is the major region controlling eye movement. The pons is a major connection point between the upper portions of the brain and the medulla and cerebellum. The medulla oblongata itself marks the division between the brain and the spinal cord. The major centers for control of respiration, cardiac activity, and vasomotor activity are located here. The cerebellum is located in the posterior fossa of the cranium, and it also has two hemispheres, which are closely coordinated to the brainstem and higher centers. The cerebellum coordinates fine motor movement, posture, equilibrium, and muscle tone.

The hemispheres of the cerebrum do not contain identical centers. Rather, the functional responsibilities of the cerebrum have been mapped as a whole. Important centers with clinical implications for you in cases such as stroke or trauma include the following: (1) speech, which is located in the temporal lobe, (2) vision, which is located in the occipital lobe, (3) personality, which is located in the frontal lobes, (4) sensory, which is located in the parietal lobes, and (5) motor, which is located in the frontal lobes. As noted previously, balance and coordination are located in the cerebellum. A last important center is called the reticular activating system (RAS), which operates in the lateral portion of the medulla, pons, and especially the mesencephalon. The RAS sends impulses to and receives messages from the cerebral cortex (the outer portion of the cerebrum). This diffuse system of interlaced cells is responsible for maintaining consciousness and the ability to respond to external stimuli (see Figure 3-9).

The brain receives about 20% of the body's total blood flow per minute. Vascular supply to the brain is provided by two systems, a physical arrangement that provides secondary supply if one system is occluded or severed. The anterior system is the carotid, and the posterior system is the vertebrobasilar. They join at the Circle of Willis before entering the structures of the brain itself. Venous drainage is via the venous sinuses and the internal jugular veins. As previously noted, there is also cerebrospinal fluid (CSF) bathing the tissues of the brain and spinal cord. Most of the intracranial CSF is found in the ventricles.

The spinal cord is 17 to 18 inches long on average in adults. It leaves the brain at the medulla and passes through an opening in the skull called the foramen magnum to enter the spinal canal. The spinal cord, which ends near the level of the first lumbar vertebra (the reason why spinal taps are done below that level), conducts impulses to and from the peripheral nervous system and locally for motor reflexes. Thirty-one pairs of nerves exit the spinal cord between adjacent vertebrae. The dorsal nerve roots carry afferent fibers, ones carrying impulses to the brain. The ventral roots carry efferent fibers, which carry impulses from the brain to the periphery. Each nerve root has a corresponding area of skin called a dermatome, to which it supplies sensation. In the field, you may be able to correlate sensory deficits to the level of a spinal cord problem. The reason why our protective motor reflexes are so fast and effective lies in the fact that the afferent and efferent impulses are coordinated in the spinal cord—they do not travel the whole way to the brain before coming back. However, because they are mediated in the spinal cord, they lack fine motor control.

The peripheral nervous system (PNS) contains 12 pairs of cranial nerves, which extend directly from the lower surface of the brain and exit through small holes in the skull, and the peripheral nerves, which exit from the spinal cord as noted previously. The nerves of the PNS control both voluntary and involuntary activities. The cranial nerves supply nervous control for the head, neck, and certain thoracic and abdominal organs. The peripheral nerves can be divided into four classes: (1) somatic sensory, afferent nerves that carry impulses concerned with touch, pressure, pain, temperature, and position, (2) somatic motor, efferent nerves that carry impulses to the skeletal (voluntary) muscles, (3) visceral (autonomic) sensory, afferent nerves that carry impulses of sensation from the visceral organs (examples being fullness in the bladder or distension of the rectum), and (4) visceral (autonomic) motor, efferent nerves that serve the involuntary cardiac muscle and the smooth muscle of the viscera and the glands.

The involuntary division of the PNS is called the autonomic nervous system, and it has two components: the sympathetic nervous system and the parasympathetic nervous system. The sympathetic system is associated with the primitive "fight or flight" response to sensory stimuli. Its major nerve roots are located near the thoracic and lumbar part of the spinal cord. Stimulation causes increased heart rate and blood pressure, pupillary dilation, rise in blood sugar, as well as bronchodilation, all responses that ready the body for stress. The neurotransmitters norepinephrine and epinephrine mediate its actions, and sympathetic activity is also closely correlated to activity in the adrenal gland medulla, tissue that is of nervous system origin and that also relies on norepinephrine and epinephrine. The parasympathetic nervous system is responsible for controlling vegetative functions such as normal heart rate and blood pressure. It is associated with the cranial nerves and the sacral plexus of nerves, and it is mediated by the neurotransmitter acetylcholine. When stimulated, it causes a decrease in heart rate, an increase in digestive activity, pupillary constriction, and a reduction in blood sugar.

4. **Define and discuss the epidemiology (including the morbidity/mortality and preventative strategies), pathophysiology, assessment findings, and management for the following neurologic problems:**

   a. **Coma and altered mental status**   pp. 287–289
   Altered mental status is extremely common, as you'll understand when you consider the wide variety of causes. Morbidity and mortality are often correlated to cause: Vigilant assessment and management on your part will optimize your patient's chances, regardless of causes. An alteration in mental status is the hallmark sign of CNS injury or illness; as such, any alteration, be it subtle or as florid as coma, requires evaluation. In coma, the patient cannot be aroused by even powerful external stimuli such as pain. The two mechanisms generally capable of causing altered mental status are structural lesions (such as tumor, trauma, degenerative disease, or another process that destroys or encroaches on the substance of the brain) and toxic-metabolic states (such as the presence of toxins including ammonia or the absence of vital substances such as oxygen, glucose, or thiamine). Causes of toxic-metabolic disturbances include anoxia, diabetic ketoacidosis, hepatic failure, hypoglycemia, renal failure, thiamine deficiency, and toxic exposure (for instance, cyanide). Some of the most common causes you'll see for altered mental status (meaning they can cause a structural lesion or a toxic-metabolic state) are the following: (1) drugs, including depressants such as alcohol, hallucinogens, and narcotics; (2) cardiovascular, including anaphylaxis, cardiac arrest, stroke, dysrhythmias, hypertensive encephalopathy, and shock; (3) respiratory, including chronic obstructive pulmonary disease (COPD), inhalation of a toxic gas such as carbon monoxide, and hypoxia; and (4) infectious, such as AIDS, encephalitis, and meningitis.

   During history taking and assessment, remember the mnemonic AEIOU-TIPS, and look for signs of these common causes: A (acidosis or alcohol), E (epilepsy), I (infection), O (overdose), U (uremia, or kidney failure), T (trauma, tumor, or toxin), I (insulin, either hypoglycemia or ketoacidosis), P (psychosis or poison), S (stroke, seizure). During physical assessment, use the AVPU method for determining level of consciousness. Unresponsive patients require especially vigilant monitoring and protection of the airway. Remember that in some cases you will not be able to determine the cause of the problem in the prehospital setting.

   Management begins with the ABCs. The initial priority is the airway; be sure to immobilize the C-spine in cases of suspected head or neck injury. Then attend to breathing, administering supplemental oxygen and assisting ventilations if needed. An unresponsive patient requires an airway adjunct. As an evaluation of circulation, check heart rate and rhythm and blood pressure. Then perform the following steps:

   • IV of normal saline or lactated Ringer's solution at a keep-vein-open rate; alternatively place a heparin lock.

- Determine blood glucose level with reagent strip or glucometer. If serum glucose is low, give 50% dextrose to mediate the hypoglycemia. Even if the patient is an uncontrolled diabetic, any transient hyperglycemia will do limited harm at most in the short prehospital period. In many cases of hypoglycemia, dextrose can be life saving, and you may see an immediate response. Glucose may also be life saving for the alcoholic patient with hypoglycemia.
- Administer naloxone if there is suspicion of narcotic overdose. (See Chapter 8, "Toxicology and Substance Abuse," for details).
- If there is suspicion of alcoholism, consider use of 100 mg thiamine (Vitamin B_1).

In chronic alcoholism, intake, absorption, and use of thiamine is impaired. Among these patients, you may see Wernicke's syndrome, a condition marked by loss of memory and disorientation that is associated with a diet deficient in thiamine. Of even greater concern is Korsakoff's psychosis, marked by memory disorder, because it may be irreversible. Thus, the of administration of thiamine as per local protocols and the judgment of medical direction may be important.

If increased intracranial pressure is possible, as in a closed head injury, hyperventilate the patient at 20 breaths per minute. The decrease in carbon dioxide causes cerebral vasoconstriction and reduces brain swelling. DO NOT over-hyperventilate, as this can decrease CO_2 to dangerously low levels. Medical direction may order use of mannitol (Osmotrol) to cause a diuresis that may shift fluid from the intravascular space through the kidneys.

b. Seizures pp. 294–299

A seizure is a temporary alteration in behavior due to a massive discharge of one or more groups of neurons in the brain. Seizures can be induced in anyone under certain stressful conditions such as hypoxia or rapidly decreasing blood glucose. Febrile seizures often occur in young children with a sudden increase in body temperature. Structural diseases of the brain such as tumors, head trauma, toxic eclampsia, and vascular disorders can also cause a seizure. Recurrent seizures without such a known cause are termed epilepsy. Epilepsy affects about 2.5 million persons, who may present with a neurological emergency or have another condition complicated by their seizure disorder. Most cases of epilepsy are idiopathic, that is, without known cause, whereas others arise secondary to damage from strokes, head trauma, tumor surgery or radiation, etc.

Assessment begins with history according to the patient or bystanders, as well as physical impression. Remember that many people think the only kind of seizure is a "grand mal," so a bystander who does not know the patient may suggest he is on drugs, or that he fainted, or give other information that is misleading. In addition, other medical conditions can present similarly to a seizure: Examples are migraine headaches, cardiac dysrhythmias, hypoglycemia, or orthostatic hypotension. Hyperventilation, as well as a number of CNS conditions, can cause stiffness in the extremities. Decerebrate movements can be caused by increased intracranial pressure. Thus, there is often more potential harm than good in administering an anticonvulsant.

The patient history should include an attempt to ascertain the following information: (1) history of seizures, and, if so, particulars of type, nature, and frequency, (2) recent history of head trauma, (3) possibility of alcohol or other drug use, (4) recent history of fever, headache, or stiff neck, (5) history of diabetes, heart disease, or stroke, and (6) current medications. During physical exam, look for evidence of head injury or injury to the tongue and for evidence of alcohol or drug abuse. Be sure to document any dysrhythmias.

Active management may not be needed for many types of seizures, including short generalized tonic-clonic seizures that have ended before you arrive. Management for most generalized seizures in process is supportive: Manage the airway, make sure the patient does not injure him- or herself, and monitor for possible hyper- or hypothermia, depending on environmental conditions. General procedures include the following: (1) assurance of scene safety, (2) maintenance of airway (DO NOT force objects between the patient's teeth or push objects into the mouth that may initiate vomiting), (3) administration of high-flow oxygen, (4) establishment of IV access, running normal saline or lactated Ringer's solution at keep-vein-open rate, (5) determination of blood glucose level, with 50% glucose given in hypoglycemia, (6) physical protection of patient from surroundings, (7) maintenance of temperature, (8) postictal positioning on left side with suction if required, (9) monitoring of cardiac rhythm, (10) consideration of an anticonvulsant if seizure is prolonged (greater than 5 minutes), (11) transport the patient in supine or lateral recumbent position in quiet, reassuring atmosphere.

Status epilepticus, two or more generalized seizures without intervening return of consciousness, can be a life-threatening emergency. The most common cause in adults with epilepsy is failure to comply with medication regimen. Status is a major emergency because it involves a prolonged period of apnea with the possibility of CNS hypoxia. The most valuable intervention is to protect the airway and to deliver 100% oxygen, preferably by BVM device. After airway and breathing have been addressed, start an IV with normal saline at keep-vein-open rate, monitor cardiac rhythm, give 25 g 50% dextrose IV push if hypoglycemia is present, give 5–10 mg diazepam IV push for an adult, and continue to monitor airway. Note that some patients will require large doses of diazepam, and this may cause respiratory depression. Depression, if significant, can be reversed with flumazenil, although this may also result in the return of seizures.

c. Syncope pp. 299–300

Syncope, or fainting, is characterized by a sudden, temporary loss of consciousness caused by insufficient blood flow to the brain, with recovery almost immediate upon supine positioning. Syncope is very common, accounting for roughly 3% of all emergency department visits. It can occur at any age. Symptoms may include prior feelings of dizziness or lightheadedness or there may be no warning at all. By definition, if return of consciousness does not occur within a few moments, the event is NOT syncope, it is something more serious. Review Table 3-2 (text page 297) for help in distinguishing between syncope and seizure.

There are three pathophysiologic mechanisms for syncope: cardiovascular, non-cardiovascular, and idiopathic. Cardiovascular causes include dysrhythmias or mechanical problems such as an abnormally functioning heart valve. Non-cardiovascular causes include metabolic, neurological, or psychiatric conditions. For instance, hypoglycemia, a transient ischemic attack (TIA), or an anxiety attack my all precipitate syncope. Idiopathic, as always, means there is no known cause even after careful evaluation. Management begins with an attempt to find and treat the underlying cause. If no cause is established, the patient should be transported to an appropriate emergency department for evaluation. Field management is somewhat similar to that for seizure: assure scene safety, maintain open airway, administer high-flow oxygen and assist ventilations as needed, check circulatory status (heart rate and rhythm, blood pressure), check and continue monitoring mental status, start IV with normal saline or lactated Ringer's at keep-vein-open rate, determine blood glucose level, monitor cardiac rhythm, and transport in reassuring environment.

d. Headache pp. 300–301

Headaches, either acute or chronic, are a tremendously common complaint: You've probably had problems with a headache at least once. Nearly 45 million Americans suffer from chronic headaches. There three general categories of headache: vascular, tension, and organic. Headaches of vascular origin include migraines and cluster headaches. Migraines occur more commonly in women, whereas cluster headaches occur more commonly in men. Migraines are typically characterized by intense, throbbing pain, sensitivity to light or sound, nausea, vomiting, and sweating. Migraines may last from several minutes to several days. They typically present as one-sided headaches and they may be preceded by an aura. Cluster headaches usually occur as a series of one-sided headaches that are sudden in onset, intense, and continue for roughly 15 minutes to 4 hours. Symptoms may include nasal congestion, drooping eyelid, and an irritated eye. Tension headaches account for a significant percentage of headaches. Most personnel in emergency medicine, have, or will, have a tension headache. Some people experience them on a daily basis. These persons may wake with a headache that worsens over the course of the day. The typical tension headache has a dull, achy pain that feels as if forceful pressure is being applied to the neck or head. The last class of headache, organic headaches, is less common. They occur in association with tumor, infection, or other diseases of the brain, eye, or other body system.

Because headaches can herald serious illness or precede a catastrophic event such as a ruptured aneurysm, it is always important to keep these possible underlying causes in mind when you speak with a patient complaining of headache. A continuous throbbing headache, particularly if over the occiput, accompanied by fever, confusion, and stiffness of the neck is classic for meningitis. Sudden onset pain, often described as "the worst pain of my life," or changes in pain pattern should all be considered possible signs of conditions as grave as intracranial hemorrhage. In general, any headache of acute onset or of changing pattern demands immediate attention on your part.

A complete and thorough history is important in evaluating the patient with headache. Questions that may evoke valuable information include the following: What were you doing when the pain started? Does anything make the pain worse (such as light, sound, or movement)? What is the quality of the pain, throbbing, crushing, tension? Does pain radiate to the neck, arm, back, or jaw? What is the severity of the pain on a scale of 1–10 and has severity changed? How long has the headache been present (is it acute or chronic)? You will see that the same line of questioning about pain is used in other settings, too, as with patients who complain of abdominal pain (Chapter 6, "Gastroenterology").

Management is supportive and generally includes the following: (1) assurance of scene safety, (2) protection of airway, (3) placement of patient in position of comfort (often accomplished by patients themselves), (4) high-flow oxygen with ventilation assistance as needed, (5) IV with normal saline or lactated Ringer's at keep-vein-open rate, determination of blood glucose, monitoring of cardiac rhythm, (6) transport with reassurance in an environment that is calm and quiet, (7) consideration of use of antiemetics or analgesics. Antiemetics that might be helpful for migraine include prochlorperazine (Compazine) and abortive agents such as sumatriptan (Imitrix).

e. Neoplasms pp. 302–304

Neoplasm is a general term for "new growth," and it is used to describe tumors that arise after birth. Neoplasms of the CNS affect about 40,000 Americans per year. These neoplasms can be divided into benign and malignant tumors based on several characteristics. The cells of a benign tumor generally resemble normal cells, grow relatively slowly, and tend to remain confined to one location. In contrast, malignant tumors of the CNS often have cells that are primitive in appearance and don't resemble normal cells, grow quickly, and may invade adjacent, healthy tissue or spread within the CNS. Both kinds of CNS tumors can be dangerous because any tumor growth can place pressure on other tissues and impair their function and because the pressure cannot be relieved by expansion of the cranial space. In adults, the cranium is rigid and fixed. Pressure exerted by a tumor causes increased intracranial pressure. There are numerous types of brain tumors, and the cause is unknown for most of them.

CNS tumors present with many signs and symptoms dependent on the size, type, and location of the tumor. It isn't your role in the field to diagnose new tumors; rather, you are more likely to have patients with previously diagnosed tumors or patients who present with problems that may reflect a CNS tumor. Common complaints among persons with undiagnosed brain tumors include the following: headache (often severe and recurrent), new onset seizures, nausea and vomiting, behavioral or cognitive changes, weakness or paralysis of one or more limbs or one side of the face, change in sensation in one or more limbs or one side of the face, new onset uncoordination, difficulty walking or unsteady gait, dizziness, double vision. Be alert for any of these signs and be sure to obtain a thorough history. In addition to the SAMPLE questions, ask the following: (1) What is the state of your general health? (2) Have you had any seizure activity, headache, or nosebleed? (3) Have you ever had surgery for removal of a brain tumor, chemotherapy, radiation therapy, holistic therapy, or any form of experimental treatment?

Management is largely supportive, with the goal of reducing anxiety and palliating symptoms. The general steps of field management have much in common with those for seizures and headaches. Assure scene safety, and protect airway. Position the patient for comfort, generally with head elevated. Use high-flow oxygen and assist ventilations as needed. Start an IV with normal saline or lactated Ringer's at keep-vein-open rate or use a saline or heparin lock. Monitor cardiac rhythm and consider narcotic analgesia if approved by medical direction.

Consider diazepam if seizures are present. Medical direction may recommend either anti-inflammatory medication (dexamethasone) and/or diuretics. Last, transport in a calm, quiet environment while reassuring the patient.

f. Abscess   p. 304

A brain abscess is a pocket of pus localized to one area of the brain. They are uncommon, accounting for 2% of intracranial masses. Signs and symptoms are similar to those of a neoplasm and include headache, lethargy, hemiparesis (weakness on one side of the body), seizures, rigidity of the neck, nausea and vomiting. Fever is frequently present, suggesting an infectious cause. Your field management is supportive and similar to that for neoplasm or meningitis.

g. Stroke   pp. 289–294

Stroke is a general term for injury or death of brain tissue, usually due to interruption of blood flow to that region of the cerebrum. The term "brain attack" is being used more frequently because of some similarities between stroke and heart attack, the latter also being due to oxygen deprivation. You should also realize that there are more treatment similarities to heart attacks. Strokes due to thromboembolic causes may be aborted or minimized with use of thrombolytic agents now used with heart attack (such as tissue plasminogen activator, tPA). The importance to you is that prompt recognition and transport of stroke patients is greater than ever. Stroke patients who may be candidates for thrombolytic therapy must receive definitive treatment within 3 hours of onset.

Strokes are the third most common cause of death and a frequent cause of considerable disability among middle-aged and elderly persons. Major risk factors include atherosclerosis, heart disease, hypertension, diabetes, abnormal blood lipid levels, use of oral contraceptives, and sickle cell disease. Strokes can be caused either by occlusion of an artery or by hemorrhage. Both interrupt blood flow to distal tissues. An occlusive stroke is any caused by blockage of the artery, resulting in ischemia to brain tissue that may progress to infarction if oxygen deprivation continues long enough. Infarcted brain tissue swells, further damaging nearby tissue that might have only a marginal blood supply itself. If swelling is sufficiently severe, herniation (protrusion of tissue through the foramen magnum, the opening at the base of the skull through which the spinal cord emerges from the cranium) can occur. Occlusive strokes are either thrombotic or embolic in origin.

Thrombotic strokes are due to a thrombus, or blood clot, that forms in and then obstructs a cerebral artery. Thrombosis is often related to atherosclerotic change in the artery. Unsurprisingly, the signs and symptoms of a thrombotic stroke are often gradual in onset. The stroke often occurs at night and is characterized by the patient waking with altered mental status and/or loss of speech, sensation, or motor function. An embolic stroke is caused by a solid, liquid, or gaseous mass that is carried to the site of obstruction from a remote site. The most common brain emboli are blood clots that often arise from diseased blood vessels in the neck (namely, the carotid artery) or from abnormal cardiac contraction. Atrial fibrillation often results in atrial dilation, a precursor to clot formation. Other types of embolli include air, tumor tissue, and fat. Typically, embolic strokes present with sudden onset of severe headaches. Hemorrhagic strokes are due to bleeding within brain tissue, and they can be categorized as intracerebral or subarachnoid (see Figure 3-20). They are discussed in detail below under intracranial hemorrhage.

Prompt and proper assessment of a stroke in progress is very important. Signs and symptoms will depend on the type of stroke and the area of the brain affected by it. Onset of symptoms may be acute, and the patient may be unconscious. You may observe stertorous breathing due to paralysis of part of the soft palate. Respiratory expirations may be puffs of air out of the cheeks and mouth. The patient's pupils may be unequal. If so, the larger pupil will be on the side of the hemorrhage. Paralysis, when present, usually involves one side of the face, one arm, or one leg. Speech disturbances may be noted, and the patient's skin may be cool and clammy.

In list form, common signs and symptoms of stroke include the following: one-sided facial drooping, headache, confusion and agitation, dysphasia (difficulty in speech), aphasia (inability to speak), dysarthria (impairment of tongue and muscles making speech difficult), vision problems such as blindness in one eye or double vision, hemiparesis (one-sided weakness), hemiplegia (one-sided paralysis), paresthesias, inability to recognize by touch, gait disturbances or uncoordinated motor movements, dizziness, incontinence, or coma.

Management of stroke emphasizes early recognition, supportive measures, prompt, rapid transport, and notification of the emergency department (see algorithm in Figure 3-21 of the textbook). Remember that aggressive airway management is vital in these patients. Other field measures include the following: (1) assurance of scene safety, including body substance isolation, (2) airway management including suction as needed, (3) ventilation assistance as needed: If the patient is apneic or breathing is inadequate, provide positive-pressure ventilation at 20/minute. Hyperventilation eliminates excessive CO_2 levels. Avoid over-hyperventilation because excessively low CO_2 levels can cause profound cerebral vasoconstriction. If breathing is adequate, give oxygen via nonrebreather mask at 15 L/minute, (4) complete a detailed patient history, (5) keep patient supine or in recovery position. If the patient has congestive heart failure, place patient in semi-upright position as needed. If patient has altered mental status and you suspect potential for airway compromise, keep him or her in left lateral recumbent, or recovery position, (6) determine blood glucose level; if hypoglycemia is present, consider 50% dextrose by IV push, (7) start an IV of normal saline or lactated Ringer's at a keep-vein-open rate or place a saline or heparin lock (avoiding dextrose solutions, which may increase intracranial pressure due to osmotic effect), (8) monitor cardiac rhythm, (9) protect paralyzed extremities, (10) reassure patient and explain all procedures as patient may be able to understand even if he or she cannot respond, and (11) transport without excessive movement or noise.

h. Intracranial hemorrhage   pp. 291–292
Hemorrhagic strokes are due to blood within brain tissue, and they can be categorized as intracerebral or subarachnoid (see Figure 3-20 in the textbook). These intracranial hemorrhages often occur with sudden onset of a severe headache. Most intracranial hemorrhages occur in a hypertensive patient when a small vessel deep within brain tissue ruptures. Subarachnoid hemorrhages most commonly result from either congenital blood vessel anomalies or from head trauma. Congenital anomalies include aneurysms and arteriovenous malformations. Aneurysms tend to be on the brain's surface and may either hemorrhage into brain tissue or into the subarachnoid space. Hemorrhage within brain tissue may tear and separate normal brain tissue. Release of blood into the ventricles containing CSF may paralyze vital centers. If blood impairs drainage of CSF, the resultant increase in intracranial pressure may cause herniation of brain tissue.

i. Transient ischemic attack   pp. 292–294
A transient ischemic attack (TIA) is a temporary manifestation of the signs and/or symptoms of stroke that is due to temporary interference with blood supply to the affected part of the brain. These symptoms may persist for a few minutes or for hours, but they almost always resolve within 24 hours. After the attack (because it reflects ischemia, not infarction), there is no evidence of brain or neurological damage. The most common cause is carotid artery disease (provoking an embolic event). Other causes can be small emboli of different origin, decreased cardiac output, hypotension, overmedication with antihypertensive medications, or cerebrovascular spasm. Part of the importance of recognizing TIAs is that they may be the precursor to a stroke. One third of TIA patients suffer a stroke soon afterward. A TIA is typically sudden in onset, with specific signs and symptoms depending on the part of the brain involved.

In the prehospital setting, it is virtually impossible to distinguish a TIA from a stroke. While taking the history, try to get the following information: previous neurological symptoms, if any; initial symptoms and their progression; changes in mental status; precipitating factors, if any; dizziness; palpitations; history of hypertension, cardiac disease, sickle cell disease, or previous TIA or stroke. Because TIAs and strokes are generally indistinguishable in the field, the management is the same. (See Stroke above.)

j. Degenerative neurological diseases   pp. 304–307
The term "degenerative neurological disease" characterizes diseases that selectively affect one or more functional systems of the CNS. Generally, they produce symmetrical and progressive involvement of the CNS, affect similar areas of the brain, and produce similar clinical signs

and symptoms. Examples discussed in the text include Alzheimer's disease, muscular dystrophy, multiple sclerosis, dystonias, Parkinson's disease, central pain syndrome, Bell's palsy, amyotrophic lateral sclerosis, myoclonus, spina bifida, and poliomyelitis. Alzheimer's disease is perhaps the most important of the degenerative disorders because of its frequency and its devastating nature. It is the most common cause of dementia in the elderly. Alzheimer's results from neuronal cell death and disappearance in the cerebral cortex, causing marked atrophy of the brain. Initially, patients have problems with short-term memory, and this usually progresses to problems with thought and intellect. Patients also develop a shuffling gait and have stiffness of body muscles. As the disease progresses, the patient develops aphasia and psychiatric problems. In its final stages, the patient may become virtually decorticate, losing all ability to think, speak, and move. Muscular dystrophy (MD) actually refers to a group of genetic diseases characterized by progressive muscle weakness and degeneration of skeletal muscle fibers. The heart and other involuntary muscles are affected in some types of MD. The most common form is Duchenne's MD. Some forms begin in childhood whereas others do not appear until midlife. Prognosis depends on the type and individual progression of the disorder. Multiple sclerosis (MS) is another common and potentially devastating degenerative disorder. It involves inflammation of certain nerve cells followed by demyelination (loss of the fatty insulation surrounding nerve fibers in the CNS). Prevalence in the U.S. is approximately 300,000–400,000 persons. Most are women who first developed symptoms between ages 20–40 years. The pathophysiology of MS involves autoimmune attack against myelin. Signs and symptoms include weakness of one or more limbs, sensory loss, paresthesias, and changes in vision. Symptoms may wax and wane over years, and they may range from mild to severe. Severe cases leave the patient so debilitated she may not be able to care for herself.

The dystonias are characterized by muscle contractions that cause twisting, repetitive movements, abnormal postures, or freezing in the middle of an action. Early symptoms include deterioration in handwriting, foot cramps, or tendency of one foot to drag after walking or running. In some cases, symptoms become more noticeable and widespread over time. In other individuals, there is little or no progression over time. Parkinson's disease is a motor system disorder also called a "shaking palsy." Parkinson's is characterized chemically by a deficiency of dopamine in the CNS, and treatment is generally aimed at increasing levels in the brain. Parkinson's is common, and you will see it. Roughly 500,000 Americans are affected, and more than 50,000 new cases are reported annually. It affects men and women equally and has an average age at onset of 60 years. It usually does not develop in persons under 40. Parkinson's is chronic and progressive, and its signs fall into four categories: tremor (which usually begins in the hand and may progress to involve the arm, a foot, or the jaw), rigidity (resistance to movement among muscles in opposing pairs), bradykinesia (slowing or loss of normal, spontaneous movement), and postural instability (with development of a forward or backward lean, stooped posture, or tendency to fall easily).

Central pain syndrome results from damage or injury to the brain, brainstem, or spinal cord, and it is marked by intense, steady pain that may be described as burning, aching, tingling, or "pins and needles." It occurs in patients who, at some point in the past, have had strokes, multiple sclerosis, limb amputation, or spinal cord injury. Pain medications generally do not provide relief, and patients often rely on sedatives or other means of keeping the CNS free from stress. One example is trigeminal neuralgia, which is caused by abnormal impulse conduction along the trigeminal nerve (cranial nerve V). It often has brief episodes of intense facial pain. The fear of a possible attack may be debilitating. Medications including carbamazepine (Tegretol) may be helpful, and surgery may be indicated for select cases.

Bell's palsy is the most common form of facial paralysis, affecting roughly 40,000 Americans yearly. It results from inflammation of the facial nerve (cranial nerve VII) and is marked by one-sided facial paralysis, inability to close the eye on the affected side, pain, tearing of that eye, drooling, hypersensitivity to sound, and impaired taste. Multiple causes exist, among them head trauma, herpes simplex virus, and Lyme disease. Treatment is usually aimed at protecting the eye. Corticosteroids may be used for inflammation when pain is severe. Most patients recover within 3 months. Amyotrophic lateral sclerosis (ALS, or Lou Gehrig's disease), affects 20,000 Americans with roughly 5,000 new cases reported each year. ALS involves progressive degeneration of the nerve cells that control voluntary movement. It is marked by weakness, loss of motor control, difficulty speaking, and cramping. Eventually a weakened diaphragm and intercostal muscles lead to breathing problems. There is currently no effective therapy and no cure, and prognosis continues to be poor, with death within 3–5 years of diagnosis (often as a result of pulmonary infection). Myoclonus refers to temporary involuntary twitching or spasm of a muscle or muscle group. It is generally considered not a disorder, but a symptom. It occurs with a variety of disorders including multiple sclerosis, Parkinson's, and Alzheimer's. Pathologic myoclonus may limit a person's ability to eat, walk, and talk. Treatment consists of medication that reduces symptoms, often antiepileptic drugs such as clonazepam, phenytoin, and sodium valproate.

Spina bifida (SB) is a congenital neural defect due to failure of one or more fetal verte-brae to close properly during development, leaving a portion of the spinal cord unprotected. Long-term effects include impairment in physical mobility, and most individuals have some form of learning disability. The three most common types are myelomeningocele, the most severe form, in which the spinal cord and meninges protrude from the opening in the spine, meningocele, in which the meninges only protrude through the spinal opening, and SB occulta, the mildest form, in which one or more vertebrae are malformed and covered only by a layer of skin. Treatment includes surgery, medication, and physiotherapy appropriate for the extent of deformity. Poliomyelitis (polio) is an infectious disease that sometimes results in per-manent paralysis. The acute disease is marked by fatigue, headache, fever, vomiting, stiffness of the neck, and pain in the hands and feet. New cases in the U.S. are rare due to routine child-hood vaccination. However, thousands of pre-vaccine polio survivors are alive today and you may see them as patients. Many of these individuals require supportive care.

Assessment of any of the degenerative disorders requires your personal impressions and history taking to determine the chief complaint. The patient may be having a flare-up of a problem or they may have an unrelated complaint. In all cases, make your assessment, inter-vene for any life-threatening problems, and learn exactly what prompted a call for EMS. Management relies on treating the chief complaint. You don't want to overlook the underly-ing condition, but you also don't want it to get in the way of recognizing and treating a more immediately serious problem. While providing care, you should keep in mind these general aspects of patients who have a disorder in this group: Mobility may be affected, and the patient may need assistance to move. Communication may be difficult. Take the time to ensure open communication with patient, family, caregivers, or bystanders. Respiratory com-promise may be a concern, particularly in exacerbations of ALS or some other conditions. Any breathing problem is a priority. Last, recognize the anxiety attendant with these disorders. Approach the patient and family with compassion. The following specific guidelines may be useful for a number of patients: Determine blood glucose; this may help you detect whether altered mental status is due to hypoglycemia. Establish an IV with normal saline or lactated Ringer's at a keep-vein-open rate. Monitor cardiac rhythm during transport.

5. Describe and differentiate the major types of seizures   pp. 295–296

Seizures can be clinically grouped as generalized or partial on a pathophysiologic basis. Generalized seizures begin with an electrical discharge in a small part of the brain but the abnor-mal activity spreads to involve the entire cerebral cortex. In contrast, partial seizures may remain confined to a small area, causing localized malfunction, or they may spread and become second-arily generalized seizures.

Generalized seizures include tonic-clonic (also commonly called grand mal) and absence seizures. A tonic-clonic seizure is a generalized motor seizure that produces a temporary loss of consciousness. Usually, it includes a tonic phase (in which muscle tone is increased) and a clonic phase (in which muscles in the extremities jerk rhythmically). In some cases, temporary paralysis of the intercostal muscles causes an interruption in breathing and cyanosis may become evident. When respirations resume, you may see copious amounts of frothy oral secretions. Incontinence is also common during a seizure, and you may note agitation or confusion, drowsiness, or even coma following a seizure, depending on the norm for that patient. Absence seizures present very differently. They are characterized by a sudden onset of a brief (typically 10- to 30-second) loss of consciousness or awareness. Loss of consciousness may be so brief that the casual observer misses it altogether. These idiopathic seizures of childhood rarely occur after age 20 years. Note that absence seizures may not respond to your normal treatment modalities.

Pseudoseizures, also called hysterical seizures, are not true electrical seizures. Rather, they represent psychiatric phenomena. The patient typically presents with sharp, bizarre movements that may be interrupted with a terse command such as "Stop it!"

Partial seizures may be either simple or complex. Simple seizures involve local motor, sensory, or autonomic dysfunction in one area of the body; there is no loss of consciousness. You should remember, however, that they may spread in area of involvement and progress to a generalized, tonic-clonic seizure. Complex seizures, which usually originate in the temporal lobe, are often characterized by an aura and focal findings such as alterations in mental status or mood. Patients in the midst of such a seizure may appear intoxicated or mentally unstable: They may be confused, stagger, have purposeless movements, or show sudden personality changes. These seizures typically last 1–2 minutes, and the patient will slowly come back to baseline after that period.

6. Describe the phases of a generalized seizure. pp. 295–296

Although patients are individuals with their own seizure patterns, many tonic-clonic seizures progress through seven phases: (1) aura, a subjective sensation that serves as a warning to those patients who experience it, (2) loss of consciousness, during the aura sensation, if there is one, (3) tonic phase, (4) hypertonic phase, during which you will see extreme muscular rigidity, including hyperextension of the back, (5) clonic phase of muscle spasms (often including the jaws) marked by rhythmic movements, (6) post-seizure, during which the patient is in a coma, and (7) postictal, during which the patient awakens.

7. Define the following:

The degenerative neurological diseases are discussed in some detail in objective 4j above, and you may wish to check that section for review on any or all of these disorders.

a. Muscular dystrophy p. 304
Muscular dystrophy (MD) is actually a group of genetic diseases characterized by progressive muscle weakness and degeneration of the skeletal or voluntary muscle fibers.

b. Multiple sclerosis p. 304
Multiple sclerosis (MS) is a disease that involves inflammation of certain nerve cells followed by demyelination; the destruction of the insulating myelin sheath is due to autoimmune activity.

c. Dystonia p. 305
The dystonias are a group of disorders characterized by muscle contractions that cause twisting and repetitive movements, abnormal posturing, or freezing in the middle of an action.

d. Parkinson's disease p. 305
Parkinson's disease is a chronic and progressive disorder of the motor system within the CNS and is characterized by tremor, rigidity, bradykinesia, and postural instability.

e. Trigeminal neuralgia pp. 305–306
Trigeminal neuralgia is due to abnormal conduction of impulses along the trigeminal nerve (cranial nerve V). The condition is an example of a central pain syndrome.

f. Bell's palsy p. 306
Bell's palsy, the most common form of facial paralysis, is a one-sided phenomenon with unknown cause, marked by inability to close the eye, pain, tearing of the eye, drooling, hypersensitivity to sound, and impairment of taste.

g. Amyotrophic lateral sclerosis p. 306
Amyotrophic lateral sclerosis (ALS), or Lou Gehrig's disease, is a progressive degenerative condition of specific nerve cells that control voluntary movement; it is marked by weakness, loss of motor control, difficulty speaking, and cramping.

h. Peripheral neuropathy pp. 276–277

Peripheral neuropathy is not considered a degenerative neurological condition; rather, it is a descriptive term that includes any malfunction or damage of the peripheral nerves. Results may include muscle weakness, loss of sensation, impaired reflexes, and malfunction of internal organs. Diabetes is one of the major causes of peripheral neuropathy involving multiple nerves (also called a polyneuropathy).

i. Myoclonus p. 306

Myoclonus is a temporary, involuntary twitching or spasm of a muscle or group of muscles. It is actually a symptom rather than a disorder. A very benign example of myoclonus is hiccups. Pathological myoclonus may be part of disorders including Alzheimer's, Parkinson's, and multiple sclerosis.

j. Spina bifida p. 306

Spina bifida (SB) is a congenital neural defect that results from failure of one or more vertebrae to close properly during fetal development. The defect may range from the asymptomatic (vertebral malformation covered by skin) to the severe (protrusion of spinal cord and meninges through an opening in the spine).

k. Poliomyelitis pp. 306–307

Poliomyelitis (polio) is a viral infectious disease characterized by inflammation of the CNS, which sometimes results in permanent paralysis.

8. Define and discuss the pathophysiology, assessment findings, and management for nontraumatic spinal injury, including:

a. Low back pain p. 308

Low back pain, defined as pain felt between the lower rib cage and the gluteal muscles, often radiating to the thighs, is an extremely common complaint but only occasionally the reason for an EMS call. Men and women are equally affected, but you should keep in mind that back pain in women over 60 years may represent the first sign of osteoporosis, an important medical condition. Vertebral fractures from causes other than osteoporosis are also possible causes. Other causes of low back pain include sciatica, which is reflected as severe pain along the path of the sciatic nerve down the back of the thigh and inner leg. Sciatica may be due to compression or trauma to the sciatic nerve or its roots, perhaps from a herniated intervertebral disk or an osteoarthritic lumbosacral vertebral bone. Sciatica may also be due to inflammation of the nerve secondary to metabolic, toxic, or infectious causes. Pain at the level of L-3, L-4, L-5, and S-1 may be due to inflammation of interspinous bursae. External to the spine are other causes of low back pain: inflammation or sprain of muscles and ligaments that attach to the spine. Most low back pain, though, is found to be idiopathic.

Assessment of back pain is based on chief complaint, history, and physical exam. When the complaint is low back pain, a precise diagnosis is likely to be difficult. Preliminary diagnosis may focus on occupational risk from repetitive lifting or exposure to machinery vibrations. Listen for clues in the history about the nature and timing of the pain and whether the current complaint is acute pain or exacerbation of a chronic condition. Your priorities in the field are to determine whether pain is due to a life-threatening or non-life-threatening condition. Note: The presence of any identifiable neurological deficit may point to a serious underlying cause, as may a gradual onset of pain consistent with degenerative disk disease or tumor growth. The location of the injury may be revealed on exam by a limited range of motion in the lumbar spine, point tenderness on palpation, alterations in sensation, pain, and temperature at a localized point, or pain or paresthesia below a point of injury. Always keep in mind that you are unlikely to be able to determine the cause of the pain in the field. Your primary goal is to look for signs of life-threatening problems and to gather historical and exam information that will be useful to the receiving physician. You will also need to decide, perhaps after consultation with medical direction, whether immobilization (and, if so, to what degree) is necessary during transport.

If there are no clear life-threatening problems requiring intervention, management is primarily aimed at minimizing pain and immobilizing as per local protocol. If there is no historical reason to suspect injury in the past or an underlying condition such as osteoporosis (which makes patients vulnerable to pathologic fracture), C-spine immobilization may still be recommended as a comfort measure during transport. Also remember that some patients will require parenteral analgesia and diazepam before they can lie on a stretcher. Consult medical direction if you feel your patient might fit into this category. Last, remember to provide ongoing assessment en route with special attention to the ABCs, vitals, and the possible presence or development of motor or sensory deficits that might indicate a critical condition capable of compromising ventilatory efforts.

b. Herniated intervertebral disk   p. 308

Intervertebral disks may rupture due to injury or due to degeneration associated with aging. Degenerative disk disease is most common in patients over 50 years of age. A herniated disk occurs when the gelatinous center of the disk extrudes through a tear in the tough outer capsule, and the resulting pain is due to pressure on the spinal cord or to muscle spasm at the site. The disks themselves are not innervated. Non-injury-related herniation may also be caused by improper lifting. Men aged 30 to 50 years are more prone to herniated disks than are women. Herniation is most common at levels L-4, L-5, and S-1, but it also may occur at C-5, C-6, and C-7. Assessment and management are discussed under low back pain in objective 8a.

c. Spinal cord tumors   p. 309

A cyst or tumor along the spine or intruding into the spinal canal may cause pain by pressing on the spinal cord, causing degenerative changes in bone, or interrupting blood supply. The specific manifestations depend on location and type of tumor or cyst. Assessment and management are discussed under low back pain in objective 8a.

10. Differentiate between neurologic emergencies based on assessment findings.   pp. 277–286

Because many signs and symptoms of neurologic dysfunction are subtle, you should use the observations made during scene size-up and formation of general impressions to look for evidence suggesting focus on the neurological system. Environmental clues may include medical equipment, medication bottles, Medic-Alert identification, alcohol bottles, etc. Note, for instance, if the patient is conscious, and, if so, is he confused or lucid? Are his posture and gait normal? Speech can give many clues, particularly if either the patient or a bystander can tell you if the speech you hear is normal for the patient. Skin color, temperature, and moisture are valuable, as is any evidence of facial drooping or muscle spasm. Mental status can then be quickly ascertained through the AVPU method. Assessment of higher cerebral functioning includes assessment of emotional status. Try to evaluate the patient's affect, thought patterns, perceptions, judgments, and memory and attention. ANY alteration from the patient's normal mental status or mood is considered significant and warrants further assessment. After that level of assessment is done, evaluate for the ABCs, including respiration pattern, effort of breathing, heart rate, rhythm, and ECG pattern. An unresponsive patient can be evaluated further with use of the Glasgow Coma Scale. Be aware that a midlevel GCS score (such as 5, 6, or 7) that drops on reevaluation has grim implications.

Scene size-up and initial history will usually make clear whether trauma is involved or not. Regardless of whether trauma is a factor, try to get information on the presence or severity of medical conditions that are risk factors for neurologic conditions, hypertension, heart disease, diabetes, atherosclerosis, as well as any chronic neurologic conditions such as epilepsy. In addition, history should try to establish whether current complaint is acute, an exacerbation of a chronic problem, or a chronic state.

Physical exam of a patient with a neurologic emergency includes the standard head-to-toe exam as well as a more detailed neurological evaluation. Full description of the exam is given on text pages 280–286. Look closely at the patient's face. The ability to smile, frown, or wrinkle the forehead gives information about the status of the facial nerve. Although slight pupillary asymmetry is normal, abnormal pupils can be an early indicator of increasing intracranial pressure. If both pupils are dilated and don't react to light, suspect brainstem injury or serious anoxia. If the pupils are dilated but still react, injury may be reversible. Most of all, remember that any patient with altered mental status and a unilaterally dilated pupil is in the "immediate transport" category. When you check the pupils, look for contact lenses. If present, they should be removed, placed in their container or saline solution, and transported with the patient.

Respiratory derangements are common with CNS illness or injury. Five abnormal breathing patterns may be commonly observed in this setting: Cheyne-Stokes respiration is a pattern marked by apnea lasting 10–60 seconds followed by gradually increasing depth and frequency of respiration. It can be seen with brain damage due to trauma or cerebral hemorrhage and with chronic hypoxia. Kussmaul's respirations are deep, rapid breaths caused by severe metabolic or CNS problems. Central neurogenic hyperventilation is caused by a lesion in the CNS and is marked by rapid, deep, noisy respirations. Ataxic respirations are poor breaths due to CNS damage causing ineffective thoracic muscular coordination. Apneustic respiration is breathing marked by prolonged inspiration unrelieved by expiration attempts and it is due to damage in the upper pons. Always remember that CO_2 has a critical effect on cerebral vessels: Increased levels cause vascular dilation, whereas low levels cause vasoconstriction. This is the basis for controlled hyperventilation in settings where some degree of vasoconstriction might minimize brain swelling.

Cardiovascular status is always important. Even if a primary cardiovascular problem is not present, CNS events are likely to cause changes to the cardiovascular system. In particular, assess heart rate, ECG rhythm, bruits over the carotid arteries, and possible presence of jugular venous distension, a sign of ineffective cardiac pumping. You should be aware that vital signs and changes in them are crucial in following the course of a neurological emergency. Note Cushing's reflex, a grouping of four characteristics in vital signs that signals increased intracranial pressure: increased blood pressure, decreased pulse, decreased respirations, and increased temperature. The earliest signs are the decrease in pulse rate and an increase in blood pressure and temperature. Review Table 3-1 (text page 285), which distinguishes vital sign patterns in shock and in increased intracranial pressure.

The exam for neurologic system status is covered in detail on text pages 282–285. Note that the components of the exam include sensorimotor evaluation (if posture is abnormal, consider whether it might be decorticate or decerebrate in nature), motor system status, and cranial nerve status.

Last, be particularly aware with elderly patients and with patients with a chronic neurological condition (such as the degenerative disorders) that it is vital to know the patient's baseline values in all areas before you can put your current findings into the context of acute changes or not. Interviewing family members or caregivers may be very helpful.

11. **Given several preprogrammed nontraumatic neurological emergency patients, provide the appropriate assessment, management, and transport.** pp. 262–310

The priorities for someone who is unconscious or clearly in urgent distress with neurologic difficulties are the same as for a patient who is affected by a potentially life-threatening emergency of another origin: Ensure adequate airway, breathing (ventilation), and circulation. This is particularly important for someone whose emergency may be originating in, or affecting, the CNS: The brain requires a constant supply of oxygen, glucose, and vitamins. After 10–20 seconds without blood flow, unconsciousness will occur. Significant deprivation of oxygen (anoxia) or glucose (hypoglycemia) can cause seizures or coma. You should always give high-flow oxygen to a patient with a neurologic emergency and give glucose to any one found to be hypoglycemic.

Neurologic injuries and illnesses usually require treatment as soon as possible to prevent progressive damage. In the case of thromboembolic stroke, this may be particularly true because therapies are coming into use that can minimize the region of brain tissue infarcted in the stroke or even prevent the progression of tissue ischemia to tissue infarction. Patients who show altered mental status and/or any clear neurologic impairment (pupillary dilation, especially unilateral, facial drooping, slurred speech, abnormal posturing—if these appear to be new or progressing findings) that may suggest TIA or stroke need immediate intervention and transport. Management of seizures and syncope often mandates prompt intervention and care, as well.

You will see many calls for complaints such as low back pain and headache. These conditions may be relatively minor or the signal of a serious underlying disorder. History suggesting new onset, severe pain, or clearly progressive pain indicates the need for aggressive assessment and management, whereas other patients with chronic pain of either origin also require full assessment but may need only supportive care.

Patients with known CNS neoplasms or degenerative neurological conditions may present with a complaint related to their underlying disease or a problem of completely different origin. Be aware that these persons are always more vulnerable to oxygen or glucose deprivation from another source (for example, cardiac disease or diabetes, respectively); in addition, remember that some patients will have airways vulnerable to compromise secondary to muscle paralysis or other neurologic causes.

CASE STUDY REVIEW

Reread the case study on pages 261 and 262 in Paramedic Care: Medical Emergencies *before reading the discussion below.*

This case study demonstrates how paramedics react to a relatively common neurological emergency: a "possible stroke patient." The case study demonstrates how initial impressions, assessment findings, and knowledge of the likely pathophysiology not only reveal diagnosis but directly guide the team in prioritizing transport and in identifying the appropriate receiving center.

Jack and Linda are dispatched to a bank with some important information already in hand: The patient is a man in his 60s with reported (presumably new-onset) neurological signs of right-sided weakness and inability to speak. Because possible stroke is a true emergency, one in which time can make a substantial difference to outcome, it is in the patient's favor that the team can respond within 3 minutes or so of the dispatch.

Their initial impression is of an elderly man sitting upright, with some assistance, in a chair. The neurological deficit of aphasia (inability to speak) appears to be confirmed on attempts to communicate with the patient, and the team realizes that the patient, although unable to speak, appears to be oriented and cooperative. Their attention then turns to airway and breathing as priorities. The man's airway is patent (at the moment), and his respirations are normal.

Blood pressure is measured in the unaffected arm, and it is hypertensive at 160/90. Chronic hypertension is a risk factor for stroke, so it is important for the team to ask about a history of hypertension and any associated medications when they get the opportunity to talk with the patient's family. If none of the bystanders knew the gentleman, and if he seemed lucid, the team might be able to solicit limited information from him via a Medic-Alert tag (if he wears one) and/or via requests for head nodding or for written responses to questions. Changes in his ability to comply with such requests might serve as a signal of decreasing mental status. The rest of his initial physical exam is largely benign except for confirmation of unilateral (right-sided) weakness. You are told that there is marked right-sided weakness, but you aren't told the extent: Does it involve the arm only, or does it also involve the face or the leg, or both? Extent of weakness, as well as any sign of additional extent, is an indicator of stroke progression and also signals that sudden airway compromise may be more likely.

Only at this point, after initial assessment, is oxygen started, a heparin lock placed in the unaffected arm, and ECG monitoring begun. The timing of the IV access and ECG monitoring is appropriate, but the team should have considered oxygen supplementation as soon as they knew the patient was unable to talk. Any time advantage in reversal of brain anoxia should be taken. On the other hand, it is a positive sign that pulse oximetry after initiation of oxygen supplementation is 99%.

You aren't told what information is elicited regarding personal medical history, but you are told that the ECG shows atrial fibrillation at a rate of 90. Atrial fibrillation is a risk factor for embolic (occlusive) stroke because small clots form in the heart and break off to enter the systemic circulation. This knowledge increases the importance of timely transport, as well as expedient consideration of appropriate facility, because current guidelines indicate that thrombolytic therapy within the first 3 hours of an embolic occlusion may well be successful in minimizing or preventing infarction of brain tissue.

Indeed, the team packages the patient carefully but expediently and transports him to a facility that can handle a "brain attack." On arrival, a hemorrhagic stroke of significant magnitude is ruled out via CT scan and the team decides to initiate therapy with tPA. The outcome is positive: The patient's aphasia resolves completely and most of his right-sided weakness reverses. The patient is discharged to a rehabilitation unit for further therapy on his hemiparesis. You don't know how or whether the man's atrial fibrillation (AF) is resolved, but you should assume that in-hospital care would have involved adjustment of medication (if he were taking any for AF) or possible electrical conversion to normal rhythm.

CONTENT SELF-EVALUATION

MULTIPLE CHOICE

A 1. Afferent nerve fibers carry messages to the central nervous system (CNS), whereas efferent fibers carry impulses from the CNS to the rest of the body.
   A. True
   B. False

C 2. The two mechanisms that generally cause altered mental status are:
   A. occlusive and hemorrhagic strokes.
   B. systemic diseases and drugs or toxic agents.
   C. structural lesions and toxic-metabolic states.
   D. head trauma and CNS disease.
   E. toxic-metabolic states and brain tumors.

B 3. Peripheral neuropathy can affect muscle activity, sensation, and reflexes, but not internal organ function.
   A. True
   B. False

E 4. The Glasgow Coma Scale assesses eye opening, verbal response, and motor response. Which correlation of score and likely outcome is incorrect?
   A. score or 3 or 4, 10% favorable outcome
   B. score of 8 or higher, 94% favorable outcome
   C. score of 5–7 that increases to 8 or higher, 80% favorable outcome
   D. score of 5–7, 50% favorable outcome in adults and 90% in children
   E. score of 5–7 that decreases by one point, 10% favorable outcome

C 5. Three interventions that may be indicated in treatment of a patient with altered mental status of unknown cause are:
   A. hyperventilation, 50% dextrose, and naloxone.
   B. mannitol (Osmotrol), 50% dextrose, and naloxone.
   C. 50% dextrose, thiamine, and naloxone.
   D. mannitol (Osmotrol), hyperventilation, and 50% dextrose.
   E. mannitol (Osmotrol), thiamine, and naloxone.

A 6. Management of a patient with a suspected stroke or a suspected TIA is the same because they can rarely be distinguished in the field.
   A. True
   B. False

C 7. If a stroke patient is apneic or breathing inadequately, controlled positive-pressure hyperventilation may be beneficial because it:
   A. causes cerebral vasoconstriction, decreasing cerebral swelling.
   B. causes a reflex increase in respiration rate.
   C. eliminates excess CO_2 levels.
   D. increases CO_2 levels toward normal range.
   E. increases the ability of brain cells to take up any available oxygen.

B 8. Among the many types of epileptic seizures, the most likely to require intervention on your part are:
   A. absence seizures.
   B. tonic-clonic seizures.
   C. petit mal seizures.
   D. simple partial seizures.
   E. complex partial seizures.

___B___ 9. Status epilepticus is considered a serious, but not life-threatening, emergency.
  A. True
  B. False

___A___ 10. If a patient with suspected syncope does not regain consciousness within a few
  moments, the event is NOT syncope, but something more serious.
  A. True
  B. False

___C___ 11. The two most common causes of headache are:
  A. vascular and organic.   D. tension and organic.
  B. vascular and neurogenic.   E. tension and neurogenic.
  C. tension and vascular.

___E___ 12. Which one of the following is NOT a degenerative neurological disorder?
  A. multiple sclerosis (MS)   D. muscular dystrophy
  B. Parkinson's disease   E. vertebral disk disease
  C. Bell's palsy

FILL-IN-THE-BLANKS

Write the word or words that best complete the statements below in the space(s) provided.

13. Stimulation of the sympathetic nervous system results in increased _heart rate_ and dilation of _bronchioles_ and _pupils_.

14. Speech is located in the _temporal_ lobe of the _cerebrum_.

15. The autonomic nervous system regulates _involuntary_ physiologic processes.

16. Tissues innervated by the sympathetic nervous system include _smooth_ and _cardiac_ muscle and some glands.

17. The diencephalon consists of the _thalmus_, the _hypothalmus_, and the _limbic_ system.

18. The neuronal processes that detect an incoming nerve impulse are the _dendrite_.

19. The peripheral nervous system consists of the _somatic nervous system_ and the _autonomic nervous system_.

20. The nervous system consists of the _central nervous system_ and the _peripheral nervous system_.

21. In outer-to-inner order, the dura mater, arachnoid membrane, and the pia mater make up the three layers of the _meninges_.

22. The multiple tips of the _axon_ allow a neuron to send an impulse to more than one other neuron.

23. Actions of the parasympathetic nervous system include decreased _heart rate_ and constriction of _bronchioles_ and _pupils_.

24. The brainstem consists of the _mesencephalon_, the _pons_, and the _medulla oblongata_.

25. Both the brain and spinal cord are bathed in _cerebrospinal fluid_.

26. The reticular activating system (RAS), in the lateral portions of the medulla, pons, and midbrain, is responsible for maintaining _conscious_ and the ability to respond to _stimuli_.

27. Vision is located in the _occipital_ lobe of the _cerebrum_.

28. Motor activity is located in _frontal_ lobes of the _cerebrum_.

29. The somatic nervous system mediates _voluntary_, _conscious_ actions.

30. The junction of two neurons is called a(n) _synapse_, and a(n) _neurotransmitter_ enables a nerve impulse to move from one neuron to another.

31. The central nervous system consists of the _brain_ and _spinal cord_.

LABEL THE DIAGRAM

The figure below shows the major parts of the brain. Label each part then match its major function(s) by placing the appropriate letter in the space provided below each label name.

32. _Thalmus_
Function(s): _H_

33. _Hypothalmus_
Function(s): _E_

34. _Pituary Gland_
Function(s): _G_

35. _Midbrain_
Function(s): _B_

36. _Pons_
Function(s): _D_

37. _Medulla Oblongata_
Function(s): _C_

38. _Cerebrum_
Function(s): _F_

39. _Cerebellum_
Function(s): _A_

Cerebral hemispheres

A. adjustment of balance and muscular coordination _Cerebellum_
B. generates involuntary somatic muscle responses, maintains consciousness _midbrain_
C. contains autonomic centers for cardiovascular, respiratory, and digestive system function _Medulla Oblongata_
D. contains centers for involuntary somatic and visceral motor activity _Pons_
E. contains centers for control of emotion, autonomic, and endocrine functions _Hypothalmus_
F. conscious thought, memory storage, and control over voluntary motor activity _Cerebrum_
G. secretes hormones responsible for regulation of endocrine glands _Pituatary Gland_
H. acts as relay and processing center for sensory information _Thalmus._

MATCHING

Write the two letters giving the cause and description of the abnormal breathing pattern in the space provided next to the name of the pattern.

__BG__ 40. Cheyne-Stokes respiration

__EH__ 41. Central neurogenic hyperventilation

__AD__ 42. Kussmaul's respiration

__CI__ 43. ataxic respirations

__FJ__ 44. apneustic respirations

A. rapid, deep respirations
B. brain damage due to trauma or cerebral hemorrhage and with chronic hypoxia
C. ineffective thoracic muscular coordination due to CNS damage
D. severe metabolic or CNS conditions
E. rapid, deep, noisy respirations involving hyperventilation
F. prolonged inspiration unrelieved by expiration attempts
G. brief period of apnea followed by increasing depth and frequency of respirations
H. lesion in the CNS
I. poor respirations
J. pattern due to damage in the upper part of the pons

Write the two letters giving the major cause and characteristic of presentation in the space provided next to the type of stroke to which they apply. A letter may be used more than once.

__AD__ 45. thrombotic stroke

__CE__ 46. intracerebral hemorrhage

__CF__ 47. embolic stroke

__BC__ 48. subarachnoid hemorrhage

A. gradual development of signs/symptoms, often first noticed on waking during night
B. congenital blood vessel abnormalities or head trauma
C. sudden onset of severe headache
D. blood clot that forms in an area of a cerebral artery narrowed by atherosclerosis
E. rupture of a small blood vessel within brain tissue
F. lodging of a blood clot, air bubble, tumor tissue, or fat in an artery that is far from its site of origin

LISTING

49. The AVPU model for mental status stands for:

A __Alert & oriented to surroundings__

V __voice__

P __pain__

U __unresponsive__

50. Assessment of a patient's cerebral function includes evaluation of emotional state. Fill in a word for each letter of the MTPJ and MA model (given on pp. 278, 279).

M mood

T thought process

P Perceptions of sourroundings

J Judgement

MA memory + attention

51. Cushing's reflex, which is associated with increasing intracranial pressure, consists of what four elements?

↑ BP

↑ temp

↓ paulse

↓ respirations

52. A mnemonic for the common causes of altered mental status is AEIOU-TIPS. Fill in one or more words for each letter of the mnemonic.

A acidosis / alcohol

E epilepsy

I infection

O overdose

U uremia

T trauma, toxin, tumor

I elnsuline

P psychosis or poison

S Stroke or seizure

53. Name the two types of occlusive strokes.

Thrombotic

Embolic

54. Name two categories of hemorrhagic strokes.

Intra ceubral

Subarchnoid

55. List the four main characteristics of Parkinson's disease.

Tremor

Rigidity

Brady kinsia

Postural Instabillity.

56. List, in increasing order of severity, the three forms of spina bifida.

Occulta

Meningocele

myelomenigocele

57. List the two common forms of vascular headache.

Migraine

cluster

SPECIAL PROJECT

Distinguishing Different Conditions in the Field

The chapter presented situations in which you might need to distinguish between very different conditions that may have somewhat similar presentations. Complete the tables below to demonstrate your knowledge of these conditions.

Scenario 1: Shock versus Increased Intracranial Pressure

As discussed in Chapter 3, one of the reasons to take vital signs every 5 minutes in patients with suspected CNS injury is that vitals may change quickly, showing signs of instability or of emergence of a diagnostic pattern. Complete the table given below to demonstrate the characteristic vital signs in shock and in increased intracranial pressure.

Vital Signs	Shock	Increased Intracranial Pressure
Blood pressure	↓	↑
Pulse	↑	↓
Respirations	↑	↓
Level of consciousness	↓	↓

Scenario 2: Syncope versus Tonic-Clonic Seizure

As discussed in Chapter 3, you may arrive on scene after an event has happened or while an event is in progress. In such cases, history from bystanders, and, when able, from the patient, may be crucial in establishing what underlying condition is present. Complete the table given below to demonstrate the different characteristics, or traits, of syncope and of a generalized tonic-clonic seizure.

Trait	Syncope	Tonic-Clonic Seizure
Starting position	standing	any position
Warning?	Pt remembers feeling of fainting	may or may not have warning preceded by Aura.
Jerking motions?	Ø	while unconscious
Return of consciousness	Immediate once supine	unconscious during seizure, drowsy afterward.

CHAPTER 4

Endocrinology

Review of Chapter Objectives

After reading this chapter, you should be able to:

1. **Describe the incidence, morbidity, and mortality of endocrinologic emergencies.** pp. 326–327, 329–330, 336–337

   Many people have endocrine disorders that involve excessive or deficient hormone production or function. The incidence of such disorders is widely variable. Some disorders are readily controlled by hormone replacement therapy; others are more complex and thus more difficult to manage. The most common of all of the endocrine disorders is diabetes mellitus, affecting at least 8 million Americans.

2. **Identify the risk factors that predispose a person to endocrinologic disease.** pp. 329, 336–337, 340, 341

   Diabetes mellitus is the most commonly encountered endocrine disorder. Among the predisposing factors that have been identified for this condition are heredity, viral infection, autoimmune antibodies, and obesity.

   Heredity is thought to be the key factor in the predisposition for Graves' disease, although autoimmune antibodies are known to trigger the excess production of thyroid hormone. Severe physiologic stress has been found to be a common triggering factor for thyrotoxicosis (thyroid storm). On the other hand, hypothyroidism or myxedema may be either congenital or acquired.

   The risk of adrenal gland disorders is increased by the administration of glucocorticoids or may be a consequence of abnormalities of the anterior pituitary gland or the adrenal cortex. Approximately half of all adrenal gland disorders are due to autoimmune disorders or may be aggravated by acute physiologic stress.

3. **Discuss the anatomy and physiology of organs and structures associated with endocrinologic diseases.** pp. 316–326

   There are eight major structures associated with the endocrine system located throughout the body: the hypothalamus, pituitary gland, thyroid gland, parathyroid glands, thymus, pancreas, adrenal glands, and gonads. The pineal gland is also part of the endocrine system.

   The hypothalamus, located deep within the cerebrum of the brain, is the junction between the endocrine system and the central nervous system. About the size of a pea, the pituitary gland is located adjacent to the hypothalamus within the cerebrum. The pineal gland is also located adjacent to the hypothalamus. The double-lobed thyroid gland is located in the neck anterior to and just below the cartilage of the larynx. The parathyroid glands are very small and are found on the posterior lateral surface of the thyroid gland. The thymus is located in the mediastinum just behind the sternum. The pancreas is located in the upper abdomen behind the stomach and between the duodenum and the spleen. The adrenal glands are somewhat triangular in shape and are located on the superior surface of the kidneys. Gonads can be found in the lower pelvis in women, with each ovary resembling an almond in size and shape. In men, the gonads are located in the scrotum.

The endocrine system is closely linked to the nervous system and plays a critical role in our ability to maintain life by regulating many bodily functions through chemical substances called hormones. The endocrine system is made up of ductless glands, which manufacture and secrete hormones that act in adjacent tissues or travel via the bloodstream to target organs or other endocrine glands to produce specific or generalized effects. Hormones regulate metabolic activity, growth and development, as well as mediate chemical reactions, maintain homeostatic balance, and initiate our adaptive response to stress.

4. Discuss the pathophysiology, assessment findings, need for rapid intervention and transport, and management of endocrinologic emergencies. pp. 326–341

As you review the anatomy and physiology of the endocrine system, it is clearly evident that the endocrine system is closely linked to the nervous system and controls a variety of physiologic processes that are essential for survival. The causes of endocrine disorders are variable and include heredity, congenital anomalies, viral infection, and autoimmune disease processes. The most commonly encountered endocrine emergencies in the prehospital setting are related to diabetes mellitus and disorders of the thyroid or adrenal glands. You should review the sections of the text which clarify the differences in clinical presentation, assessment, and management of these disorders.

5. Describe osmotic diuresis and its relationship to diabetes mellitus. p. 329

Osmosis is the tendency for water molecules to migrate across a semi-permeable membrane so that the concentrations of particles approach equivalence on both sides. When blood glucose levels rise above 180 mg/dL, no more glucose can be reabsorbed through the renal tubules and glucose begins to be lost (or "spill") into the urine. This causes the osmotic pressure, or concentration of particulates, to rise inside the kidney tubule to a level higher than that of the blood. Water follows glucose into the urine to cause a marked water loss termed osmotic diuresis that is the basis for the polyuria (excessive urination) associated with untreated diabetes.

6. Describe the pathophysiology of adult and juvenile onset diabetes mellitus. pp. 329–330

Juvenile onset or Type I diabetes mellitus is a serious disease characterized by very low production of insulin by the beta cells of the pancreas. In many cases, there is no insulin being produced. It is called juvenile onset diabetes because of the average age of the patient at the time of diagnosis. Type I diabetes is also known as insulin-dependent diabetes because patients require regular injections of insulin to control their disease. Heredity appears to be an important factor in determining which people will develop Type I diabetes. The cause of Type I diabetes is not clear. Other factors attributed to triggering juvenile onset diabetes are viral infection, an autoimmune response, or genetically determined premature deterioration of beta cells. The immediate cause of Type I diabetes is the destruction of pancreatic beta cells.

Type II diabetes mellitus, also known as non-insulin-dependent diabetes, is responsible for almost 90 percent of all cases of diabetes. Type II diabetes usually begins in later life and is often associated with obesity, so it is known as adult onset diabetes. Type II diabetes is associated with a moderate decline in insulin production accompanied by a marked decrease in the utilization of the insulin within the body. The cause is not clearly understood, although obesity is believed to play a role in its development. Increased weight, along with the increased size of fat cells, causes a relative deficiency in the number of insulin receptors, thus making the fat cells less responsive to insulin. Type II diabetes is usually managed through a combination of diet, exercise, and the administration of medications to reduce either blood glucose or enhance the efficiency of insulin. Occasionally insulin administration is required.

7. Differentiate between the pathophysiology of normal glucose metabolism and diabetic glucose metabolism. pp. 327–329

Metabolism, which means "to change," is a term used to refer to all of the chemical and energy transformations within the body. Two kinds of change take place in the cell. One kind builds complex molecules from simple ones (anabolism), such as the synthesis of glycogen from glucose. The other kind breaks down complex molecules into simpler ones (catabolism), such as occurs with the breakdown of glucose into carbon dioxide, water, and energy (in the form of ATP). When materials are abundant after meals and the glucose is high, insulin enables cells to use glucose directly and to store energy as glycogen, protein, and fat. Insulin stimulates glucose pathways. In contrast, glucagon, the dominant hormone during periods of low blood glucose, stimulates catabolic pathways to produce usable energy from the body's stores.

The rate at which glucose can enter the cell is dependent upon insulin levels. Insulin combines with insulin receptors on the surface of the cell membrane, allowing glucose to enter the cell by increasing the permeability of the cell membrane. The rate at which glucose can be transported into the cells can be accelerated tenfold by insulin.

Sometimes the body cannot use glucose as its primary energy source, as is the case in patients with diabetes mellitus. Without insulin, the amount of glucose that can be transported into the cells is far too small to meet the body's energy demands. Without insulin, the glucose remains in the bloodstream, resulting in hyperglycemia. Carbohydrate depletion is also seen in other conditions, such as a high-fat, low-carbohydrate diet or starvation (which can be associated with some eating disorders). Under these conditions, the body slowly switches from glucose to fat as the primary energy source. Adipose cells break down fats into their component free fatty acids, and the blood concentration of these acids rises considerably.

Most of the fatty acids are used directly by the body's cells as an energy source. The liver takes in some, where the catabolism of fatty acids produces acetoacetic acid. When more acetoacetic acid is released by the liver than can be effectively utilized by body cells, it accumulates in the bloodstream along with two other closely related substances, acetone and β-hydroxybutyric acid. The three substances are collectively called ketone bodies. Their presence in excessive quantities is called ketosis.

8. **Describe the mechanism of ketone body formation and its relationship to ketoacidosis.** pp. 328, 330–332

When the body's carbohydrate stores begin to become depleted, small amounts of glucose can be formed by the breakdown of protein and fat through the process of gluconeogenesis. The byproducts of amino acid breakdown include carbon dioxide and water and the formation of urea. The breakdown of fat results in the formation of carbon dioxide, water, and ketone bodies.

The normal blood ketone level in humans is low because ketones are usually metabolized as rapidly as they are formed. If there are low levels of glucose stored in the cells, the ability of the body to oxidize the ketones is soon exceeded and ketones begin to build up in the bloodstream, resulting in a condition known as ketosis. This results in an increased amount of acid in the body fluids. The resulting metabolic acidosis is often severe and can be fatal.

9. **Discuss the physiology of the excretion of potassium and ketone bodies by the kidneys.** pp. 328–329

Whenever the flow rate of fluid inside the tubules of the kidney rises, as in osmotic diuresis, an increase in excretion of potassium occurs. This leads to the potential for significant hypokalemia and its effects, such as potentially life-threatening cardiac dysrhythmias. In ketotic states, ketone bodies are excreted through respiration and will also spill into the urine.

10. **Describe the relationship of insulin to serum glucose levels.** pp. 315, 323–324

Insulin is a glucagon antagonist and lowers the blood glucose level by promoting energy storage. Insulin increases the rate at which various body cells take up glucose by changing the permeability of the cell membranes. These changes also make the cell more permeable to potassium, magnesium, and phosphate ions, as well as many amino acids. Because the liver rapidly breaks down insulin, the hormone must be secreted constantly.

Homeostasis of blood glucose is remarkably effective. In non-diabetics, when blood glucose is high, as after a meal, the beta cells of the pancreas release insulin. Insulin enables cells to use glucose directly as well as to store energy as glycogen, protein, and fat. If you were to draw a venous blood sample to measure fasting blood glucose levels, you'd find the level in healthy individuals is usually between 80–90 mg glucose/dL blood. In the first 60–90 minutes after a meal the level will increase to approximately 120–140 mg/dL before dropping off to near-fasting levels as insulin is released to move the glucose from the bloodstream into the cells. Conversely, when blood glucose levels are low, the alpha cells of the pancreas release glucagon to raise the blood glucose level.

11. Describe the effects of decreased levels of insulin on the body.   pp. 329–333

Insulin deficiency contributes to the development of hyperglycemia. Without insulin to facilitate the movement of large glucose molecules across cell membranes, the blood glucose level rises even as the intracellular level of glucose plummets. At the same time, the alpha cells of the pancreas release glucagon to increase blood glucose by stimulating the breakdown of glycogen, as well as stimulating the breakdown of body proteins and fats with subsequent chemical conversion to glucose (gluconeogenesis).

12. Describe the effects of increased serum glucose levels on the body.   pp. 333, 336

With a rise in blood glucose levels, as is the case in Type I diabetes, the body's cells cannot take up circulating glucose. Glucose then spills into urine, leading to a large water loss, via osmotic diuresis, and significant dehydration. This can lead to significant loss of potassium and hypokalemia.

13. Discuss the pathophysiology, assessment findings, and management of the following endocrine emergencies:

a. nonketotic hyperosmolar coma   pp. 332–333

This condition is a complication of Type II diabetes due to inadequate insulin activity and is marked by high blood glucose, marked dehydration, and decreased mental function.

Development of the coma is slower than with ketoacidosis. Early signs include increased urination and thirst. Later signs may include orthostatic hypotension, dry skin, and tachycardia.

This condition is difficult to distinguish from ketoacidosis in the field. Field management focuses on maintaining ABCs and fluid resuscitation.

b. diabetic ketoacidosis   pp. 330–332

Diabetic ketoacidosis is a serious, potentially life-threatening complication of diabetes mellitus. It occurs when profound insulin deficiency is coupled with increased glucagon activity.

The onset is slow, lasting from 12 to 24 hours. In its early stages, the signs and symptoms include increased thirst, excessive hunger, urination, and malaise. Increased urination results from the osmotic diuresis accompanying glucose spillage into the urine. Intensified thirst is caused by the body's attempt to replace the fluids lost by increased urination. Nausea, vomiting, marked dehydration, tachycardia, and weakness characterize diabetic ketoacidosis. The skin is usually warm and dry. Coma is not uncommon. The breath may have a sweet or acetone-like character due to the increased ketones in the blood. Very deep, rapid respirations, called Kussmaul's respirations, also occur. Kussmaul's respirations represent the body's attempt to compensate for the metabolic acidosis produced by the ketones and organic acids present in the blood. It may be complicated by several electrolyte imbalances. The most significant is decreased potassium. Decreased potassium (hypokalemia) can lead to serious dysrhythmias or even death.

The approach used with the patient suffering from diabetic ketoacidosis is essentially the same as with any unconscious patient. You should first complete your initial assessment of airway, breathing, and circulation. You will then complete your focused history and physical exam. Pay particular attention to the presence of a Medic-Alert bracelet and/or insulin in the refrigerator. Also, obtain a history from bystanders. The fruity odor of ketones occasionally can be detected on the breath. If possible, complete the rapid test for blood glucose.

It is not uncommon for patients in ketoacidosis to have blood glucose levels well in excess of 300 mg/dL. The field management of such cases is focused on maintenance of ABCs and fluid resuscitation to counteract the patient's dehydration. Treatment should include drawing a red top tube (or the tube specified by local protocols) of blood. Following this, you should administer one to two liters of normal saline per protocol. If transport time is lengthy, the medical control physician may request intravenous or subcutaneous administration of regular insulin.

If the blood glucose level cannot be quickly determined, draw a red top tube of blood for analysis and start an IV of normal saline. Following this, administer 50 ml (25 grams) of 50 percent dextrose solution. This additional glucose load will not adversely affect the ketoacidotic patient because it is negligible compared to the total quantity present in the body. If the patient is alcoholic, consider administering 100 mg of thiamine. Transportation to an appropriate facility should be expedited.

c. hypoglycemia pp. 333, 336

Hypoglycemia, or low blood glucose, is a potentially life-threatening medical emergency. Sometimes called insulin shock, it can occur if a patient accidentally or intentionally injects too much insulin, eats an inadequate amount of food after taking insulin, or has overexercised and burned up all available glucose. Untreated, the insulin will cause the blood glucose to drop to a very low level. The longer the period of hypoglycemia persists, the greater the risk that the brain cells will be permanently damaged or even killed.

The signs and symptoms of hypoglycemia are many and varied. An abnormal mental status is the most important and often the earliest sign. In the earliest stages of hypoglycemia, the patient may appear restless or impatient or complain of hunger. As the blood sugar falls lower, he or she may display inappropriate anger or display a variety of bizarre behaviors. Physical signs may include diaphoresis and tachycardia. If the blood sugar falls to a critically low level, the patient may sustain a hypoglycemic seizure or become comatose. In contrast to diabetic ketoacidosis, hypoglycemia can develop quickly. When encountering a patient behaving bizarrely, you should always consider hypoglycemia.

In suspected cases of hypoglycemia, perform the initial assessment quickly. Inspect the patient for a Medic-Alert bracelet. If possible, determine the blood glucose level. If the blood glucose level is noted to be less than 60 mg/dL, draw a red top tube of blood and start an IV of normal saline. Next, administer 50–100 milliliters (25–50 grams) of 50 percent dextrose intravenously. If the patient is conscious and able to swallow, complete glucose administration with orange juice, sodas, or commercially available glucose pastes.

If the blood glucose cannot be obtained and if the patient is unconscious, you should start an IV of normal saline and administer 50–100 milliliters (25–50 grams) of 50 percent dextrose. Expedite transport to the nearest medical facility. If you suspect alcoholism, administer 100 mg of thiamine prior to the administration of dextrose.

d. hyperglycemia pp. 329, 330–332

Diabetes mellitus results from either inadequate amounts of circulating insulin or inadequate utilization of insulin. This means that there is an excess of blood glucose while there is an intracellular deficit. In diabetes, glucose builds up in the bloodstream, especially after meals. The blood glucose level rises higher and returns to normal more slowly in the diabetic than in the non-diabetic. An oral glucose tolerance test uses this phenomenon in the diagnosis of diabetes. The diabetic's inadequate insulin level and impaired glucose tolerance are partly due to the decreased entry of glucose into the cells, thus leaving more glucose in the bloodstream.

The second cause of hyperglycemia in the diabetic results from difficulties with the function of the liver. When blood glucose levels are high, insulin secretion is normally increased and the breakdown of glycogen is decreased. In the diabetic, however, insulin secretion is decreased, and the alpha cells secrete glucagon to stimulate glycogenolysis by the liver, thus raising the blood glucose level.

In Type I diabetes the decreased insulin secretion is accompanied by a steady accumulation of glucose in the blood. Hyperglycemia acts like an osmotic diuretic and glucose "spills over" into the urine (glycosuria) pulling large amounts of water with it (polyuria). The body's attempt to dilute the concentration of glucose in the bloodstream results in intracellular dehydration and stimulates thirst (polydipsia). As the cells become glucose-depleted, they begin to use proteins and fats as an energy source resulting in weight loss and the formation of harmful byproducts, such as ketones and organic free fatty acids. The body's response to this state of cellular starvation is to trigger hunger in the patient (polyphagia). If the acids and ketones continue to collect in the blood, severe metabolic acidosis occurs and coma ensues, resulting in serious brain damage or death.

Type II diabetes does not usually result in diabetic ketoacidosis. It can, however, develop into a life-threatening emergency termed hyperglycemic hyperosmolar nonketotic (HHNK) coma. In Type II diabetes, when blood glucose levels exceed 600 mg/dL, the high osmolality of the blood causes an osmotic diuresis and marked dehydration of body cells. However, sufficient insulin is produced to prevent the manufacture of ketones and the complications of metabolic acidosis. In this respect, the condition differs from diabetic ketoacidosis.

e. thyrotoxicosis   pp. 336–338

Thyrotoxic crisis, more commonly known as "thyroid storm," is a life-threatening medical emergency which can be fatal within as little as 48 hours if not treated. It is usually associated with severe physiologic (trauma, infection, uncontrolled diabetes mellitus, etc.) or psychological stress. You will also encounter thyroid storm from an accidental or intentional overdose of thyroid hormone. Many patients with thyrotoxicosis have underlying Graves' disease (hyperthyroidism).

The signs and symptoms associated with thyroid storm reflect the patient's profound hypermetabolic state and increased adrenergic response. The patient may be hyperthermic (with temperatures as high as 105°) and tachycardic (especially common are atrial tachydysrhythmias), with a high pulse pressure and dyspnea. Mental status changes range from agitation and restlessness to delirium and coma. Nausea, vomiting, and diarrhea are also often present. Death often follows heart failure and profound cardiovascular collapse.

Field management is focused on supportive care with oxygenation, ventilatory assistance, fluid resuscitation, and cardiac monitoring, along with expedited transport for definitive care to block the high circulating levels of thyroid hormones.

f. myxedema   pp. 338–339

Inadequate levels of the thyroid hormones in adults produce hypothyroidism or myxedema, which results in a generalized decrease in metabolism. While it may occur in males or females of any age, it is most commonly seen among middle-aged females or as a consequence when surgery or radiation is used to treat hyperthyroidism.

This disorder tends to have a gradual onset, and the initial signs and symptoms tend to be quite subtle and include hoarse voice and slow speech, facial bloating, weakness, cold intolerance, lethargy, and fatigue as well as altered mental states, particularly depression. Additionally, the skin and hair are quite dry and coarse in texture. Patients with hypothyroidism are treated with replacement thyroid hormone, usually synthetic T_4 agents such as levothyroxine (Synthroid).

Rarely do these patients require emergency treatment for their hypothyroidism unless it progresses to myxedema coma; however, you will encounter many patients who take thyroid replacement hormones.

Myxedema coma, a life-threatening complication of hypothyroidism, is not uncommon in colder climates but is unusual in warm ones. It is most often seen in older patients who have pulmonary or vascular disease. Other contributing factors include a history of thyroid disease, exposure to cold, infection, trauma, or drugs that suppress the central nervous system such as sedatives and hypnotics. The mortality rate associated with myxedema coma is high.

Myxedema coma usually has a gradual onset, with lethargy and depression that progresses to coma. Other signs and symptoms include extreme hypothermia (temperatures as low as 75°F are not uncommon), low amplitude bradycardia, carbon dioxide retention, and profound respiratory depression.

Emergency management of myxedema coma is focused on maintenance of the ABCs and, as always, careful monitoring of the patient's cardiac and oxygenation status; most patients will require intubation and ventilatory assistance. Active rewarming is contraindicated due to the risk of cardiac dysrhythmias and the potential to cause vasodilatation, which may contribute to cardiovascular collapse. Although it is appropriate to initiate intravenous access, care must be taken to limit fluids since fluid and electrolyte imbalance is common. Follow local protocols or contact medical control for specific orders based on your patient's presentation.

g. Cushing's syndrome   pp. 340–341

Chronic high levels of glucocorticoids result in the development of Cushing's syndrome or hyperadrenalism. Cushing's syndrome may occur as a result of long-term glucocorticoid (steroid) therapy, or by abnormalities of the adrenal glands, or by a pituitary tumor triggering excessive secretion of adrenocorticotropic hormone (ACTH), which stimulates the adrenals to produce excessive amounts of glucocorticoids.

Presenting signs and symptoms include: weight gain, particularly through the trunk of the body, face, and neck, with a typical "moon-faced" appearance and often a "buffalo hump" due to the fat deposits in these areas; skin changes, such as the thinning of the skin to an almost transparent appearance, a tendency to bruise easily, delayed healing from even minor wounds, and the development of facial hair among women; increased vascular sensitivity; hypertension; mood swings and memory impairment or decreased ability to concentrate.

Treatment involves removing the cause, such as the surgical removal of a tumor, or adjusting the dosage of glucocorticoids. While it is unlikely that you would encounter a patient with an acute hyperadrenal crisis, you are very likely to encounter patients who exhibit signs and symptoms of Cushing's syndrome. These patients have a higher incidence of cardiovascular disease, hypertension, and stroke than the general population and are prone to infection. When performing your assessment, be alert for the signs mentioned above which are associated with high glucocorticoid levels. Pay particular attention to skin preparation when starting intravenous lines, due to the fragility of these patients' skin and their susceptibility to infection. Your observations noted in your patient care report and relayed to the receiving hospital staff may contribute to the early diagnosis and treatment of this disorder, especially in those patients who do not have a primary care provider whom they see on a regular basis.

h. adrenal insufficiency, or Addison's disease p. 341

Most commonly, adrenal insufficiency, or Addison's disease, is an idiopathic autoimmune disorder causing atrophy of the adrenal glands and resulting in the inadequate production of the adrenal hormones, such as cortisol, aldosterone, and androgens. Other causes include pituitary or hypothalamic dysfunction, adrenal hemorrhage, infections, such as tuberculosis, acquired immunodeficiency syndrome (AIDS), or sudden cessation of long-term or high-dose therapy with synthetic glucocorticoids.

Chronic adrenal insufficiency is characterized by progressive weakness, fatigue, decreased appetite, and weight loss. Hyperpigmentation of the skin and mucous membranes is one of the earliest signs. The hyperpigmentation tends to be most significant in sun-exposed areas, joints, and pressure points. Patients with Addison's disease are prone to hypotension, hypoglycemia, hyponatremia, and hyperkalemia. About half of the patients will have gastrointestinal problems such as nausea, vomiting, or diarrhea, which will exacerbate the electrolyte imbalances and increase the potential for cardiac dysrhythmias.

Acute adrenal insufficiency, known as Addisonian crisis, is a life-threatening medical emergency characterized by profound hypotension and shock, which can be rapidly fatal. It is most commonly seen in those patients with Addison's disease who've been exposed to stress such as acute infection, trauma, dehydration, or emotional duress. It has been suggested that adrenal insufficiency should be considered in any patient with unexplained cardiovascular collapse. Vomiting and diarrhea tend to increase the volume depletion and subsequent hypotension. It is not uncommon for patients to report abdominal pain, which tends to mimic an acute abdomen. Fever, weakness, and confusion are also common.

Lifelong replacement hormone therapy and careful monitoring of electrolyte levels are used to treat chronic adrenal insufficiency. Most of this is provided by the primary care physician. Patient education is critical to maintenance of well-being. All patients with Addison's disease are advised to wear a Medic-Alert tag in addition to carrying an identification card detailing their current medication regimen and physician's phone number.

Emergency management is focused on maintenance of the ABCs and, as always, careful monitoring of the patient's cardiac and oxygenation status as well as blood glucose level. Hypoglycemia poses its own threat to the patient's well-being, so blood glucose levels should be assessed and 25–50 grams of 50% dextrose should be administered to patients with levels less than 50 mg/dL or those with altered mental status. Obtaining a baseline 12-lead EKG is important due to the potential for dysrhythmias related to electrolyte imbalance. Fluid resuscitation should be aggressive. Follow your local protocol or contact medical control for specific orders based on your patient's presentation. Immediate transport to an appropriate facility is imperative since definitive treatment includes the administration of glucocorticoids and/or mineralocorticoids in conjunction with correcting other electrolyte or hormonal abnormalities.

14. Describe the actions of epinephrine as it relates to the pathophysiology of hypoglycemia. p. 333

Hypoglycemia, or low blood sugar, reflects high insulin and low glucose levels. Regardless of the cause, when insulin levels are high, glucagon may be ineffective in raising blood glucose levels. In prolonged fasts, almost half the glucose normally produced through gluconeogenesis is of renal origin. This activity is stimulated by epinephrine.

15. Describe the compensatory mechanisms utilized by the body to promote homeostasis when hypoglycemia is present. pp. 315, 323–324

When blood glucose levels fall, the alpha cells of the pancreas secrete glucagon. Glucagon stimulates the breakdown of glycogen into glucose for release into the bloodstream. This process, called glycogenolysis, takes place throughout the body but occurs primarily in the liver. In addition to stimulating the breakdown of glycogen, glucagon also stimulates the breakdown of proteins and fats with subsequent conversion to glucose. This process of producing sugar from nonsugar sources is called gluconeogenesis. Both of these processes contribute to the maintenance of homeostasis by raising blood glucose levels.

16. Differentiate among different endocrine emergencies based on assessment and history. pp. 326–341

As you proceed through your course, you will encounter a variety of real and simulated patients with endocrinologic disorders and emergencies. Use the information provided in this chapter of your text, as well as the application of this information as demonstrated by your instructors, preceptors, and mentors to enhance your own ability to differentiate endocrinologic emergencies.

17. Given several scenarios involving endocrine emergency patients, provide the appropriate assessment, management, and transportation. pp. 315–341

Throughout your classroom, clinical, and field training, you will encounter a variety of real and simulated patients with endocrinologic emergencies. Use the information provided in this chapter of your text, as well as the application of this information as demonstrated by your instructors, preceptors, and mentors to enhance your ability to assess, manage, and transport patients with endocrinologic emergencies.

CASE STUDY REVIEW

Reread the case study on pages 313–315 in Paramedic Care: Medical Emergencies *before reading the discussion below.*

This case study draws attention to the assessment and management of a commonly encountered patient presentation, altered mental status, which is subsequently determined to be due to the potentially life-threatening endocrine emergency, hypoglycemia.

Shauna and Steve arrive at the scene of an "unknown medical emergency." Prior to their entry into the house, they are joined on scene by two police officers. Many jurisdictions have dispatch protocols in place that specify dual dispatch of EMS and law enforcement personnel for calls of an unknown nature or those where there has been or is a potential for violence.

As is sometimes the case at emergency scenes, the patient may not have placed the call for service. Whenever possible, it is helpful in those situations where the 911 call has been placed by a third-party caller to be able to interview that individual to obtain information about the situation on your arrival on scene. In this case, Mrs. Spencer is a concerned neighbor who is able to provide a great deal of information about the usual residents of this home.

The scene size-up and bystander-provided information raise a high index of suspicion about potential dangers, and the police enter the house first to secure the scene. Only after the scene is declared safe do Shauna and Steve enter. It is important to always remember that there is no benefit to be gained by risking your own personal safety. There is truth to the adage that "fools rush in."

Shauna begins her initial assessment of the patient even as she approaches the teenager identified by Mrs. Spencer as Mark McKenzie. Although he is conscious, his responses to Shauna are incoherent. The overturned furniture and disarray on the scene, along with Mark's confusion, lead Shauna and Steve to consider hypoglycemia or drug use as possible causes for the situation. Sudden changes in mental status or bizarre behavior should always make you consider hypoglycemia. Mark's confusion and apparent violent behavior, along with his tachycardia and diaphoresis, are very typical manifestations of hypoglycemia. The decision to gently restrain Mark is based on his lack of appropriate interaction with his environment as well as concern for his own safety and the safety of all of the personnel on the scene.

Routine assessment of oxygen saturation via pulse oximetry and blood glucose level determination via a glucometer reflects the standard of care for any patient presenting with an altered mental status. Most EMS agencies also routinely obtain pre-treatment venous blood samples for analysis at the hospital when dealing with patients presenting with altered mental status.

The glucometer reading of "LOW" indicates a blood glucose level that is less than 50 mg/dL, confirming the presumptive diagnosis of hypoglycemia. Prompt and careful administration of 50 percent dextrose intravenously is the treatment of choice. It is imperative that this medication is administered into a patent IV line in a large vein. Localized venous irritation is likely when small veins are used, and if the dextrose should extravasate, tissue necrosis is common.

Mark's prompt improvement in response to the administration of dextrose is fairly typical. It is not uncommon for diabetics to have no recall of the events that transpired while they were hypoglycemic. The arrival of Mark's mother on scene allows the EMS personnel to get more information about Mark's usual health status. It is not uncommon for diabetics to have some variation in their usual level of control when their insulin dosages have been changed. Although it makes good sense for diabetics to wear some type of medical alert device on their bodies, it is not uncommon for adolescents to be non-compliant with that practice. Follow your agency's protocols regarding "refusal of transport."

CONTENT SELF-EVALUATION

MULTIPLE CHOICE

_____ 1. Which of the following is an exocrine gland?
   A. pineal
   B. thymus
   C. salivary
   D. parathyroid
   E. adrenal

_____ 2. The term describing the sum of cellular processes that produce energy and molecules needed for growth and repair is:
   A. anabolism.
   B. catabolism.
   C. metabolism.
   D. homeostasis.
   E. physiology.

_____ 3. The gland that is the connection between the endocrine system and the central nervous system is the:
   A. pituitary.
   B. hypothalamus.
   C. thymus.
   D. pineal.
   E. thyroid.

_____ 4. Diabetes insipidus is a disorder associated with carbohydrate metabolism that is similar to diabetes mellitus.
   A. True
   B. False

_____ 5. Antidiuretic hormone plays a role in maintaining fluid balance by increasing water reabsorption.
   A. True
   B. False

_____ 6. All of the following are hormones secreted by the anterior pituitary gland EXCEPT:
   A. growth hormone.
   B. oxytocin.
   C. prolactin.
   D. adrenocorticotropic hormone.
   E. thyroid-stimulating hormone.

_____ 7. In children, the thymus secretes a hormone that is critical to the maturation of T-lymphocytes, which play a significant role in:
   A. maintaining blood calcium levels.
   B. cell-mediated immunity.
   C. cellular metabolism.
   D. carbohydrate metabolism.
   E. gluconeogenesis.

_____ 8. All of the following are pancreatic hormones EXCEPT:
   A. polypeptide.
   B. glucagon.
   C. somatostatin.
   D. cortisol.
   E. insulin.

_____ 9. Homeostasis of blood glucose is controlled by insulin and:
   A. polypeptide.
   B. glucagon.
   C. somatostatin.
   D. cortisol.
   E. thymosin.

_____ 10. The substance that the alpha cells of the pancreas secrete when blood glucose levels fall is:
   A. polypeptide.
   B. glucagon.
   C. somatostatin.
   D. cortisol.
   E. insulin.

_____ 11. The substance secreted by the beta cells of the pancreas when blood glucose levels rise is:
   A. polypeptide.
   B. glucagon.
   C. somatostatin.
   D. cortisol.
   E. insulin.

_____ 12. Insulin's primary function is to:
   A. metabolize glucose at the cellular level.
   B. free glucose from muscle storage sites.
   C. transport glucose across the cell membrane.
   D. store glucose at the cellular level.
   E. enhance the function of glucagon.

_____ 13. The production of glucose by the processes of glycogenolysis and gluconeogenesis is triggered by:
   A. polypeptide.
   B. glucagon.
   C. somatostatin.
   D. cortisol.
   E. insulin.

_____ 14. All of the following are hormones secreted by the adrenal glands EXCEPT:
   A. epinephrine.
   B. cortisol.
   C. somatostatin.
   D. norepinephrine.
   E. aldosterone.

_____ 15. Glucocorticoids play a role in maintaining blood glucose levels by promoting gluconeogenesis and:
   A. decreasing glucose utilization.
   B. increasing glucose utilization.
   C. promoting salt and fluid retention.
   D. decreasing salt and fluid retention.
   E. potentiating the effects of catecholamines.

_____ 16. Catecholamines such as epinephrine and norepinephrine are hormones secreted by the adrenal medulla.
   A. True
   B. False

_____ 17. The primary function of aldosterone is to:
   A. regulate sodium and potassium excretion.
   B. regulate calcium and magnesium excretion.
   C. promote gluconeogenesis.
   D. inhibit gluconeogenesis.
   E. stimulate glucocorticoid production.

_____ 18. Diabetes mellitus is caused by the inadequate production or activity of:
   A. polypeptide.   D. cortisol.
   B. glucagon.   E. insulin.
   C. somatostatin.

_____ 19. Osmotic diuresis, a characteristic of untreated diabetes, contributes to the development of:
   A. polydipsia and polyphagia.   D. polyuria.
   B. polydipsia and polyuria.   E. polyphagia.
   C. polyuria and polyphagia.

_____ 20. All of the following are signs and symptoms of diabetic ketoacidosis EXCEPT:
   A. abdominal pain.   D. cold, clammy skin.
   B. deep rapid respirations. E. tachycardia.
   C. decreased mental function.

_____ 21. Diabetic ketoacidosis, characterized by high blood glucose and metabolic acidosis, occurs as a result of all of the following EXCEPT:
   A. profound insulin deficiency.   D. physiologic stress.
   B. increased glucagon activity.   E. overexertion.
   C. cessation of insulin injections.

_____ 22. Kussmaul's respirations are a primary compensatory mechanism for reducing acidosis in the patient with diabetic ketoacidosis.
   A. True
   B. False

_____ 23. The most important sign or symptom associated with hypoglycemia is:
   A. tachycardia.   D. polydipsia.
   B. cool, clammy skin.   E. polyphagia.
   C. altered mental status.

_____ 24. Hyperglycemic hyperosmolar nonketotic acidosis differs from diabetic ketoacidosis because significant production of ketone bodies is prevented by the action of:
   A. polypeptide.   D. cortisol.
   B. glucagon.   E. insulin.
   C. somatostatin.

_____ 25. Even in the absence of a blood glucose level, altered mental status in a known diabetic should always be treated with 50 percent dextrose.
   A. True
   B. False

_____ 26. All of the following are signs and symptoms associated with thyrotoxic crisis EXCEPT:
   A. high fever.   D. delirium.
   B. bradycardia.   E. vomiting.
   C. hypotension.

_____ 27. Potential causes for myxedema coma include all of the following EXCEPT:
   A. excessive thyroid medication.   D. cold environment.
   B. infection.   E. CNS depressants.
   C. trauma.

_____ 28. Signs and symptoms associated with myxedema coma include all of the following EXCEPT:
   A. hypothermia.   D. CO_2 retention.
   B. decreased mental status.   E. seizures.
   C. low amplitude bradycardia.

_____ 29. Long-term exposure to excess glucocorticoids or abnormalities to either the adrenal cortex or pituitary gland may cause hyperadrenalism.
   A. True
   B. False

_____ 30. Addison's disease is characterized by high corticosteroid activity that causes major disturbances in water and electrolyte balance.
   A. True
   B. False

MATCHING

Write the letter of the term in the space provided next to the appropriate definition.

   A. homeostasis   F. oxytocin
   B. hormone   G. calcitonin
   C. anabolism   H. gluconeogenesis
   D. catabolism   I. glycogenolysis
   E. antidiuretic hormone   J. Addisonian crisis

_____ 31. crisis form of shock associated with adrenocortical insufficiency that is characterized by profound hypotension and electrolyte imbalance

_____ 32. phase of metabolism associated with building molecules of higher complexity

_____ 33. hormone that increases water reabsorption by the kidneys

_____ 34. conversion of protein and fat to form glucose

_____ 35. hormone responsible for lowering blood calcium levels

_____ 36. phase of metabolism associated with the breakdown of complex molecules

_____ 37. hormone that causes uterine contraction and lactation

_____ 38. breakdown of glycogen to form glucose

_____ 39. chemical substance released to control or affect processes in other organs or body systems

_____ 40. the natural tendency of the body to keep the internal environment and metabolism at a steady, normal level

SPECIAL PROJECT

Label the Diagram

Write the names of the endocrine glands marked A through I in the figure shown and then list at least **one** *of the hormones secreted by each gland.*

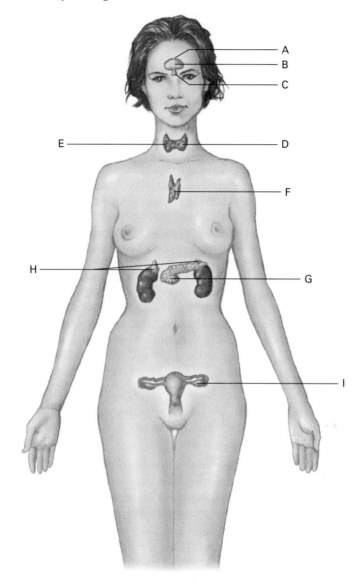

A. _____

B. _____

C. _____

D. _____

E. _____

F. _____

G. _____

H. _____

I. _____

CHAPTER 5

Allergies and Anaphylaxis

Review of Chapter Objectives

After reading this chapter, you should be able to:

1. Describe the incidence, morbidity, and mortality of anaphylaxis.   **p. 347**

Anaphylaxis results from an exposure to a particular substance that sets off a chain of biochemical events that can ultimately lead to shock and death. While the exact incidence is unknown, an estimated 400 to 800 deaths annually in the United States are attributed to anaphylaxis. Two of the most common fatal causes of anaphylaxis are attributed to injected penicillin and stings from bees and wasps (*Hymenoptera*). Between 100 and 500 deaths per year are attributed to penicillin, while 25 to 40 persons die each year from *Hymenoptera* stings. Overall, the incidence of anaphylaxis seems to be declining due to better recognition and treatment, particularly the availability of numerous potent antihistamines.

2. Identify the risk factors most predisposing to anaphylaxis.   **p. 350**

Anaphylaxis is the fastest and most severe form of immediate hypersensitivity reaction. Some persons have an allergic tendency. This allergic tendency is genetically passed from parent to child and is characterized by the presence of large quantities of IgE antibodies.

3. Discuss the anatomy and physiology of the organs and structures related to anaphylaxis.   **pp. 347–349**

The immune system is a complex system responsible for combating infection. Components of the immune system can be found in the blood, the bone marrow, and the lymphatic system. The immune response is a complex cascade of events that occurs following activation by an invading substance.

Following exposure to a particular antigen, large quantities of IgE antibodies are released. These antibodies attach to the membranes of basophils and mast cells, causing them to release histamine, heparin, and other chemicals into the surrounding tissue. The release of these chemical mediators causes a response in the cardiovascular, respiratory, and gastrointestinal systems as well as in the skin.

4. Describe the prevention of anaphylaxis and appropriate patient education.   **pp. 357–358**

Many severe allergic or anaphylactic reactions can be prevented. Patients with a history of anaphylaxis should be educated about avoidance, recognition, and treatment. For some allergies, such as to foods or medications, it may be possible to avoid subsequent exposures. Patients susceptible to anaphylaxis should always wear some sort of identification, such as a Medic-Alert device, to specify their allergy should they be found unresponsive. Many patients with severe allergies also carry an emergency kit, such as an EpiPen, to manage anaphylaxis.

In some cases, the severity of an allergic reaction may be diminished through a process called desensitization. Desensitization involves the administration of very small amounts of the antigen to the patient in a series of injections. The amount of antigen in each injection is gradually increased to a point where the body's immune response to the allergen is blunted and thus anaphylactic reactions are averted.

5. Discuss the pathophysiology of allergy and anaphylaxis.   pp. 347, 351

The signs and symptoms associated with allergy and anaphylaxis are due to the physiologic changes triggered by the chemical mediators of the immune response that are released from the basophils and mast cells. Histamine is the primary mediator of all allergic reactions. It is a potent substance that causes bronchoconstriction, vasodilation and increased vascular permeability, and increased intestinal motility. Other chemical substances are also released that have effects similar to or synergistic with histamine, such as SRS-A (slow-reacting substance of anaphylaxis), which results in an asthma-like attack or asphyxia.

6. Describe the common routes of substance entry into the body.   pp. 350–351

Allergens can enter the body through various routes including oral ingestion, inhalation, topically, and through injection or envenomation. The vast majority of anaphylactic reactions result from injection or envenomation.

7. Define allergic reaction, anaphylaxis, antigen, antibody, and natural and acquired immunity.   pp. 346–349

An allergic reaction is an exaggerated immune response to a foreign protein or other substance, while anaphylaxis is an unusual or exaggerated allergic reaction to a foreign protein or other substance.

An antigen is any substance that is capable, under appropriate conditions, of inducing a specific immune response. An antibody is a member of a unique class of chemicals that are manufactured by specialized cells of the immune system. The antibody is the principle agent of a chemical attack on an invading substance. Following exposure to an antigen, antibodies are released from cells of the immune system. The antibodies attach themselves to the invading substance so it can be removed from the body by other cells of the immune system.

Natural immunity refers to the immunity that is present at birth; also called innate immunity, it is genetically determined. Acquired immunity is immunity that develops over time and results from exposure to an antigen.

8. List common antigens most frequently associated with anaphylaxis.   pp. 347–348

Any substance that is capable, under appropriate conditions, of inducing a specific immune response is known as an antigen. Most antigens are proteins. The following agents are among those that commonly trigger anaphylaxis: antibiotics, foods, or insect stings. Refer to Table 5-1 on text page 348 for a more complete list.

9. Discuss human antibody formation.   pp. 347–349

Antibodies are a unique class of chemicals that are manufactured by specialized cells of the immune system, called B cells. Another name for antibodies is immunoglobulins (Igs), and there are five different classes: IgA, IgD, IgE, IgG, and IgM. Following exposure to an antigen, antibodies are released from cells of the immune system. The antibodies attach themselves to the invading substance to facilitate removal of the substance from the body by other cells of the immune system. This response is known as humoral immunity.

If the body has never been exposed to a particular antigen, the response of the immune system is different than if it has been previously exposed. The initial response to an antigen is called the primary response. Following exposure to a new antigen, several days pass before both the cellular and humoral components of the immune system respond. Generalized antibodies (IgG and IgM) are released first.

Simultaneously other components of the immune system begin to develop antibodies specific to the new antigen. The cells also develop a memory of the particular antigen and, if there is a subsequent exposure to this same substance, the immune system response is much faster. This is known as the secondary response. As part of this secondary response, antibodies specific for the offending antigen are released. Antigen-specific antibodies are much more effective in facilitating removal of the offending antigen than the generalized antibodies released during the primary response.

10. Describe the physical manifestations of anaphylaxis. pp. 351–354, 356–357

The signs and symptoms of anaphylaxis begin within 30 to 60 seconds following exposure for the vast majority of patients. The more rapid the onset, the more severe the patient presentation. Respiratory manifestations of anaphylaxis include laryngeal edema and bronchoconstriction. Cardiovascular symptoms include tachycardia plus massive vasodilation resulting in profound hypotension. The combination of respiratory and cardiovascular signs will lead to a rapid deterioration of the patient's mental status. Generalized flushing and urticaria are common, as is angioedema about the head, face, and neck. Nausea, vomiting, and diarrhea may accompany hypermotility of the gastrointestinal tract.

11. Identify and differentiate between the signs and symptoms of allergic reaction and anaphylaxis. p. 356

Allergic reactions can range from a mild skin rash to a severe life-threatening multisystem response. Allergic reaction, also known as hypersensitivity, takes two forms, delayed or immediate. Delayed hypersensitivity is the result of cellular immunity and does not involve antibodies. It may occur hours to days after exposure and is very common. Delayed hypersensitivity usually presents as a skin rash and is often due to exposure to certain drugs and chemicals, for instance, poison ivy. Other signs and symptoms may include mild bronchoconstriction, mild intestinal cramps, or diarrhea, while the patient's mental status and vital signs will remain normal.

Immediate hypersensitivity is antibody-mediated immunity and often has a genetic link. The range of clinical presentation is widely variable. Examples of these reactions include hay fever, drug and food allergies, eczema, and asthma. Allergens can enter the body by various routes, but as a rule, those that enter by injection tend to have more rapid and more severe effects. Immediate hypersensitivities may be merely annoying, like the itching eyes and runny nose of hay fever, or may pose a real and immediate life threat, as seen in the anaphylactic reaction described in the case study at the beginning of this chapter.

The signs and symptoms of anaphylaxis begin within seconds following exposure. The more rapid the onset of symptoms, the more severe the patient presentation. Respiratory manifestations of anaphylaxis include laryngeal edema and bronchoconstriction. Cardiovascular symptoms include tachycardia plus massive vasodilation resulting in profound hypotension. A rapid deterioration of the patient's mental status accompanies the cardiovascular collapse. Generalized flushing and urticaria are common, as is angioedema about the head, face, and neck. Nausea, vomiting, and diarrhea may accompany hypermotility of the gastrointestinal tract. Refer to Table 5-3 on text page 356 for a comparison of signs and symptoms of allergic reactions and anaphylaxis.

12. Explain the various treatments and pharmacological interventions used in the management of allergic reactions and anaphylaxis. pp. 354–357

The first priority in the management of allergic reactions and anaphylaxis is to establish and maintain the patient's airway. Administer oxygen immediately along with ventilatory support as needed. You should be prepared to intubate, recognizing that laryngeal edema may change the size and appearance of the airway.

Establish vascular access as soon as possible and be prepared to run crystalloid solutions wide open if the patient is hypotensive.

Epinephrine is the drug of choice for severe allergic reaction and anaphylaxis. In mild to moderate cases, administer 0.3–0.5 mg of 1:1,000 epinephrine subcutaneously; while in severe reactions and anaphylaxis, administer 0.3–0.5 mg of intravenous 1:10,000 epinephrine. Remember that the effects of epinephrine wear off quickly, so be prepared to repeat boluses in 3 to 5 minutes. It may be necessary to establish a continuous epinephrine infusion.

Antihistamines, such as diphenhydramine, are widely used for the management of allergic reactions due to their ability to block histamine receptors. The usual dosage is 25–50 mg given either intravenously or intramuscularly. It may also be helpful to administer beta agonist agents via hand-held nebulizer to help reverse bronchospasm. Adult patients should receive 0.5 ml of albuterol in 3 ml of normal saline.

As is always the case, your management approach should always be dictated by local protocols. Other medications that may be used to manage severe anaphylaxis include corticosteroids, such as SoluMedrol, to suppress the inflammatory response or vasopressors, such as dopamine, to enhance cardiac output. You'll recall that adequate fluid resuscitation prior to initiating vasopressor therapy is important.

13. Correlate abnormal findings in assessment with the clinical significance in the patient with an allergic reaction or anaphylaxis. pp. 351–354

The central physiological action in severe allergic reaction and anaphylaxis is the massive release of histamine and other chemical mediators of the immune system. The resultant bronchospasm, airway edema, peripheral vasodilation, and increased capillary permeability can take a patient from his or her usual state of health to the brink of death in mere seconds. This chemically caused transformation is readily evident in the patient's clinical presentation: air hunger, dyspnea, angioedema, tachycardia, and hypotension. Your timely intervention is imperative to your patient's survival.

14. Given several preprogrammed and moulaged patients, provide the appropriate assessment, care, and transport for the allergic reaction and anaphylaxis patient. pp. 346–358

Throughout your classroom, clinical, and field training, you will encounter a variety of real and simulated patients with allergic reactions or anaphylaxis emergencies. Use the information provided in this chapter of your text, as well as the application of this information as demonstrated by your instructors, preceptors, and mentors to enhance your ability to assess, manage, and transport these patients.

CASE STUDY REVIEW

Reread the case study on pages 345 and 346 in Paramedic Care: Medical Emergencies *before reading the discussion below.*

This case study draws attention to the typical presentation and management for a patient experiencing severe anaphylaxis.

The majority of fatal anaphylaxis cases in the United States are attributed to injections, usually of penicillin. It is for this reason that patients receiving injections in an outpatient setting are asked to remain on site for at least 20 to 30 minutes afterward to insure the availability of emergency care should the need arise. In this case, the injection was an immunization received just 15 minutes earlier. The patient's immediate response was a red rash and generalized itching that quickly progressed to marked respiratory compromise and cardiovascular collapse. The clinic staff had administered oxygen via a nasal cannula and was setting up an IV.

With the arrival of Steve and Beth on-scene, appropriate emergency care was quickly initiated; the nasal cannula was replaced with high-flow oxygen via nonrebreather mask, keeping an ET kit readily accessible. Beth established vascular access and initiated fluid resuscitation to correct massive vasodilation, while Steve administered epinephrine subcutaneously to counteract the immune system response. Although the patient showed improvement within 2 minutes of the epinephrine administration, Steve knew that the medication wears off quickly and was prepared to administer IV 1:10,000 epinephrine in case the improvement did not continue. Diphenhydramine was also administered to block the histamine receptors. All of these efforts were effective in reversing the anaphylaxis, and the patient was treated in the ER with corticosteroids to suppress the immune response and additional IV fluids and released within 2 hours.

Subsequent questioning at the hospital revealed that this patient had received a tetanus injection at the clinic and that he had a similar reaction with a prior tetanus immunization. This situation highlights the importance of patient education about the potential for repeat and possibly more severe allergic reactions. It also underscores the importance for every health care professional to carefully question patients about allergies or untoward responses to medication prior to administering any drug.

CONTENT SELF-EVALUATION

MULTIPLE CHOICE

_____ 1. The type of immunity resulting from a direct attack of a foreign substance by specialized cells of the immune system is known as:
  A. humoral.   D. acquired.
  B. cellular.   E. genetic.
  C. natural.

_____ 2. The unique class of chemicals that are manufactured by specialized cells of the immune system to attack invading foreign proteins is:
  A. allergens.   D. antibodies.
  B. antigens.   E. pathogens.
  C. toxins.

_____ 3. Any substance that is capable, under appropriate conditions, of inducing a specific immune response is a(n):
  A. immunoglobulin.   D. antibody.
  B. antigen.   E. pathogen.
  C. toxin.

_____ 4. The type of immunity that is present at birth and has no relation to a previous exposure to a particular antigen is:
  A. humoral.   D. acquired.
  B. cellular.   E. genetic.
  C. natural.

_____ 5. The type of immunity that develops over time as a result of exposure to an antigen is:
  A. humoral.   D. acquired.
  B. cellular.   E. genetic.
  C. natural.

_____ 6. An allergic reaction is best defined as an exaggerated, sometimes potentially life-threatening response by the immune system to a foreign substance.
  A. True
  B. False

_____ 7. All of the following are common allergens EXCEPT:
  A. insect stings.   D. seafood.
  B. drugs.   E. radiology contrast materials.
  C. antibodies.

_____ 8. The vast majority of anaphylactic reactions occur as a result of:
  A. inhalation.   D. topical exposure.
  B. ingestion.   E. genetics.
  C. injection.

_____ 9. The antibody most commonly associated with hypersensitivity reactions is:
  A. IgA.   D. IgG.
  B. IgD.   E. IgM.
  C. IgE.

_____ 10. The primary chemical mediator of an allergic reaction is:
   A. heparin.   D. basophil.
   B. histamine.   E. the mast cell.
   C. SRS-A.

_____ 11. All of the following are physiologic effects associated with the release of the chemical mediators of anaphylaxis EXCEPT:
   A. bronchodilation.   D. increased vascular permeability.
   B. vasodilation.   E. secretion of gastric acids.
   C. increased intestinal motility.

_____ 12. Urticaria, a wheal and flare reaction characterized by red raised bumps that appear on the skin, is due to:
   A. bronchodilation.   D. decreased vascular permeability.
   B. vasodilation.   E. secretion of gastric acids.
   C. increased intestinal motility.

_____ 13. The first line parenteral drug for the management of anaphylaxis is:
   A. oxygen.   D. methylprednisolone.
   B. diphenhydramine.   E. albuterol.
   C. epinephrine.

_____ 14. The first priority when responding to a patient with an anaphylactic reaction is to:
   A. protect the airway.   D. assure scene safety.
   B. administer diphenhydramine.   E. establish vascular access.
   C. stabilize the cervical spine.

_____ 15. Hypotension that is seen in severe anaphylaxis is due to:
   A. internal hemorrhage.   D. vasodilation.
   B. inadequate oxygenation.   E. gastrointestinal hypermotility.
   C. bradycardia.

MATCHING

Write the letter of the drug in the space provided next to the phrase that best describes its action.

   A. dopamine
   B. epinephrine
   C. diphenhydramine
   D. methylprednisolone
   E. albuterol

_____ 16. Beta agonist that reverses bronchospasm

_____ 17. Blocks histamine receptors

_____ 18. Suppresses inflammatory response

_____ 19. Sympathetic agonist that improves cardiac output

_____ 20. Potent vasopressor to support blood pressure

SPECIAL PROJECT

Completing Tables

A. *Complete the following table by listing the common systemic signs and symptoms associated with allergies and anaphylaxis.*

System	Signs and Symptoms
Skin	
Respiratory system	
Cardiovascular system	
Gastrointestinal system	
Nervous system	

B. *Complete the following table by listing the actions associated with each drug.*

Drug	Actions
Albuterol	
Diphenhydramine	
Dopamine	
Epinephrine	
Methylprednisolone	

CHAPTER 6

Gastroenterology

Review of Chapter Objectives

After reading this chapter, you should be able to:

1. Describe the incidence, morbidity, and mortality of gastrointestinal emergencies.   p. 363

Gastrointestinal (GI) emergencies account for over 500,000 emergency visits and hospitalizations annually. Of that total, more than 300,000 are due to GI bleeding. These numbers are expected to increase over time due to the trends of delay in seeking treatment until over-the-counter medication no longer controls symptoms and of the aging of the American population. You will see GI emergencies in your practice, and it is likely that a large proportion will involve older persons. The number of patients over age 60 years in this patient population as risen from roughly 3% to over 45% in only a few years.

2. Identify the risk factors most predisposing to gastrointestinal emergencies.   p. 363

Many of the most common risk factors are self-induced by patients, and they include excessive alcohol and tobacco consumption, stress, ingestion of caustic substances, and poor bowel habits. Because of the various risk factors and possible causes of GI emergencies, it is particularly important that you know how to complete a thorough focused history and examination before making a field diagnosis and how to assess the seriousness of the emergency and possible prevention strategies to minimize organ damage.

3. Discuss the anatomy and physiology of the organs and structures related to gastrointestinal diseases.   pp. 368–369, 376

The GI tract is a long tube that extends from the mouth to the anus and is divided structurally and functionally into different parts. In general, the GI system is divided into the upper and lower GI tracts. The upper GI tract includes the mouth, esophagus, stomach, and duodenum, whereas the lower GI tract includes the remainder of the small intestine and the large intestine, rectum, and anus. In the upper GI tract, food is ingested and preliminary physical and chemical digestion is begun. In the lower GI tract, digestion of food is completed, nutrients are absorbed into the body, and remaining fiber, intestinal bacteria, and other materials are eliminated through the anus as feces. In addition, three additional organs, the liver, gallbladder, and pancreas, are intimately associated with the GI system both structurally (through connections with the duodenum) and functionally. The vermiform appendix, a blind sac found at the junction of the small and large intestines, does not have any apparent physiologic role in GI function but is important to you because of the inflammatory condition called appendicitis, which you will see in patients in the field.

4. **Discuss the pathophysiology of abdominal inflammation and its relationship to acute pain.** pp. 363–365

Sudden onset, or acute, pain can be caused by a variety of mechanisms, one of which is inflammation. Inflammation of hollow organs such as the appendix or gallbladder produces pain that is characteristically poorly localized and crampy in nature (visceral pain). When inflammation is widespread within the abdomen, as happens after an inflamed appendix ruptures, inflammation of the peritoneal membrane (peritonitis) results in pain that is usually localized and sharp in nature (somatic pain). It is important for you to become familiar with the different types of pain because they often represent progressive stages in an inflammatory condition—for example, appendiceal pain that changes from visceral to somatic pain over time.

5. **Define somatic, visceral, and referred pain as they relate to gastroenterology.** pp. 363–365

Somatic pain is characteristically sharp and localized, and it originates in the peritoneal membrane or within elements of the wall of the abdominal cavity, such as skeletal muscle. Bacterial irritation, which is common after perforation of the gut or rupture of the appendix or gallbladder, causes somatic pain where the degree of extension of irritation through the abdominal cavity is often paralleled in the physical extent of the abdomen in which pain is perceived. Visceral pain is typically crampy and vague in character and poorly localized; it is commonly due to inflammation, distention, or ischemia in the walls of the GI tract (which is hollow) or in the capsule of a solid organ such as the liver. Referred pain is not a type of pain; rather, it is the term applied to any pain that is felt in a site other than the site of origin. Appendicitis is often first felt as periumbilical pain.

6. **Differentiate between hemorrhagic and nonhemorrhagic abdominal pain.** pp. 364–365, 367

Recall that many GI emergencies are hemorrhagic. If hemorrhage results from perforation or rupture of an organ, pain will often be sudden in onset, somatic in nature, and extend in location as blood spreads through the abdominal cavity. Hemorrhage within the GI tract may initially produce visceral pain that is more characteristic of a nonhemorrhagic process such as inflammation or ischemia. Hemorrhage that is extensive enough to cause abdominal distention implies serious volume loss and will also be reflected in altered vital signs. Finally, pain from a dissecting aortic aneurysm (a grave, non-GI surgical emergency) is often felt between the shoulder blades.

7. **Discuss the signs and symptoms and differentiate between local, general, and peritoneal inflammation relative to acute abdominal pain.** pp. 363–365

Local inflammation within the GI tract often produces visceral pain associated with sympathetic nervous system stimulation (which typically results in nausea, vomiting, diaphoresis, and tachycardia). General inflammation within the abdomen often includes bacterial or chemical irritation of the peritoneum (the origins of peritonitis) and is thus associated with increasingly widespread somatic pain. Peritonitis (inflammation of the peritoneum) often represents the end stage of a generalized inflammatory or hemorrhagic process; as such, it is often associated with the most significant physical signs including altered vitals or overt shock. Because pain associated with peritonitis is often very severe, it is typical to find the patient lying with knees to chest as this position minimizes stretch on the already inflamed peritoneum.

8. **Describe the questioning technique and specific questions when gathering a focused history in a patient with abdominal pain.** pp. 365–367

Questioning is done with the SAMPLE technique (Symptoms, Allergies, Medication, Past medical history, Last oral intake, and Events leading to the current complaint). Specific questions about the present illness typically use the OPQRST-ASPN mnemonic to gather information about the abdominal pain:
- Onset of pain (sudden or slow)
- Provocation or palliation of pain in terms of position or activity such as walking
- Quality (or nature) of the pain

- Region where pain is felt, along with any radiation of pain (For instance, radiation of pain among different locations implies similar neural pathways as referred pain and may give clues to origin of problem.)
- Severity of pain at the moment and over time
- Time over which pain has been felt (Note that any patient with pain lasting over 6 hours is considered a surgical emergency and requires transport to an appropriate facility for evaluation.)
- Associated Symptoms, such as vomiting (if yes, ask about appearance of vomitus), change in bowel habits (if "diarrheal," inquire whether stool may suggest hemorrhage via foul-smelling, tarry appearance or obvious blood), or lost appetite
- Pertinent Negatives such as absence of change in GI tract function associated with positives such as pelvic pain, change in urinary habits, or positive cardiovascular history. (Remember that diaphragmatic irritation with pain felt in neck or shoulder may reflect inferior myocardial infarction.)

9. **Describe the technique for performing a comprehensive physical examination on a patient complaining of abdominal pain.** p. 367

Always start with the least invasive step, visual inspection. This includes checking patient appearance and positioning as well as visually inspecting the abdomen for signs of distention or discoloration. Be sure to get a complete set of baseline vital signs early in the process. Changes in vitals along with alterations in mental status may indicate early shock due to hemorrhage or other processes. Auscultation and percussion often do NOT provide useful information in the field; however, if you do auscultate, be sure to do so before palpating in order to avoid perturbation in abdominal sounds. Palpation with gentle pressure should start in the LEAST affected area and move toward the point of greatest pain. Remember to immediate stop palpation if you feel any pulsation. Further palpation may cause rupture of the affected blood vessel or organ.

10. **Discuss the pathophysiology, assessment findings, and management of the following gastroenterological problems:**

Upper gastrointestinal bleeding pp. 369–370
The six most common causes of hemorrhage in the upper GI tract are (in descending order) peptic ulcer disease, gastritis, variceal rupture, Mallory-Weiss syndrome (esophageal laceration, generally secondary to vomiting), esophagitis, and duodenitis. Note that ulcers and gastritis account for 75% of cases (with 50% due to ulcers). Irritation and erosion of the GI lining is the most common pathophysiologic basis for bleeding, and involvement of the stomach lining underlies 75% of upper GI bleeds. Because most such cases involve chronic, low-level hemorrhage, many patients can be cared for on an outpatient basis. However, brisk upper GI bleeds may be life threatening. Assessment findings that can help to distinguish the severity of the bleed include presence and severity of hematemesis (vomiting of blood) and/or melena (passage of partially digested blood represented as dark, tarry stools). Look for subtle signs of shock and manage accordingly. Besides shock, another potentially grave complication of some bleeds is airway compromise due to aspiration of vomitus (when vomiting is present). Be sure to support the airway, and beware of vomiting in patients who are lying in a supine position. A patient with pain characteristic of peritonitis, especially with discoloration or bulging of the abdomen, may have a life-threatening blood loss. General management centers on airway, oxygenation, and circulatory status. Position to minimize risk of aspiration, provide high-flow oxygen, and start two large-bore IV lines (one with blood tubing and one for volume replacement with normal saline). Base fluid resuscitation on patient condition and response to treatment.

Lower gastrointestinal bleeding pp. 376–377
Hemorrhage from the lower GI tract is most common in association with chronic medical conditions and the anatomic changes of advancing age. The most common causes include diverticulosis, colorectal lesions, and inflammatory bowel disease. Remember that lower GI bleeds rarely result in the massive hemorrhage that can be associated with esophageal or stomach pathology. Assessment should establish whether the problem is new in onset or chronic (be sure to look for scars from previous surgical procedures). Questions about stool or inspection of stool may show

melena, which usually indicates a slow lower GI bleed, or bright red blood, which indicates severe hemorrhage with rapid passage through the intestines or a source in the distal colon. Distal GI causes include hemorrhoids and rectal fissures. Be sure to assess for abdominal signs such as discoloration or bulging and maintain ongoing check for signs of early shock. General management centers on the patient's physiologic status. Watch airway and oxygenation closely, and use oxygen if necessary. Establish IV access and fluid resuscitation based on patient's findings or shift in findings over time. If there are any signs of significant blood loss, be sure one IV line is capable of use for blood transfusion.

Acute gastroenteritis   pp. 372–373
Acute gastroenteritis involves inflammation of the stomach and intestines associated with sudden onset vomiting, diarrhea, or both. It is very common; the underlying inflammation causes erosion of the mucosal and submucosal layers of the GI tract with blood loss and damage to the intestinal villi. Triggers can include alcohol or tobacco use, use of nonsteroidal anti-inflammatory agents, stress, and GI or systemic infection. The most common and striking finding is copious volumes of watery diarrhea secondary to damage to the intestinal lining. Diarrhea may contain blood. In general, patients are often febrile and suffering from general malaise as well as nausea and vomiting. Watch for any signs of early shock such as altered mental status, development of pale, clammy skin, or changes in vitals. Abdominal tenderness is common; distention is uncommon unless significant amounts of gas are in the intestines. In cases of severe dehydration, watch for problems such as cardiac arrhythmia secondary to electrolyte disturbance. Management is supportive and palliative, with any needed support for airway (position to minimize odds of aspiration), oxygenation, or circulation. Fluid resuscitation via oral or IV route may be indicated. Be sure you take appropriate precautions during patient care to prevent spread of any possible infectious disease.

Colitis   pp. 377–378
Colitis is a general term for inflammation of the large intestine. Ulcerative colitis, which you may see in the field, is an inflammatory bowel disease that frequently affects relatively young people (with average age of 20 to 40 years at onset). Mild disease may only affect the distal colon, and it may present in the field with bloody diarrhea and discomfort. More severe disease may affect the entire colon, and this may present with severe, bloody diarrhea, electrolyte disturbances, or even hypovolemic shock. Management is tied to the patient's condition and includes appropriate support of oxygenation and circulation. If the patient has bouts of nausea and vomiting, beware of possible aspiration and airway compromise. Any patient who presents with a lower GI bleed or colicky, visceral-type pain should be transported for diagnostic evaluation.

Gastroenteritis   pp. 373–374
Gastroenteritis, inflammation of the stomach and intestines, is characterized by longer-term changes in the mucosa, thus distinguishing it from acute gastroenteritis. Gastroenteritis is usually due to microbial infection, with viral infection most common. However, patients with bacterial infection are usually the sickest. Common findings are fever, nausea, vomiting, diarrhea, lethargy, and, in the most severe cases, shock. Infection with *H. pylori* (the most common infectious cause in the U.S.) commonly presents with heartburn, abdominal pain, and the presence of gastric ulcers. Management includes appropriate infection precautions and patient care centered on monitoring of ABCs and transport. When outbreaks are associated with natural disaster or other possible contamination of water supply, be sure to protect yourself by use of proper sanitation and protection of water and food supplies.

Diverticulitis   pp. 380–381
Diverticulitis represents inflammation secondary to infection of diverticula, the outpouchings of intestinal mucosa and submucosa common in older Americans. Diverticulitis frequently starts with occlusion of a diverticulum by fecal material followed by bacterial infection. Complications include colonic hemorrhage or perforation. Common presenting signs of diverticulitis include low-grade fever, nausea and vomiting, and point tenderness on palpation. Because roughly 95% of cases

involve the sigmoid colon, another name for this condition is "left-sided appendicitis." Management is supportive, with attention to the ABCs. Signs of shock suggest significant hemorrhage.

Appendicitis pp. 385–386

Appendicitis is inflammation of the vermiform appendix. You will encounter acute appendicitis in the field, most commonly in older children and young adults. Untreated appendicitis can result in rupture with subsequent peritonitis. The pathophysiology has parallels to that of diverticulitis: The appendix becomes obstructed with fecal material, and the resultant inflammation and infection cause the characteristic discomfort, which may present initially as periumbilical, visceral pain, but later becomes the well-known somatic, right lower quadrant pain. Somatic pain or signs of peritonitis suggest significant inflammation with ischemia or infarction of the appendix or appendiceal rupture, respectively. Other findings such as fever, anorexia, and nausea or vomiting relate to the stage of appendiceal inflammation. Exam findings range from vague abdominal discomfort on palpation (in early cases) to clear peritonitis. Management during transport centers on positioning for comfort, managing airway to avoid aspiration, and establishing IV access. Monitor as you would for bowel obstruction and be aware of any early signs of shock.

Ulcer disease pp. 374–376

Peptic ulcers, created secondary to mucosal erosion by gastric acid, can occur anywhere in the GI tract and are particularly common in the duodenum and stomach. You will see ulcer cases and GI problems complicated by the presence of peptic ulcers. Pathophysiology includes genetic predisposition (seen as positive family history) as well as risk factors such as stress, use of nonsteroidal anti-inflammatory drugs, acid-stimulating products such as alcohol and nicotine, and chronic infection with *H. pylori*. The common mechanism is a breach of the mucous layer that protects the mucosa from the acid secreted in the stomach. Findings can vary widely. Chronic pain is typically worst when the stomach is empty and is relieved by eating or drinking coating liquids such as milk. Acute pain, particularly when somatic in character, may suggest rupture of the ulcer with hemorrhage into the abdomen. Bleeds manifest similarly to other upper GI hemorrhages and are handled similarly. In severely ill patients, appearance suggests severity of distress (such as lying still with knees drawn to chest), and there are often signs of shock. Management depends on physiologic status and involves monitoring of ABCs with appropriate intervention for possible or overt shock.

Bowel obstruction pp. 382–385

Bowel obstruction involves partial or complete blockage of a portion of the small or large intestine. Rapid diagnosis and treatment are essential to avoid complications such as bowel infarction. The four most common causes are hernias, intussusception, volvulus, and adhesions. The most common site is the small intestine due to smaller diameter and greater length and motility of intestinal loops. Chronic obstruction is often due to a progressive process such as tumor growth or adhesions. Acute obstruction may be due to ingestion of a foreign body or incarceration and strangulation of a hernia or loop of intussuscepted bowel. Findings suggestive of obstruction include pain (which is often diffuse and visceral in nature) and vomiting. The character of the vomitus (for example, feces-like material) may suggest the approximate site of the obstruction. Significant ischemia or infarction is suggested by findings of early or overt shock. Visual inspection may reveal distention, peritonitis, or free air within the abdomen. Ask about scars that indicate prior surgery and look for discoloration that may indicate the presence of free blood in the abdominal cavity. Palpation may be useful in localizing discomfort but beware of any but light pressure because heavier pressure may cause rupture of the obstructed segment. Treatment depends on the patient's physiologic status, with attention and support of the ABCs. Remember to place one IV line capable of blood transfusion if there are any indications of significant hemorrhage.

Crohn's disease pp. 378–380

Crohn's disease, like ulcerative colitis, is an inflammatory bowel disease. However, the pathologic inflammation can occur anywhere in the GI tract from the mouth to the rectum. After inflammation damages the mucosa and submucosa, granulomas form that further damage the wall of the GI tract. Patients with Crohn's frequently have narrowing of damaged segments, occasionally to the point of complete obstruction. Other findings include diarrhea and intestinal or perianal abscesses or fistulas. Because of the variety of sites involved in different patients, as well as the variety of complications due to progressive damage, prehospital diagnosis is nearly impossible. You should remember that an acute flare-up of symptoms accompanied by absence of bowel sounds suggests intestinal obstruction, which is a surgical emergency. Because significant hemorrhage is unusual, however, hypovolemic shock is infrequent among these patients. Prehospital management is largely palliative, with specific monitoring and support of the ABCs. Evidence of obstruction or shock calls for high-flow oxygen and circulatory support including IV access and fluid resuscitation.

Pancreatitis   p. 388

Pancreatitis is inflammation of the pancreas. The four main pathologic types are metabolic, mechanical, vascular, and infectious. Metabolic causes (specifically alcoholism) account for over 80% of cases. Alcohol causes deposition of platelet plugs in the acini. As flow of digestive secretions from the pancreas is impaired, digestive enzymes become activated while within the pancreas, damaging pancreatic tissue. Progression of this chronic damage can lead to hemorrhage, which presents as sudden onset nausea, vomiting, and severe pain that is in the left upper quadrant and may radiate to the back or the epigastric region. Mechanical pancreatitis is due to gallstones or elevated serum lipids. As digestive secretions accumulate behind the obstruction, pancreatic tissue damage occurs, edema develops, and blood flow is secondarily impaired, causing further damage due to ischemia. Mechanical pancreatitis is often acute in onset. Vascular causes of pancreatitis include thromboembolism and ischemia secondary to shock. Findings of mild pancreatitis include visceral pain, often epigastric in location, abdominal distension, nausea and vomiting, and elevated blood amylase and lipase. Findings in severe pancreatitis include refractory hypotensive shock, blood loss, and respiratory failure. As with other conditions involving hemorrhage, management of severe pancreatitis centers on support of ABCs including use of high-flow oxygen and appropriate IV access.

Esophageal varices   pp. 370–372

A varix is a swollen vein, and esophageal varices (plural) are usually due to hypertension in the portal system. Varices are subject to rupture and hemorrhage, and mortality in these cases exceeds 35%. The most common cause is liver damage secondary to alcohol consumption (via cirrhosis of the liver and portal hypertension). The other common cause is ingestion of caustic substances, which damage the esophagus directly and eventually cause rupture of an esophageal vein. Initial presentation of rupture features painless bleeding with evolution of signs of hemodynamic instability. Hematemesis can be both forceful and large in volume. Clotting time increases as high portal pressure backs up blood into the spleen, destroying platelets. Because tamponade isn't possible in the prehospital setting, management centers on rapid transport with care focusing on aggressive airway management (including orotracheal intubation if needed), use of high-flow oxygen, and IV fluid resuscitation.

Hemorrhoids   pp. 381–382

Hemorrhoids are small masses of swollen veins in the rectum or anus (internal and external hemorrhoids, respectively). Most are of unknown origin and occur in midlife, although some result from recognizable causes such as pregnancy or portal hypertension. In addition, external hemorrhoids can be caused by heavy lifting with straining. Although hemorrhoids frequently bleed during defecation, particularly in the setting of constipation, significant hemorrhage is rare. The typical cause for your call will be distress over the presence of bright red blood with defecation. The physical findings are usually benign, with hemodynamic stability and absence of signs of shock (skin is warm and dry, tachycardia is consistent with anxiety). Emotional assurance and monitoring for continued physiologic stability (due to possibility that bleeding is first sign of a lower GI bleed) is usually sufficient during transport. Either signs of significant bleeding or bleeding hemorrhoids in an alcoholic patient warrant closer monitoring and transport for immediate care.

Cholecystitis   pp. 386–388

Roughly 90% of cases of cholecystitis, inflammation of the gallbladder, are due to gallstones. Cholecystitis caused by stones can be acute or chronic. In both cases, the basic pathophysiology involves obstruction of the flow of bile by gallstones, with resultant inflammation of the gallbladder. Bacterial infection can also cause chronic cholecystitis. An acute attack is characterized by right upper quadrant pain, often with referred pain in the right shoulder. The right subcostal region may be tender due to muscle spasm. Sympathetic nervous stimulation may cause pale, cool, clammy skin. Prehospital care centers on palliation of distress and monitoring of ABCs with use of oxygen if needed and with establishment of IV access.

Acute hepatitis   pp. 389–390

Acute hepatitis, inflammation of the liver, can result from any injury to liver cells associated with an infectious or inflammatory process. Viral hepatitis is most common, and alcoholic hepatitis secondary to cirrhosis is also common. Symptoms range from mild manifestations to overt liver failure and death, and mortality is high due to the wide range of potential causes. You will find that presentation often parallels severity of hepatitis: Common complaints include right upper quadrant tenderness not relieved by eating or antacids and development of clay-colored stools (this secondary to decreased bile production). If bilirubin retention exists, scleral icterus and jaundice may be present. Palpation may reveal liver enlargement, and fever may be due to infection or tissue necrosis. Presence of cool, clammy, diaphoretic skin suggests hemorrhage of a hepatic lesion. Secure ABCs and establish IV access. Be particularly careful in consideration of use of any pharmacologic agent because liver failure may impair drug metabolism. Never forget to use personal protective equipment and to use body substance isolation precautions.

11. **Differentiate between gastrointestinal emergencies based on assessment findings.**   pp. 365–367

Assessment includes initial size-up, SAMPLE focused history with attention to current complaint, personal medical and family history, and physical examination. History of present illness will reveal whether condition is acute, chronic, or an acute flare-up of a chronic problem. The relation of pain (if any) with last oral intake may suggest ulcers (in which eating typically relieves pain) or, in contrast, cholecystitis (where pain may worsen after eating, particularly a fatty meal). The presence of chest pain rather than abdominal pain (or in addition to abdominal pain) may mean a condition has generated referred pain: Examples include gastroesophageal reflux (heartburn), gastric or duodenal ulcers, or cholecystitis. A change in nature of pain from visceral to somatic may infer a progression of abdominal pathology. Always remember before starting the physical exam that the majority of GI emergencies entail bleeding from the upper or lower GI tract: Watch for signs of hemorrhage in vitals (and changes in vitals) and on visual inspection of the abdomen, as well as examination of any vomitus or stool.

12. **Given several preprogrammed patients with abdominal pain and symptoms, provide the appropriate assessment, treatment, and transport.**   pp. 363–390

Care of any hemorrhagic case entails close monitoring of ABCs with attention to airway (minimizing risk of aspiration of any vomitus), breathing (high-flow oxygen is often indicated), and circulation (establishment of one or two IV lines with ability for blood transfusion where appropriate, and fluid resuscitation as needed). Although there are some conditions such as Crohn's disease in which bleeding rarely leads to hypovolemic shock, you should always be prepared to treat shock. Cases that seem to represent progressive, nonhemorrhagic conditions such as appendicitis, cholecystitis, or diverticulitis should also be monitored for stability and signs of acute events such as rupture or hemorrhage. Last, be aware that GI emergencies often present in older patients with coexisting morbid conditions and monitor cardiopulmonary status and other organ function carefully. Take close note of conditions such as alcoholism, consider GI problems associated with them (such as hepatitis, pancreatitis, or esophageal varices), and adjust assessment and treatment accordingly.

CASE STUDY REVIEW

Reread the case study on pages 361 and 362 in Paramedic Care: Medical Emergencies *before reading the discussion below.*

This case study demonstrates how paramedics react to a life-threatening emergency of unknown origin, treat each critical problem as it appears with focus on the ABCs, and transport the patient to an appropriate emergency facility. In addition to noting how the teams react to the patient's presentation and assessment, note how clues to the GI origin of his condition emerge from the assessment and history known to the ED staff.

George and Stephanie's dispatch is one you will encounter often, the "unknown medical emergency." Although the study doesn't say which equipment they are transferring for use in the house, you know they should be prepared to support the basic ABCs (airway, breathing, circulation) in a patient who may be gravely ill and have cardiopulmonary compromise either as part of the primary complaint or secondary to shock of some type.

The only information they get on the scene is from a hysterical spouse, and it is nonspecific except for the mention of blood. George and Stephanie consider the possibility of self-inflicted injury or violence, as well as accidental trauma, and call for police backup, which arrives with little delay. By the time the deputy sheriff arrives, the team is ready to enter the house, having donned appropriate protective gear (because of the blood) and gathered equipment useful in trauma and medical settings.

Their readiness means there is no further delay in initiating critical care and assessment. The patient has his spine immobilized and is then moved to a position that is protective of his airway and allows assessment. The first findings, about respirations and pulse, indicate the man is physiologically unstable; the same is inferred from an apparently large volume of blood found on the floor. Note that the team instinctively looks for sites of external hemorrhage and finds none.

The paramedics' next actions go to the central focus of any severe emergency: the ABCs. As they attempt to stabilize the airway through intubation, the patient vomits. Ready suction prevents aspiration of the vomitus and provides a clue to the GI origin of the hemorrhage: The vomited material turns out to be bright red blood. Intubation in the face of the intact gag reflex and active vomiting is achieved with rapid sequence intubation, and oxygen supplementation is begun with a bag-valve unit. IV access is secured, and an initial fluid bolus is given. The scenario doesn't give the bore of the needle, but you should assume one or two IV lines will be established as soon as possible, with at least one line of caliber sufficient to support blood transfusion.

Vital signs confirm that the patient is physiologically unstable (tachycardia, but no sign of dysrhythmia yet) and in hypovolemic shock (tachycardia, depressed blood pressure), and the physical finding of diminished breath sounds with rales at the bases suggests that the patient may have already aspirated blood. Even if aspiration hasn't occurred, the pulmonary findings indicate compromised function.

You don't know whether the wife gave any historical information or not, and you don't know whether she came to the hospital in a separate vehicle. If she were capable of giving any historical information, one of the team members should have questioned her at the home or while en route about the patient's medical history, particularly whether he had any GI conditions or co-morbid conditions (such as alcoholism) that may have led to GI hemorrhage. (Note that the patient was middle-aged, not elderly, which may increase the importance of asking about co-morbid conditions because you cannot assume any age-related organ dysfunction.)

The history is revealed at the nearby emergency facility, when staff recognize the patient as a man with alcohol-induced problems that they have previously treated: The co-morbid conditions of portal hypertension and liver failure are identified. Initial assessment by the surgical resident reveals the cause of the life-threatening upper GI hemorrhage, a ruptured esophageal varix. The ED staff further supports treatment of shock and rushes the patient for definitive therapy of the bleed in the surgical suite.

George and Stephanie close the call by learning more about the pathophysiology of the underlying conditions and the probable trigger for the variceal rupture (forceful vomiting in the setting of portal hypertension). The attending physician also lets them know that the rapidity and correctness of their care may have saved the patient's life.

CONTENT SELF-EVALUATION

MULTIPLE CHOICE

_____ 1. Which of the following statements about gastrointestinal (GI) emergencies is NOT true?
   A. GI emergencies account for about 5% of all annual visits to the emergency department.
   B. The majority of GI emergencies entail GI hemorrhage.
   C. The number of GI emergencies is expected to rise, in part due to aging of the population.
   D. The risk factors for GI emergencies are well known, and most (such as familial predisposition to GI conditions) are out of control of the patient.
   E. The number of GI emergencies is expected to rise, in part due to delays in seeking treatment by patients who treat themselves as long as symptoms allow.

_____ 2. Risk factors for GI disease include excessive use of alcohol and tobacco, stress, ingestion of caustic substances, and poor bowel habits.
   A. True
   B. False

_____ 3. All of the following statements about physical examination of the abdomen are true EXCEPT:
   A. Visual inspection should always be done first.
   B. Palpation should always precede auscultation.
   C. Of auscultation, percussion, palpation, and visual inspection, palpation may be most likely to produce a lot of useful information.
   D. Discoloration of the skin (specifically, ecchymosis) may indicate where hemorrhage has occurred into the abdominal cavity.
   E. Abdominal distension may be an ominous sign, suggesting either free air in the abdomen or loss of a large amount of circulating volume.

_____ 4. Three organs intimately associated with the GI tract are the:
   A. teeth, tongue, and epiglottis.
   B. appendix, gallbladder, and parotid gland.
   C. cystic duct, the bile duct, and the common bile duct.
   D. appendix, the rectum, and the anus.
   E. liver, pancreas, and gallbladder.

_____ 5. The chief function of the upper GI tract is digestion, whereas the chief functions of the lower GI tract are absorption of nutrients and excretion of wastes.
   A. True
   B. False

_____ 6. Major causes of upper GI hemorrhage include all of the following EXCEPT:
   A. gastritis.   D. peptic ulcers.
   B. rupture of an esophageal varix.   E. Mallory-Weiss syndrome.
   C. gastroenteritis.

_____ 7. Severe, potentially life-threatening upper GI hemorrhage is common with:
   A. variceal and hemorrhoidal rupture and bleeding.
   B. peptic ulcer disease and Crohn's disease.
   C. esophageal varices and hepatic cirrhosis.
   D. esophageal varix rupture and esophageal Mallory-Weiss tears.
   E. eroded gastric ulcers and eroded ulcerative colitis lesions.

_____ 8. Blood is indicated by melena, stool containing small or large amounts of bright red blood, and hematochezia, dark, tarry, foul-smelling stool.
   A. True
   B. False

_____ 9. Of acute gastroenteritis and gastroenteritis, gastroenteritis is the more likely to be caused by microbial infection.
   A. True
   B. False

_____ 10. Conditions that routinely call for the paramedic to take infectious precautions include:
   A. hepatitis and cirrhosis.
   B. peptic ulcer disease and gastroenteritis.
   C. cholecystitis and pancreatitis.
   D. gastroenteritis and appendicitis.
   E. hepatitis and gastroenteritis.

_____ 11. Patients with peptic ulcer disease typically have worsening of pain after eating, whereas patients with cholecystitis typically have relief of pain after eating.
   A. True
   B. False

_____ 12. Any patient who presents with lower GI bleeding or colicky abdominal pain should be transported to the emergency department for evaluation.
   A. True
   B. False

_____ 13. Conditions that typically have lesions in the rectum and anus include:
   A. diverticulosis and hemorrhoids.
   B. ulcerative colitis and Crohn's disease.
   C. ulcerative colitis and hemorrhoids.
   D. volvulus and intussusception.
   E. hernias and hemorrhoids.

_____ 14. Among the most common causes of bowel obstruction are:
   A. intestinal tumors, volvulus, and hernias.
   B. intussusception, volvulus, and hemorrhoids.
   C. adhesions, hernias, and intestinal tumors.
   D. hernias, volvulus, and adhesions.
   E. appendicitis, volvulus, and diverticulitis.

_____ 15. Acute pancreatitis is most commonly caused by:
   A. excessive use of alcohol and tobacco.
   B. gallstones and excessive use of alcohol.
   C. infectious GI disease and gallstones.
   D. drug toxicity and excessive use of alcohol.
   E. vascular disease causing ischemia and gallstones causing obstruction of the pancreatic duct.

MATCHING

Write the letter of the type of pain in the space provided next to the appropriate description of the pain.

   A. somatic   D. radiated
   B. peritonitis   E. referred
   C. visceral

_____ 16. pain originating in the walls of hollow organs that is typically produced by the processes of inflammation, distension, or ischemia

_____ 17. pain perceived in a location other than the one from which it originates

_____ 18. pain frequently characterized by the patient as sharp and well localized

_____ 19. condition caused by presence of free blood or GI contents within the abdominal cavity, which is typically perceived by the patient as somatic pain that is eased in a knee-chest position

_____ 20. pain frequently originating in the capsules of solid organs and typically perceived by the patient as sharp or tearing in character

_____ 21. pain between the shoulder blades that may be produced by a dissecting abdominal aorta

_____ 22. pain that an appendicitis patient may perceive when the inflamed appendix ruptures

_____ 23. pain that seems to the patient to move from one location to another

Write the letter of the signs or symptoms in the space provided next to the condition to which they apply.

    A. epigastric pain, abdominal distension, and nausea and vomiting
    B. colicky, lower left quadrant pain, low-grade fever, nausea, and vomiting
    C. blood loss, refractory shock, and respiratory failure
    D. upper right quadrant tenderness, fever, nausea, and vomiting

_____ 24. hepatitis

_____ 25. mild pancreatitis

_____ 26. diverticulitis

_____ 27. severe pancreatitis

FILL-IN-THE-BLANKS

28. Define the SAMPLE history format by filling in the missing terms:

S _____

A _____

M _____

P _____

L _____

E _____

29. Any case of abdominal pain lasting over _____ in duration is considered a surgical emergency and should be transported to an appropriate facility.

30. Upper GI hemorrhage is defined as bleeding in the GI tract proximal to the

_____ _____ _____ , whereas lower GI

hemorrhage is defined as bleeding in the GI tract distal to it.

SPECIAL PROJECT

History Taking

Examine the responses noted in a patient's history of her present illness and fill in the type of question beside the response. Question types are drawn from the OPQRST-ASPN history format discussed on text pages 365 and 366.

For the previous half hour to hour, pain has been constant and close to a 9 (out of 10) in intensity. _____

Nausea without vomiting has been present, along with no appetite, since the discomfort began. _____

Patient remembers it was about 10:00 PM when she first realized her abdominal pain was significant (7 hours ago). _____

Pain is now constant and sharp like a knife. _____

Pain was poorly localized last evening, but became localized to the right lower quadrant overnight; however, it has become generalized over the abdomen within the last half hour or so. _____

Patient first noticed some vague, generalized discomfort yesterday afternoon at some point before dinnertime. _____

Currently, there is almost nothing that relieves the pain. Patient does best when lying very still with knees drawn toward chest. _____

There is no pain associated with urination, and no pain has been perceived outside of the abdomen. _____

Consider the patient's history of present illness given above with the information placed in the order below. Then give a probable field diagnosis:

Patient first noticed some vague, generalized discomfort yesterday afternoon at some point before dinner. Nausea without vomiting has been present, along with no appetite, since the discomfort began.

Patient remembers it was about 10:00 PM when she first realized her abdominal pain was significant (roughly 7 hours ago). Pain was poorly localized last evening, but became localized to the right lower quadrant overnight; however, it has become generalized over the abdomen within the last half hour or so. There is no pain associated with urination, and no pain has been perceived outside of the abdomen.

For the previous half hour to hour, pain has been constant and close to a 9 (out of 10) in intensity. Pain is now constant and sharp like a knife. Currently, there is almost nothing that relieves the pain. Patient does best when lying very still with knees drawn toward chest.

Probable field diagnosis: _____

CHAPTER 7

*

Urology and Nephrology

Review of Chapter Objectives

After reading this chapter, you should be able to:

1. **Describe the incidence, morbidity, mortality, and risk factors predisposing to urologic and nephrologic emergencies.**   pp. 395–396, 409, 413, 419, 421

   Renal (kidney) and urologic (urinary tract) disorders are very common, affecting about 20 million Americans, so you will definitely see emergencies related to these disorders in the field. The seriousness of these disorders is demonstrated by two statistics: Roughly 250,000 Americans have the most severe form of long-term kidney failure (end-stage failure) and require either dialysis or transplantation to live. More than 50,000 Americans die annually from some form of kidney disease. Some emergencies are not necessarily life threatening but are very painful to experience and common in the population: Over 500,000 persons are treated annually for kidney stones. Persons most at risk for severe kidney problems include older patients, persons with diabetes mellitus, persons with chronic hypertension, and individuals with more than one risk factor. The two risk factors most significant for end-stage renal failure are hypertension and diabetes, which account for more than half of all cases. The risk factors for kidney stones are very different. Some kinds of stones follow a familial pattern, suggesting genetic predisposition. Other risk factors include physical immobilization, use of certain medications (anesthetics, opiates, and psychotropic drugs), and metabolic disorders such as gout. Finally, urinary tract infection, which accounts for over 6 million office visits yearly, has identified risk factors: female gender, paraplegic persons and others (notably some persons with diabetes) with nerve disruption to the bladder, pregnancy, and regular use of instrumentation such as catheters.

2. **Discuss the anatomy and physiology of the organs and structures related to urologic and nephrologic diseases.**   pp. 396–403

   The two major organs of the urinary system are the kidneys and the urinary bladder. Two major structures are the ureters and the urethra. The kidney is the critical organ of the urinary system: The kidneys perform the vital functions of the urinary system, which include:
   - Maintenance of blood volume with proper balance of water, electrolytes, and pH
   - Retention of key substances such as glucose and removal of toxic wastes such as urea
   - Major role in regulation of arterial blood pressure
   - Control of the development of red blood cells

   The first two roles are achieved through the production of urine in the kidneys. The kidneys' role in regulation of blood pressure is achieved in part through control of the body's fluid volume. In addition, they produce an enzyme called renin, which acts to activate a hormone (chemical messenger) called angiotensin, which is part of a hormonal pathway that acts to retain water in the body (increase blood pressure).

   The structural and functional unit within the kidney is the nephron, and each kidney contains about 1 million nephrons, establishing the functional reserve that most people take for granted. Blood is filtered into the first part of the nephron, the glomerulus, and then moves through a length of specialized tubule. As the fluid moves through the parts of the tubule, movement of water and some materials out of the tubule and into the blood occurs (reabsorption), as does movement of some materials out of blood and into the tubule (secretion). The kidneys can maintain an exquisitely fine control over the relative activity of reabsorption and secretion for virtually every substance that is filtered into the glomerulus. The ability of the kidney to retain glucose, excrete wastes such as urea, and thus perform all of its vital roles is extraordinary, and life depends upon it. When kidney function is too low or nonexistent, an individual will die unless the function is replaced through artificial dialysis or through kidney transplantation. The final role of the kidney, control over development of red blood cells, is achieved through production and release of a hormone called erythropoietin, which stimulates red blood cell synthesis in the bone marrow.

Each ureter runs from a kidney to the bladder, and urine moves out of the kidney through them to reach the bladder. Because ureters are very small in internal diameter, they can become blocked by internal objects such as kidney stones. The bladder is a muscular sac that expands to hold urine. During urination, stored urine is eliminated from the bladder (and the body) through the tube called the urethra.

In women, the structures of the urinary system and the reproductive system are completely separate. In men, however, reproductive fluid (semen) is also eliminated from the body through the urethra. Thus, consideration of symptoms of urinary tract trouble in men is sometimes more complex than consideration of the same problem in women. For instance, infection in a man's urethra can come directly through sexual activity.

The genitourinary systems of men include some specifically reproductive organs and structures: the testes (the primary male reproductive organs, which produce testosterone and sperm cells) and tubing called the epididymis and vas deferens, through which sperm cells leave the testes and move toward the urethra. Sperm leaves the vas deferens to enter the urethra as it passes through the substance of the other male reproductive organ, the prostate gland, which produces fluid that mixes with sperm to produce semen, the male reproductive fluid. The prostate will be important to you in field work because it surrounds the first part of the male urethra. Prostate enlargement, which occurs routinely with age, can compress the urethra to the point of closure. This can result in retention of urine and a medical emergency call.

3. Define referred pain and visceral pain as they relate to urology.   **p. 404**

Visceral pain and referred pain have the same underlying pathophysiology as they do in the setting of GI emergencies. In the setting of urology, visceral pain usually arises in the walls of hollow structures such as the ureters, bladder, and urethra or the male vas deferens or epididymis. Visceral pain is characteristically described as aching or crampy and feels deeply internal within the body and poorly localized. Visceral pain can mark the first presentation of both kidney stones and urinary tract infection (although both are better known for somatic pain patterns that arise later). Referred pain, which is felt in a location other than the one of origin, has some notable urologic examples. Pyelonephritis, inflammation within the kidney, is often referred to the neck or shoulder.

4. Describe the questioning technique and specific questions the paramedic should use when gathering a focused history in a patient with abdominal pain.   **pp. 405–406**

Recall Chapter 6, "Gastroenterology," where you learned about the focused history relating to abdominal pain that might be GI in origin. The technique is similar when the GI system is not the focus of attention. For instance, initial questioning still follows the OPQRST format (shown below with some specific questions in parentheses):

- Onset of pain (Sudden or slow? Activity at the time?)
- Provocation or palliation of pain (Pain on urination, inability to void or void normally, and palliation with walking all may suggest urinary tract origin.)
- Quality of the pain (Visceral pain is common with urinary emergencies; a change to somatic pain, particularly flank pain, may suggest ureteral obstruction by a stone.)

- Region where pain is felt, along with any radiation of pain (Listen for suggestions of referred/radiated pain; in postpubertal women, be sure to get menstrual history and follow-up comments suggesting OB/GYN problems)
- Severity of pain currently and over time (Most urinary conditions don't cause the abrupt switch to somatic pain—with increase in severity—seen with a ruptured appendix, for instance.)
- Time over which pain has been felt. (Note that any patient with pain lasting over 6 hours is considered a surgical emergency and requires transport to an appropriate facility for evaluation.) When in doubt, consider case a potential surgical emergency and treat/transport as such.

Additional questions center on:

- Previous history of similar event (Note that kidney stones and infections may be recurrent problems; family history may also be helpful.)
- Nausea/vomiting (Because nausea and vomiting can be caused purely by autonomic nervous system discharge, this is not necessarily a sign localizing to GI system; nausea and vomiting is common with severe pain associated with kidney stones.)
- Changes in bowel habits (Diarrhea may suggest a GI condition; constipation may be less helpful as a clue to the origin of a problem.)
- Weight loss (Loss over hours to days suggests dehydration, whereas longer-term loss suggests chronic illness of GI dysfunction.)
- Last oral intake, include beverages (Learning this is necessary for possible surgical cases; timing of a meal may also suggest acute onset problem or aggravation of an existing one.)
- Chest pain (Consider MI but also consider referred pain; note that diabetic persons may not have typical pain pattern during MI due to neuropathy.)

5. Describe the technique for performing a comprehensive physical examination of a patient complaining of abdominal pain. pp. 406–408

The physical exam includes overall impressions as well as examination of the abdomen. Elements include both patient appearance and posture/activity. Walking often suggests urinary origin: Walking that relieves pain may suggest a kidney stone, and walking hunched up in a febrile person complaining of back pain may suggest kidney infection. Additionally, altered level of consciousness in the absence of fever may suggest hemorrhage and evolution of hypovolemic shock. Hemorrhage should lead you to consider GI or reproductive (OB) emergencies. Patients undergoing dialysis may have chronic changes in mental status during dialysis; try to discern whether the level you see is the norm for that person or represents an acute or subacute change. Also consider the apparent state of the patient's health and his or her personal appearance, which can often give leads to a chronic condition or one of acute onset. Skin color and appearance can suggest chronic anemia (pale, cool, dry skin), shock (pale, clammy skin), or fever (dry, flushed).

Examination of the abdomen was covered in Chapter 6 and in objective 5 of this chapter. Percussion may be very useful in the setting of urology: Pain on percussion of the flanks may suggest kidney inflammation and infection, and pain on percussion of the pelvic rim may suggest problems in the bladder. Remember that pregnancy may also be found during physical examination as you palpate above the pelvic rim. A ruptured ectopic pregnancy may be suggested by lower quadrant pain that increases with palpation and evidence of hemorrhage. In older men, palpation above the pelvic rim may reveal the enlarged, fluctuant mass of an obstructed bladder due to prostatic hypertrophy. In all men, exam includes examination of the scrotum and penis. Urethral discharge may suggest infection. Scrotal masses may be painful (such as infectious epididymitis) or nonpainful (testicular cancer, which is most common in young men, or a varicocele). Ask questions about acute or longer-term presence of any mass. For men with an apparently obstructed bladder, find out when they last urinated and whether there had been any change in pattern.

Generally, nephrologic and urologic emergencies don't produce acute abnormalities on exam, unlike GI emergencies. However, pain from an inflamed or infected kidney may be felt in the flank, and pelvic pain may suggest bladder origin or a reproductive problem in either a man or woman. Always consider possible miscarriage from either an ectopic pregnancy or an intrauterine one in girls and women of childbearing age.

6. Define acute renal failure. p. 409

Acute renal failure is defined as a sudden (over a period of a day or days) drop in urine output to less than 400–500 ml per day. Low urine output is oliguria, whereas no urine output is anuria.

7. Discuss the pathophysiology of acute renal failure. pp. 409–411

There are three types of acute renal failure (ARF) based on pathophysiology: prerenal, renal, and postrenal. You may see all three types in the field. Remember that acute renal failure may be reversible if recognized and treated early enough.

- Prerenal ARF is due to insufficient blood flow to the kidneys. This type accounts for 40–80% of cases, and it is the most likely to be reversible if perfusion is restored. Common causes in the field include cardiac failure (often an MI), hemorrhage, dehydration, shock, and sepsis, as well as anomalies of a renal artery or vein.
- Renal ARF is due to a pathologic process within the kidney tissue itself. The three general causes are damage to small vessels and/or glomeruli, tubular cell damage, and interstitial damage. In each type, nephron function is lost.
- Postrenal ARF is due to obstruction at some point distal to the kidneys: both ureters, the bladder outlet, or the urethra. Postrenal ARF may be reversible if the obstruction is identified and removed before permanent kidney damage occurs.

8. Recognize the signs and symptoms related to acute renal failure. pp. 411–412

Timing of voiding difficulty can provide vital information: A normal history with sudden onset inability to void may suggest distal obstruction, whereas feeling ill over a number of days with some decrease in voiding may suggest chronic renal problems with an acute aggravation: Ask for renal history. Some triggers of acute renal failure may be obvious: dehydration secondary to diarrhea, hemorrhage, shock, sepsis. Visual inspection may reveal cool, pale, moist skin (which suggests shunting of blood to core, including kidneys, if shock is absent) and edema in hands, feet, or face. Physical findings may reveal the trigger for the failure: A distended, discolored abdomen may suggest severe intra-abdominal hemorrhage with hypoperfusion to kidneys.

9. Describe the management of acute renal failure. pp. 412–413

Because acute renal failure can cause life-threatening metabolic complications (consider the key role of the kidneys in regulation of fluid volume, electrolytes, and pH), provide close monitoring and support of the ABCs. High-flow oxygen should be used, and patient positioning and IV fluid resuscitation are important. In general, you want to protect fluid volume and cardiovascular function to minimize damage due to renal hypoperfusion and eliminate or reduce exposure to any potentially nephrotoxic drug.

Drug information may be available from medical direction; likewise, specific advice for care of dialysis patients may also be obtained before or during transit.

10. Integrate pathophysiological principles and assessment findings to formulate a field impression and implement a treatment plan for the patient with acute renal failure. pp. 409–413

If onset is acute and without evidence of distal obstruction, prerenal ARF may be suggested. Be sure to treat any identifiable potential trigger condition and aggressively protect fluid volume and oxygenation. Always remember that prerenal ARF may be reversible if you act quickly and correctly; this is still true in patients with chronic renal failure. Quick action may also preserve remaining function if renal causes are suspected. Renal causes may require the hospital setting for definitive treatment, but the treatment staples are the same as for prerenal. If history or exam suggests postrenal obstruction, be sure to get as much information as possible for use by hospital staff. For instance, known cancer in the abdomen or pelvis may suggest bilateral ureteral obstruction. Advanced age in men may suggest acute renal retention secondary to prostate enlargement, and history in boys or men of recent sexual activity, recreational drugs, or parties may suggest the possible presence of a foreign body in the urethra.

11. Define chronic renal failure. p. 413

Chronic renal failure is inadequate kidney function due to the permanent loss of nephrons (usually representing a loss of at least 70–80% of total nephrons). When metabolic instability sets in (around 80% loss), the condition is termed end-stage renal failure, and either dialysis or kidney transplantation is required to survive.

12. Discuss the pathophysiology of chronic renal failure. pp. 413–414

The three processes that can underlie chronic renal failure are the same as those producing acute renal failure: damage to small blood vessels or glomeruli, tubular cell injury, and damage to interstitial tissue. In each case, surviving nephrons adapt by structural changes that increase function, but these changes damage the nephrons themselves over time, leading to greater loss of nephron numbers. Common causes of damage to blood vessels and glomeruli include systemic hypertension, atherosclerosis, diabetes, and systemic lupus erythematosus, an autoimmune disease. Causes of tubular cell injury include nephrotoxic drugs and heavy metals and distal obstruction with backup of urine into the kidney. Finally, interstitial damage can be caused by infections including pyelonephritis and tuberculosis.

13. Recognize the signs and symptoms related to chronic renal failure. pp. 414–416

All of the kidney's major functions are deranged or lost in chronic renal failure. The general syndrome of signs and symptoms associated with chronic failure is termed uremia or uremic syndrome, so-called for the characteristic buildup of the waste urea. Clinical elements of uremia are found in Table 7-4 on text page 415. They include peripheral and pulmonary edema, hypertension, hyperkalemia and acidosis, congestive heart failure and accelerated atherosclerosis, headache, impaired mental status, seizures, muscle irritability, anorexia/nausea/vomiting, ulcers and GI bleeding, glucose intolerance due to cellular resistance to insulin, jaundice, uremic frost, pruritus, easy bleeding, chronic anemia, and vulnerability to infection. In addition, children and young adults may show poor growth and development, including delayed sexual maturation.

14. Describe the management of chronic renal failure. pp. 416–419

Long-term management will focus on dialysis (either hemodialysis or peritoneal dialysis, dependent on individual circumstances) or transplantation.

15. Integrate pathophysiological principles and assessment findings to formulate a field impression and implement a treatment plan for the patient with chronic renal failure. pp. 413–419

Immediate management is similar to that for acute renal failure: Focus on close monitoring and support of the ABCs with high-flow oxygen, positioning to support blood flow to internal organs and brain, and administration of IV fluid if hypovolemia is suggested. Chief prevention strategies are protection of fluid volume and cardiovascular function with correction of major electrolyte disturbances as merited by individual findings and the philosophy of erring on the side of conservative treatment. Close monitoring of the ECG may give you time to adjust and respond to cardiac problems caused by fluid overload or electrolyte disturbances. Life-threatening conditions should always be treated and lesser conditions or complications noted for consideration by the receiving staff. Where possible, be sure your impressions clearly note which conditions have been chronic (or the norm) for the patient and which findings represent acute changes. As indicated and allowed by medical direction, fluid lavage may be considered for patients who use peritoneal dialysis.

16. Define renal dialysis. pp. 416–419

Renal dialysis is artificial replacement of some of the kidneys' vital functions. Two different technologies, hemodialysis and peritoneal dialysis, are widely used. Both rely on the physiologic principles of osmosis and equalization of osmolarity across a semipermeable membrane. As blood flows over such a membrane, many critical substances such as urea and sodium, potassium, and hydrogen ions move from blood into the hypo-osmolar solution, the dialysate, thus reducing the concentrations in blood. The overall effect is to lessen or eliminate temporarily volume overload and toxically high blood concentrations of electrolytes, urea, and other substances.

In hemodialysis, the patient's blood is passed through a machine containing a semipermeable membrane. Vascular access is established through a permanent anastamosis of an artery and vein in the forearm. If such a fistula is not possible, an indwelling catheter may be placed in the internal jugular vein. In peritoneal dialysis, the peritoneal membrane is used as the semipermeable membrane and dialysate solution is introduced into, and then removed from, the abdominal cavity via an indwelling catheter.

17. Discuss the common complications of renal dialysis.   pp. 417–418

Complications common to both forms of dialysis include physiologically destabilizing shifts in blood volume and composition and blood pressure during and shortly after dialysis. Other complications common to both forms include shortness of breath or dizziness and neurologic abnormalities ranging from headache to seizure or coma. Hypotension may represent dehydration, hemorrhage, or infection. Shortness of breath or chest pain may reflect cardiac dysrhythmias, ischemia, or even MI. In many cases the neurologic abnormalities represent shifts in the chemical milieu of the brain. Seizures are usually responsive to benzodiazepines.

Complications specific to hemodialysis include bleeding at the needle puncture site, local infection, and stenosis or obstruction of the internal fistula. Under normal flow conditions, you will hear or feel a bruit or thrill. Leading complications requiring hospitalization include thrombosis, infection, and development of an aneurysm. The latter are particularly common in patients in whom artificial graft material was used to construct the fistula. The most common complications in patients undergoing peritoneal dialysis include infection in the catheter or tunnel containing the catheter, or in the peritoneum itself. Because the incidence of peritonitis is roughly one episode per year, you may find the signs of peritonitis in this patient group.

18. Define renal calculi.   p. 419

Renal calculi (calculus, singular) are crystal aggregations in the kidney's urine collecting system. The same condition is referred to as nephrolithiasis. Although overall morbidity and mortality are low, brief hospitalizations are common for patients because of the severity of the pain as stones move through the renal pelvis, ureter, bladder, and urethra.

19. Discuss the pathophysiology of renal calculi.   p. 420

Some kinds of stones form as part of a systemic metabolic disorder such as gout (excess uric acid) or primary hyperparathyroidism (excess calcium). Most stones, however, form due to a more general imbalance between the amount of water flowing through the kidney tubing and the mineral ions, uric acid, and other relatively insoluble substances that are dissolved in that water. Trigger events for stone formation include change in diet, activity, or climate, all of which can alter water conservation or the amount of one or more such substances in the blood and, thus, the filtrate. Calcium stones are the most common and are most frequently seen in men aged 20 to 30 years. This type of stone is likely to recur and is likely to be found in a family history. Struvite stones are also common; their formation is often related to chronic urinary tract infection or frequent bladder catheterization. Perhaps because of the tie to infection, these stones are more common in women. Struvite stones can grow to fill the renal pelvis; in such cases, they present a "staghorn" appearance on X-rays. The less common stones are made of uric acid or cystine. Uric acid stones can occur in the presence of gout (about 50% of cases); they are also more common men and tend to occur in families. Cystine stones are the least common, and they are associated with excess cystine in filtrate. There is probably at least a partial genetic predisposition, and they are known to occur in families.

20. Recognize the signs and symptoms of renal calculi.   p. 420

The assessment almost always focuses on pain as the chief complaint; the pain associated with kidney stones is generally conceded to be among the most severe known, ranking up there with labor pain. Typical history is a vague onset of discomfort in the flank progressing within an hour or so to an extremely sharp pain that may remain in the flank or radiate downward toward the pelvis or scrotum in men. Migrating pain suggests that the stone is in the lowest third of the involved ureter. Stones that lodge low in the ureter or within the bladder wall characteristically cause bladder symptoms such as frequency, urgency, and painful urination. In women these symptoms may make it difficult to distinguish stones from an infection. Physical exam will almost always reveal someone in considerable distress, often agitated and walking restlessly. High blood pressure and tachycardia may correlate with the degree of pain. Skin is typically cool, clammy, and pale due to autonomic discharge. Abdominal exam may be difficult to perform or assess given patient restlessness and muscle guarding secondary to pain.

21. Describe the management of renal calculi. p. 421

Management, as always, begins with the ABCs. Position for comfort, but be ready for vomiting, particularly if pain is severe or last oral intake recent. IV access may be needed for analgesic administration (if needed and appropriate per local protocol) or fluid to promote urine formation and movement of the stone through the urinary tract.

22. Integrate pathophysiological principles and assessment findings to formulate a field impression and implement a treatment plan for the patient with renal calculi. pp. 419–421

The common pathophysiology for all types of stones rests on an imbalance of water and relatively insoluble substances in the kidney filtrate. The type and size of stone, as well as current site in the urinary tract, may be discerned from personal and family history, as well as physical examination. Assessment for treatment (prior to and during transport) focuses on nature, site, and severity of pain. A urine sample may reveal blood in the presence of any type of stone. A urine sample may be particularly valuable from a woman patient because of inclusion of infection in the differential diagnosis, especially when bladder symptoms are present. Because passage of the stone is the ultimate goal, IV fluid may be beneficial as soon as it can be started as it promotes urine formation. Analgesia may be necessary, dependent on the individual patient and local protocol.

23. Define urinary tract infection. p. 421

Infection of the urinary tract implies infection in the urethra, bladder, or kidney, or the prostate gland in men. Urinary tract infections (UTI) are extremely common, accounting for about 6 million office visits per year, and you will see them in the field.

24. Discuss the pathophysiology of urinary tract infection. pp. 421–422

Because bacteria usually enter via the urethra, infections are more common in women (who have a much shorter urethra), paraplegic patients or others who require catheterization, and diabetic persons who have neuropathy involving the bladder. UTIs are generally divided into those affecting the lower urinary tract (namely, urethritis, cystitis, and prostatitis) and those of the upper urinary tract (pyelonephritis). Lower UTIs are much more common because of bacterial entrance via the urethra and NOT commonly via the bloodstream. Sexually active females may be at higher risk due to indirect factors (use of contraceptives vaginally and unintentional introduction of enteric flora into the urethra), and direct sexual transmission of infection can occur in males. Pyelonephritis usually occurs due to an infection that ascends through the urinary tract. The infectious inflammation can affect the interstitium, nephrons, or both. Incidence is highest during pregnancy and among the sexually active, paralleling the epidemiology of lower UTIs. Intrarenal abscesses can result, and rupture with spillage of contents into adjacent perirenal fat can cause formation of a perinephric abscess. Note that the likely pathogens are distinctly different in community-acquired and nosocomial infections.

25. Recognize the signs and symptoms related to urinary tract infection.   pp. 422–423

The typical triad of a lower UTI consists of painful urination, frequent urge to urinate, and difficulty in beginning and continuing flow. Pain frequently is visceral in character before voiding, progresses to severe, burning pain during and after urination, and then receding to visceral pain again. Many women will have a past medical history of such episodes, which may or may not have been diagnosed and treated. Vitals generally reflect those of someone in pain, with slight tachycardia and an increase in blood pressure. Exam will probably show tenderness over the pubis and cool, clammy skin. Patients with pyelonephritis typically have a fever and feel more generally ill. Their pain is typically in the flank or lower back with occasional reference to the neck or shoulder. Pain tends to be somewhat more somatic in character: moderately severe or severe and constant. The triad of lower urinary tract symptoms may or may not be present. (If not, ask whether they have been present recently.) The exam of a patient with pyelonephritis will be more striking, with a restless and ill appearance, warm, dry skin if fever is present, and possible tenderness over the flank. Lloyd's sign, tenderness on percussion of the lower back at the costovertebral angle, indicates pyelonephritis.

26. Describe the management of a urinary tract infection.   p. 423

Management centers on monitoring and support of the ABCs. Positioning may help the patient with severe pain; be prepared in case the patient vomits. Analgesics are usually unnecessary; severely painful cases of pyelonephritis may be the exception. As with renal stones, hydration to increase and dilute urine flow is generally helpful. Use of IV fluid eliminates the risk of vomiting and satisfies treatment guidelines for possible surgical cases.

27. Integrate pathophysiological principles and assessment findings to formulate a field impression and implement a treatment plan for the patient with a urinary tract infection.   pp. 421–423

Lower UTIs typically arise from infection that has entered via the urethra and has damaged tissue in the lower urinary tract. Hydration increases urine formation and promotes a more dilute urine (in a patient with normal renal function), and so it may help ease the symptoms of urgency, frequency, and pain in the patient with a lower UTI. Lack of systemic signs indicates that normal monitoring of ABCs is probably sufficient before and during transport. Patients with pyelonephritis (upper UTI) are more likely to show fever and other signs of systemic infection. IV hydration is also indicated for the same reasons and because IV access may be needed if physiologic instability develops or the patient is deemed later to be a surgical case. Transport for diagnosis and definitive treatment (appropriate antibiotic therapy) provides the link to long-term care.

28. Apply epidemiology to develop prevention strategies for urologic and nephrologic emergencies.   pp. 396, 409

Urinary tract infections, which include genitourinary infections in men, are the most typical urologic emergency. IV hydration promotes formation of a dilute urine that will help to eliminate bacteria within the urinary tract and decrease the triad of symptoms typically associated with lower UTIs: pain, frequency, and urgency. In elderly men, pain or poor urination may frequently be due to obstruction by an enlarged prostate: In these cases, the enlarged bladder will be felt on exam. Hydration is also useful for patients with pyelonephritis. ABCs should always be supported. Because UTIs, particularly lower UTIs, are more common among diabetic patients with neuropathy, it is also wise to assess diabetic status for signs of instability while monitoring ABCs as in all other patients. Remember to relay all relevant information on fetal age, presence of any complications, etc., in pregnant women presenting with UTIs to the receiving facility so they can arrange appropriate OB support.

Prevention strategies are probably most critical for the nephrologic emergencies directly involving kidney function (acute and chronic renal failure) and indirectly involving function (renal calculi with possible obstruction of the distal urinary tract). Prevention strategies in patients with acute renal failure (ARF), particularly cases that may be prerenal in origin, center on protection of fluid volume (usually through IV fluid) and support of cardiovascular function. Close monitoring of the ABCs is critical because of the possibility of metabolic derangements secondary to renal failure. Although reversibility is less likely with renal and postrenal ARF, the same strategies are important. Avoidance of nephrotoxic drugs is important, as is alleviation of postrenal obstruction as soon as possible.

29. Integrate pathophysiological principles to the assessment of a patient with abdominal pain. pp. 404–408

Abdominal pain is questioned in similar ways whether or not the system of origin (GI, urinary tract, reproductive) is suspected from the initial size-up or complaint. The distinction of visceral and somatic pain may be useful in discerning cause, as is any referred pain pattern. For instance, most urologic/nephrologic emergencies typically feature visceral pain. However, renal stones are notorious for severe, somatic pain when they lodge somewhere in the distal urinary tract. Although the presence of nausea and vomiting is generally not helpful (if not due to GI disturbance, it is frequently due to autonomic discharge), presence of diarrhea suggests GI origin. Similarly, pain associated with urination suggests urinary tract origin.

30. Synthesize assessment findings and patient history information to accurately differentiate between pain of a urologic or nephrologic emergency and that of another origin. pp. 404–408

As noted in Chapter 6, many GI emergencies feature hemorrhage, and discernment through vital signs and physical exam of likely hemorrhage is an important first step in looking for system of origin. Examination of vomitus or diarrhea is also helpful. Gross examination of urine may not be helpful; however, gross blood is consistent with kidney stone in an otherwise appropriate presentation, and cloudiness of urine may represent the large numbers of white cells that may be present in pyelonephritis. Remember the typical pain patterns: GI emergencies often start with visceral pain (frequently located higher than in urinary tract conditions) and progress to somatic pain if an inflamed or damaged structure ruptures; postrupture peritonitis is not unusual. In contrast, most urologic/nephrologic emergencies feature visceral pain felt in the pelvis or male scrotum. Somatic-like pain felt in the flank, shoulder, or neck may suggest a kidney stone. Tenderness in the lower back at the costovertebral angle may suggest pyelonephritis, particularly if systemic signs of infection are present. If the urinary system appears likely, be sure to address the issue of renal function. Prevention strategies to prevent further loss of nephrons are vital to implement expediently.

31. Develop, execute, and evaluate a treatment plan based on the field impression made in the assessment. pp. 402–423

Because acute renal failure can cause life-threatening metabolic complications (consider the key role of the kidneys in regulation of fluid volume, electrolytes, and pH), close monitoring and support of the ABCs are essential. High-flow oxygen should be used, and positioning and IV fluid resuscitation are important. In general, you want to protect fluid volume and cardiovascular function to minimize damage due to renal hypoperfusion and eliminate or reduce exposure to any potentially nephrotoxic drug. The same applies to an acute problem in a patient with chronic renal failure. It is always important to prevent nephron loss, even in patients who already have compromise. In patients with renal calculi, it is important to promote urine formation and flow in an effort to move the stone through the distal urinary tract. In urinary tract infections (either lower or upper), IV hydration may promote formation of dilute urine that will flush some microbes from the urinary tract and relieve some of the pain, frequency, and urgency that might be present. Monitoring of the ABCs and support of any acute complications is always mandated.

CASE STUDY REVIEW

Reread the case study on page 394 in Paramedic Care: Medical Emergencies *before reading the discussion below.*

This case study demonstrates how paramedics react to a stressful medical emergency involving severe pain of unknown origin. In addition to noting how the team reacts to the patient's presentation and assessment, note how clues to the nephrologic origin of his condition emerge from the assessment and history.

Rachel and Jack receive a call that is nonspecific but concerning: A man has fallen and cannot get up. Jack and Rachel have almost no information before arriving at the scene. They do not know the age of the patient, whether traumatic injury is involved, the nature of the underlying cause of the fall. In their first moments at the house they realize that they are dealing with a relatively young, apparently healthy man who is having an acute episode of severe pain and apparently is not getting up because of the pain.

Their initial actions center on historical questions about the pain and on an initial physical assessment. The patient tells them that the pain was of sudden onset and is very severe. His concerns about the possible cause of his problem give them an immediate clue: He tells them there is a family history of kidney stones, that his brother had one recently, and could he be suffering from one. At the time this information is received, a urine specimen is obtained that appears to have blood in it.

You aren't told whether there are any significant findings on physical exam, so the assumption is that the exam was largely benign. You do know that the patient's vital signs are consistent with pain and stress: a relatively high blood pressure (at least if the patient isn't chronically hypertensive), tachycardia, and brisk respirations.

The team secures IV access and starts oxygen supplementation and transports to the emergency department, where a diagnostic IVP shows complete ureteral obstruction due to an apparent radiopaque renal stone. Treatment centers on rest, gentle analgesia, and IV fluid to promote urine formation and flow. Finally, a visible stone is passed, David's pain subsides, and he can go home.

Although you aren't told about predischarge counseling, you do know that calcium-containing stones, the most common kind, tend to appear in men of approximately his age group, tend to run in families, and tend to recur in an affected individual. The patient should learn about the pathophysiology of stones and any dietary, physical, or other lifestyle modifications that might help reduce the likelihood of recurrence.

CONTENT SELF-EVALUATION

MULTIPLE CHOICE

_____ 1. The major functions of the urinary system include all EXCEPT:
A. maintenance of blood volume.
B. control of development of white blood cells.
C. regulation of arterial blood pressure.
D. maintenance of the balance of electrolytes and blood pH.
E. removal of many toxic wastes from the blood.

_____ 2. BUN, or blood urea nitrogen, and creatinine are both measured in blood as part of assessment of kidney function.
A. True
B. False

_____ 3. The enzyme that is produced by the kidney and is part of the physiologic response to low blood pressure is called:
A. aldosterone.　　　　　　　　　　D. renin.
B. angiotensin.　　　　　　　　　　 E. progesterone.
C. erythropoietin.

_____ 4. The urethra in men is much shorter than it is in women, and this is one reason why there is a gender difference in the incidence of lower urinary tract infections.
A. True
B. False

_____ 5. Sperm cells are eliminated from a man's body after they move out of the testicles and pass through the following structures in first-to-last sequence:
A. vas deferens, epididymis, urethra.
B. ureter, epididymis, vas deferens, urethra.
C. epididymis, vas deferens, urethra.
D. epididymis, vas deferens, prostate gland, urethra.
E. vas deferens, epididymis, prostate gland, urethra.

_____ 6. Typical questions to ask when obtaining a focused history related to abdominal pain include all of the following EXCEPT:
A. previous history of similar event?
B. sudden or gradual unintended weight loss?
C. presence of chest pain?
D. last oral intake?
E. last date of sexual activity, if sexually active?

_____ 7. Indications that a woman's abdominal pain might be of obstetric (pregnancy-related) origin include all of the following EXCEPT:
A. known pregnancy or last menstrual period not in immediate past.
B. frequency and urgency of urination.
C. indications of intra-abdominal hemorrhage.
D. presence of blood in the vagina and on the vulva.
E. palpation of the uterus above the pelvic rim.

_____ 8. Patients most at risk for kidney disorders are the elderly, persons with diabetes mellitus, hypertension, or both, and patients with more than one risk factor.
A. True
B. False

_____ 9. Oliguria is defined as low urine output (roughly 400–500 ml daily or less), whereas anuria is complete absence of urine output.
A. True
B. False

_____ 10. The two factors responsible for more than half of all cases of end-stage renal failure are:
A. damage due to nephrotoxic drugs and other substances and hypertension.
B. pyelonephritis and diabetes mellitus.
C. diabetes mellitus and hypertension.
D. infections and glomerulonephritis.
E. atherosclerosis and hypertension.

_____ 11. Common elements of uremic syndrome include all of the following EXCEPT:
A. peptic ulcer.   D. hypoglycemia.
B. hyperkalemia and metabolic acidosis.   E. chronic anemia.
C. easy bleeding and bruising.

_____ 12. Always be alert for development of physiologic instability in patients with chronic renal failure, regardless of initial presentation.
A. True
B. False

_____ 13. All of the following statements about kidney stones are true EXCEPT:
   A. Renal calculi and nephrolithiasis are synonymous terms for kidney stones.
   B. Brief hospitalization for kidney stones is common because of the severity of pain while a stone is being passed.
   C. Immobilization and use of opiates and psychotropic drugs are risk factors for stones.
   D. Calcium and uric acid stones tend to run in families, suggesting a genetic link.
   E. Calcium stones are associated with chronic urinary tract infection or frequent bladder catheterization.

_____ 14. Male patients with kidney stones rarely have referred pain in the testicle on the affected side.
   A. True
   B. False

_____ 15. Risk factors for urinary tract infection include all of the following EXCEPT:
   A. female gender.
   B. pregnancy.
   C. advanced age.
   D. persons requiring routine bladder catheterization.
   E. persons with conditions causing urinary stasis.

MATCHING

Write the letter of the medical specialty in the space provided next to its definition.

A. nephrology
B. urology

_____ 16. the medical specialty pertaining to the kidneys

_____ 17. the surgical specialty pertaining to the urinary system

Write the letter of the description of the cause of acute renal failure (ARF) in the space provided next to the appropriate type of ARF.

A. injury to the nephrons, interstitial tissue, or both
B. hypoperfusion due to hypovolemia or compromised cardiovascular function
C. obstruction of both ureters or at the level of the bladder neck or urethra

_____ 18. prerenal ARF

_____ 19. postrenal ARF

_____ 20. renal ARF

Write the letter of the organ or structure in the space provided next to the infection/inflammation that can affect that organ or structure.

A. urethra
B. prostate gland
C. urinary bladder
D. kidney

_____ 21. cystitis

_____ 22. pyelonephritis

_____ 23. urethritis

_____ 24. prostatitis

Fill-in-the-Blanks

Use the following list of terms relating to the structure and physiology of the kidney to fill in the blanks in the following statements. Note that NOT all terms will be used. One or more may be used multiple times.

secretion	nephron	filtrate
Bowman's capsule	distal tubule	descending loop of Henle
reabsorption	ascending loop of Henle	proximal tubule
urine	glomerulus	
water	sodium and chloride ions	

25. The successive parts of the nephron tubule are the _____ ,

    the _____ , the _____ ,

    and the _____ .

26. Filtration, the first process in formation of urine, occurs when blood is filtered through the

    capillaries of the glomerulus and into _____ . This fluid,

    called _____ , then passes into the proximal tubule.

27. The hormone aldosterone increases reabsorption of _____

    and _____ in the distal tubule and collecting duct.

28. In the process of _____ , substances such as potassium and

    hydrogen ions are transported from the blood into the tubule.

29. Fill in the blanks below to show the components of the OPQRST focused history about pain.

    O _____

    P _____

    Q _____

    R _____

    S _____

    T _____

Use the following list of terms relating to dialysis to fill in the blanks in the statements below. Note that NOT all terms will be used. One or more may be used multiple times.

infection	semipermeable membrane
artificial graft	arteriovenous fistula
filtrate	peritonitis
dialysate	

30. Two components necessary for either form of dialysis are a(n)

    _____ and a(n) _____ .

31. In peritoneal dialysis, the peritoneum is used as the _____ .

32. In hemodialysis, vascular access is achieved through a(n)

    _____ connecting an artery and vein or a(n)

    _____ .

33. _____ is a complication common to both kinds of dialysis.

LABEL THE DIAGRAMS

Supply the missing labels for the figure showing the major organs and structures of the urinary system by writing the appropriate letters in the spaces provided.

A. urethra

B. urinary bladder

C. ureter

D. kidney

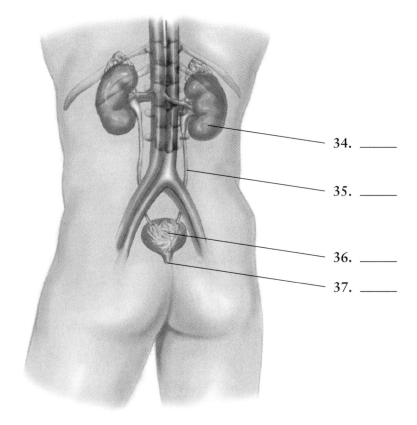

34. _____

35. _____

36. _____

37. _____

Supply the missing labels for the figure showing the the internal structure of the kidney by writing the appropriate letters in the spaces provided.

A. medulla

B. pyramid

C. cortex

D. papilla

E. hilum

F. renal pelvis

G. renal capsule

38. _____

39. _____

40. _____

41. _____

42. _____

43. _____

44. _____

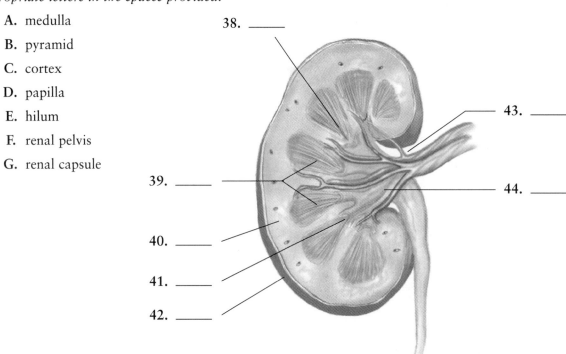

SPECIAL PROJECT

Making the Call

You are called to the home of a patient who is familiar to you as an individual with end-stage renal failure. The call is for "passing out" during home peritoneal dialysis. When you reach the residence, the middle-aged man is awake and alert and has finished his dialysis session. When asked about the recent event, he says he does not usually faint during dialysis although he commonly feels dizzy.

He says he has felt more tired over the past few days and that he is experiencing more abdominal discomfort during his dialysis sessions. He denies recent illness or injury to his abdomen, although he says he thinks he may have had a low-grade fever on the preceding evening. He admits to more soreness around the catheter entrance site than normal but says he isn't in constant pain and is fairly comfortable as he moves around in the house.

His vital signs are normal.

During your visual inspection of the man's abdomen you note the end of a catheter protruding with obvious reddening, swelling, and discharge around the entrance site.

1. Based on what you know about peritoneal dialysis, what equipment is visible and invisible beneath the skin of the patient's abdomen?

2. Based on the history and physical findings, what is the probable nature of the underlying problem?

3. What equipment or bodily structures may be affected by the problem?

4. What precautions, if any, should you take during transport of this patient to an appropriate medical facility?

Chapter 8
✳
Toxicology and Substance Abuse

Review of Chapter Objectives

After reading this chapter, you should be able to:

1. **Describe the incidence, morbidity, and mortality of toxic and drug abuse emergencies.** **p. 429**

    Toxicological emergencies are defined as those relating to exposure to a toxin, which is a chemical substance that causes adverse effects within the exposed individual. The term toxin includes drugs and poisons. Over the years, both the number and severity of toxicological emergencies has increased, so this is an area with which you must become familiar and must take steps to remain current in your knowledge. The estimated number of poisonings is over 4 million per year (and the term poisonings *excludes* drug overdoses). Roughly 10% of all EMS calls involve toxic exposures. About 70% of all accidental poisonings involve children under the age of 6 years; however, these poisonings tend to be relatively mild, accounting for only 5% of fatalities. Adult poisonings and drug overdoses are less frequent but they account for over 90% of hospital admissions for toxic exposures and 95% of the fatalities in this category.

2. **Identify the risk factors most predisposing to toxic emergencies.** **p. 429**

    Age is an important risk factor: About 70% of all accidental poisonings involve children under the age of 6 years. A child who has had an accidental ingestion has a 25% chance of another, similar ingestion within one year. Intentional exposure as a form of drug experimentation or suicide is common in older children and young adults. Although adult poisonings and overdoses are less frequent, they account for 90% of hospital admissions for exposure to a toxic substance and 95% of fatalities. Among adults, most poisonings and drug overdoses are intentional. For instance, 80% of all attempted suicides involve a drug overdose. Interpersonal violence is a second risk factor: Poisoning in an older child can be the result of an intentional act by a parent or caregiver. Third, specific settings and situations make accidental poisoning more likely: Exposure in an industrial workplace or on a farm is increasingly common. Finally, use of medications is itself a risk factor. Most often, accidental exposures among older children and adults represent hypersensitivity reactions or dosage errors when taking prescribed medications.

3. **Discuss the anatomy and physiology of the organs and structures related to toxic emergencies.** **pp. 430, 431**

    Agents that are ingested through the mouth are exposed to the teeth, tongue, and mucous membranes of the mouth, as well as the throat and esophagus, before entering the stomach. As with intentionally ingested foods, agents remain in the stomach for a period of time before they pass into the small intestine (length of time depends on amount of stomach contents, whether contents are liquid or solid, etc.). Most absorption into the bloodstream takes place during passage of the agent through the small intestine.

Agents that are inhaled pass through the nose (possibly also the mouth), pharynx, trachea, and other, increasingly small airways before reaching the alveoli of the lungs. Absorption is largely at the distal end of the respiratory tree, the alveolar-capillary interface, which is the normal site for gas exchange (typically oxygen and carbon dioxide). Because the epithelial lining of the airways is relatively delicate, local effects can occur through tissue irritation in these medial structures.

With surface absorption, the agent must pass through the skin or mucous membranes to which it has been applied in order to enter the body and cause local or systemic effects (the latter if agent is absorbed into bloodstream).

In cases of injection, the needle passes through the skin and subcutaneous tissues to reach a vein. The amount and depth of skin and subcutaneous tissue varies widely on different body sites. Typically, skin is thin and there is little subcutaneous tissue at sites with easy venous access such as the forearms and hands, as well as the comparable sites on the lower extremities. Be aware that drug addicts who have sclerosed readily available veins may have the ability to inject substances successfully into very small and usually inaccessible vessels.

4. Describe the routes of entry of toxic substances into the body. pp. 430–431

There are four routes of entry into the body: ingestion, inhalation, surface absorption, and injection. Ingestion via the mouth is the most common route of entry for toxic exposure. Inhalation of a poison into the lungs results in rapid absorption from the alveolar air into the blood. Causative agents are in the form of gases, vapors, fumes, or aerosols. Surface absorption applies to cases in which entry is through the skin or mucous membranes. Injection applies when the toxic agent is injected under the skin, into muscle, or directly into the bloodstream.

5. Discuss the role of Poison Control Centers in the United States. pp. 429–430

Poison Control Centers assist in the treatment of poison victims and provide information on new products and new treatment recommendations. They are usually based in major medical centers serving large populations, and many have computer systems that allow staff to rapidly and accurately access information. Centers are available to you 24 hours a day, 7 days a week: Take the time to memorize the telephone number of the Center serving your area. Your Center can help you determine the potential toxicity for your patient when you give them the following information: type of agent, amount and time of exposure, and physical condition of the patient. With this information, you may be able to start the current, definitive treatment in the field. The Center can notify the receiving facility before you get the patient there.

6. Discuss the pathophysiology, assessment findings, need for rapid intervention and transport, and management of toxic emergencies. pp. 429–468

- *Pathophysiology:* With each route of entry, there is a general pattern of possible toxic effects depending on the type and amount of agent involved: Immediate effects involve the tissues exposed to the toxic agent during entry. Delayed, systemic effects are related to absorption into the bloodstream and circulation throughout the body. In ingestion, corrosive agents can cause immediate injury through burns of the lips, oral mucous membranes, tongue, throat, and esophagus. Delayed effects can arise from absorption via the small intestine into the blood with effects on distant organs and tissues. In inhalation, immediate injury can occur from irritation of the airways resulting in extensive edema and damaged tissue. Delayed, systemic effects occur when the agent travels through the bloodstream and interacts with distant organs and tissues. In surface absorption, immediate injury can occur in the involved skin or mucous membranes. Delayed effects again relate to absorption into the bloodstream. With injection, immediate injury is seen as irritation at the injection site, usually visible as red, irritated, edematous skin. Delayed, systemic effects are again due to distribution throughout the body via the bloodstream.
- *Assessment:* Certain basic principles of assessment apply to most toxicological emergencies. For instance, maintain a high index of suspicion that a poisoning or drug overdose may have occurred. During scene size-up, look for potential dangers to yourself and other rescuers, such as a threat of violence from suicidal patients and the threat of accidental injection from used needles that may be hidden on the patient's person or at the scene. In cases with chemicals and

hazardous materials, it is crucial that you use the proper clothing and equipment. Be sure that such articles are distributed to team members who have been trained in their use.

Assessment of the patient begins with a history if the patient appears to be able to give one. Critical questions include what kind of toxin the patient was exposed to and when exposure occurred (so you have clues for likelihood of immediate or delayed effects or both). Physical involves a rapid head-to-toe exam with full vital signs.

- *Time needs:* In accordance with your local protocols, relay information to Poison Control. Generally speaking, you never want to delay initiation of supportive or definitive care or transport because of delays in sending information to, or receiving information from, Poison Control. Time is of the essence, literally. Ongoing assessment is particularly important for this group of patients because they can deteriorate rapidly. Repeat initial assessment and vitals every five minutes for critical or unstable patients and every fifteen minutes for stable patients. Specific assessment findings are given for each type of agent.
- *General management:* The preliminary steps of management include securing rescuer safety and removing the patient from any toxic environment. Support ABCs as you would with any other patient, keeping in mind that damage may have occurred to the mouth, pharynx, and/or airway in inhalation injury, and to the mouth and pharynx in ingestion incidents. The direct access to the cardiovascular system that occurs with injection cases may also complicate support of the ABCs.

The first management step specific to toxicological emergencies is decontamination, that is, minimization of toxicity by reducing the amount of toxin absorbed into the body. Decontamination involves three steps: The first is reduction of intake of toxin (steps will be route-specific, such as removal from fume-filled atmosphere in inhalation, removal of clothes and cleansing of skin in surface absorption, removal of stinger in injection, etc.).

The second step is reduction of absorption after toxin is in the body, and this usually applies to ingestion incidents. The most common method entails use of activated charcoal to bind molecules of the toxin to it and prevent absorption into the bloodstream. Gastric lavage (stomach pumping) is of limited use as a step to reduce absorption. Lavage must be done within about one hour of exposure to be effective, and its possible complications (aspiration and perforation) are significant. Lavage is uncommon except in specific circumstances, for example, when the toxin doesn't bind to activated charcoal or when the toxin has no antidote. The third step in decontamination is enhanced elimination of toxin from the body. Cathartics enhance gastric mobility and thus may shorten the time the toxin is in the GI tract. Know the limitations in use of cathartics in your area, especially among pediatric patients, in whom they can induce severe electrolyte disturbances. Whole bowel irrigation with use of a gastric tube seems to be effective and carries few potential complications; however, its use is limited to only a few centers.

The third management step specific to toxicological emergencies is use of an antidote, a substance that neutralizes the specific toxin and counteracts its effects in the body. As you can see in Table 8-1 on text page 434, there are not many antidotes, and few are 100% effective. Your best guide is to be thoroughly knowledgeable with your local protocols, the directions given by the Poison Control Center, and by counsel given by Medical Control.

7. **List the most common poisonings, pathophysiology, assessment findings, and management of poisoning by ingestion, inhalation, absorption, injection, and overdose.** pp. 430–468

Ingestion is the most common route of poisoning that you will see. Frequently ingested poisons include household products, petroleum-based agents such as gasoline and paint, cleaning agents such as alkalis and soaps, cosmetics, drugs (prescription, non-prescription, and illicit), plants, and foods. Some poisons can remain in the stomach for several hours, which may permit removal of the poison from the stomach and the body before systemic absorption can occur via passage through the small intestine. In at least one case, ingestion of aspirin, removal from the stomach is difficult because the ingested tablets bind together to form one large bolus. Useful questions for historical assessment include: (1) What did you ingest? (Obtain samples or containers whenever possible) (2) When did you ingest the substance? (3) How much did you ingest? (4) Did you drink any alcohol? (5) Have you attempted to treat yourself? (including induction of vomiting) (6) Have you been under mental health care, and, if so, why? (answer may indicate potential for suicide) (7) What is your weight? Physical exam is especially important because history may be unavailable or unreliable. Your exam should provide physical evidence of intoxication and discover co-morbid conditions that may affect treatment or response. Pay particular attention to skin, eyes, mouth, chest, circulation status, and abdomen (review text page 435). Be aware that a patient may have ingested multiple substances. Management centers on prevention of aspiration, intubation where necessary (RSI may be required to avoid patient's clamping down on tube), use of high-flow oxygen, and IV access for volume replacement and possible IV drug administration. Remember that it is always important to have ongoing cardiac monitoring and reassessment of vital signs.

Toxic inhalations can be self-induced or due to accidental exposure. Commonly inhaled poisons include toxic gases, carbon monoxide, ammonia, chlorine, freon, toxic vapors, fumes, or aerosols (from products such as paint and other hydrocarbons, glue, etc.), carbon tetrachloride, methyl chloride, tear gas, mustard gas, amyl nitrite, butyl nitrite, and nitrous oxide. Inhaled toxins primarily cause direct injury in the respiratory system, and these problems may be most severe in patients who inhaled a chemical or propellant concentrated in either a paper or plastic bag.

Given the pathophysiology of inhaled toxins, you should look for signs/symptoms related to three major systems: the central nervous system (dizziness, headache, confusion, hallucinations, seizures, or coma), the respiratory system (tachypnea, cough, hoarseness, stridor, dyspnea, retractions, wheezing, chest pain or tightness, rales or rhonchi), and the heart (dysrhythmias). Management starts with protecting yourself from any toxins in the atmosphere and removal of the patient from the injurious environment. Follow these guidelines: Wear protective clothing, use appropriate respiratory protection, and remove the patient's contaminated clothing. Then you can perform the initial assessment, history, and physical examination focusing on the central nervous system, respiratory, and cardiac systems. Support ABCs as you would with any other patient, keeping in mind that damage may have occurred to the mouth, pharynx, and/or airway as a direct, immediate injury. Contact medical direction and your Poison Control Center according to your particular protocols.

For **surface absorption,** the most common contacts are with poisonous plants such as poison ivy, poison sumac, and poison oak. Many toxic chemicals can be absorbed through the skin. Organophosphates, which are used as pesticides, are easily absorbed through the skin and mucous membranes, as is cyanide. The signs and symptoms vary widely depending on the toxin involved. Whenever you suspect surface absorption, take the following general steps: (1) wear protective clothing; (2) use appropriate respiratory protection; (3) remove the patient's contaminated clothing; (4) perform initial assessment, history, and physical exam; (5) initiate supportive measures; and (6) contact Poison Control Center and medical direction.

Females in the insect class *Hymenoptera,* honeybees, hornets, yellow jackets, wasps, and fire ants, are common causes of **injection injury.** In addition, spiders, ticks, snakes, and certain marine animals are known causes of toxic exposure by injection. In addition to intentional injections, most poisonings by injection involve bites and stings from insects and animals. Be alert for the possibility of allergic reactions or anaphylaxis. Over time, beware of delayed systemic reactions. General principles of field management include the following: (1) protection of all rescue personnel because the culprit organism may still be in the area; (2) removal of the patient from danger of repeated injection (particularly in the case of yellow jackets, wasps, or hornets); (3) whenever possible and safe, obtain the injury-causing organism and bring it to the emergency department; (4) perform initial assessment and rapid physical exam; (5) prevent or delay further absorption of the poison; (6) initiate supportive measures as needed; (7) watch for anaphylaxis; (8) transport as rapidly as possible; and (9) contact Poison Control Center and medical direction per protocols.

8. **Define the following terms:**

   a. **Substance or drug abuse**   p. 461

      Substance or drug abuse is use of a pharmacological product for purposes other than medically defined reasons.

b. Substance or drug dependence
p. 461

Substance or drug dependence is the same thing as addiction: Physiological dependence exists if discontinuance of the drug would cause adverse physical reactions. Psychological dependence exists if discontinuance of the drug would cause the presence or increase in tension or emotional stress.

c. Tolerance
p. 461

Tolerance is a phenomenon associated with continued use of a drug; it implies that the user must take increasingly large doses of the drug in order to achieve the same effect.

d. Withdrawal
p. 462

Withdrawal refers to alcohol or drug discontinuance in which the patient's body reacts severely when deprived of the abused substance.

e. Addiction
p. 461

Addiction is the same thing as dependence: Addiction can have a physiological or psychological component or both.

9. List the most commonly abused drugs (both by chemical name and by street names). pp. 464–465

The most commonly abused drugs include: (1) alcohol in its fermented and distilled forms; (2) barbiturates such as phenobarbital and thiopental; (3) cocaine (both crack and rock forms); (4) narcotics/opiates such as heroin, codeine, meperidine, morphine, hydromorphone, pentazocine, methadone, Darvon, and Darvocet; (5) marijuana and hashish (also called grass or weed on the street); (6) amphetamines such as Benzedrine, Dexedrine, and Ritalin (called speed on the street); (7) hallucinogens including LSD, STP, mescaline, psilocybin, and PCP (also called angel dust); (8) sedatives from different chemical families such as Seconal, Valium, Librium, Xanax, Halcion, Restoril, Dalmane, and phenobarbital; and (9) the benzodiazepines, Valium, Librium, Xanax, Halcion, Restoril, Dalmane, Centrax, Ativan, and Serax.

10. Describe the pathophysiology, assessment findings, and management of commonly used drugs. pp. 438–452, 461–468

In addition to the specific drugs discussed in objective 11 below, it is notable that many groups of drugs produce definable toxic syndromes. Knowledge of these syndromes is useful because it helps you cluster information for compounds that produce similar clinical pictures. (1) Anticholinergic toxidrome is caused by belladonna alkaloids, atropine, scopolamine, synthetic anticholinergics, and incidental anticholinergics such as antihistamines, tricyclic antidepressants, and phenothiazines. Signs and symptoms include dry skin/mucous membranes, blurred near vision, fixed dilated pupils, tachycardia, hyperthermia and flushing, lethargy, and CNS signs, respiratory failure, and cardiovascular collapse. Management is as described for the tricyclics in objective 11. (2) Narcotic toxidrome is due to illicit drugs such as heroin and opium, prescription narcotics such as meperidine and methadone, and combination medications including narcotic agents such as hydromorphone, diphenoxylate (Lomotil), and oxycodone. Assessment findings include CNS depression, pinpoint pupils, slowed respirations, hypotension, positive response to naloxone. Note that pupils may be dilated and excitement may predominate the clinical picture. Management is described in objective 11 below. (3) The sympathomimetic toxidrome is caused by aminophylline, amphetamines, caffeine, cocaine, ephedrine, dopamine, methylphenidate (Ritalin), and phencyclidine. Features include CNS excitation, hypertension, seizures, tachycardia (hypotension with caffeine). Management is discussed in objective 11.

11. List the clinical uses, street names, pharmacology, assessment findings, and management for patients who have taken the following drugs or been exposed to the following substances:

a. Cocaine
pp. 462–464

Cocaine has sympathomimetic effects, and assessment findings include CNS excitation, dilated pupils, hyperactivity, hypertension, seizures, tachycardia, and hypotension if taken with caffeine. Benzodiazepines may be required for seizures or diazepam 5–10 mg can be given as a seizure precaution; beta blockers are contraindicated because their unopposed alpha receptor stimulation can cause cardiac ischemia, increased hypertension, and hyperthermia. General measures include ABCs, respiratory support and oxygenation, ECG monitoring, IV access, and treatment of any life-threatening dysrhythmia.

b. Marijuana and cannabis compounds p. 465

Marijuana and related compounds can be smoked (inhaled) or taken orally, and pertinent signs and symptoms include euphoria, dry mouth, dilated pupils, and altered sensation. Management centers on ABCs, reassurance and speaking in a quiet voice, and ECG monitoring if indicated.

c. Amphetamines and amphetamine-like drugs pp. 463, 465

Amphetamines are CNS stimulants that can be taken orally or injected. Assessment findings include exhilaration, hyperactivity, dilated pupils, hypertension, psychosis, tremors, and seizures. Management centers on ABCs, oxygenation and ECG monitoring, IV access, treatment of any life-threatening dysrhythmia, and diazepam 5–10 mg as a seizure precaution. Diazepam and haloperidol in combination may be useful in controlling hyperactivity.

d. Barbiturates pp. 463, 464

The barbiturates, which are CNS depressants, can be taken orally or injected. Signs and symptoms include lethargy, emotional lability, incoordination, slurred speech, nystagmus, coma, hypotension, and respiratory depression. Management focuses on ABCs and respiratory support with oxygenation, IV access, ECG monitoring, and contact with Poison Control. Alkalinization of urine and diuresis may improve elimination of barbiturates from the body.

e. Sedative-hypnotics p. 465

Sedative-hypnotics are generally taken orally, and they are also CNS depressants. Assessment findings include altered mental status, hypotension, slurred speech, respiratory depression, shock, bradycardia, and seizures. Management centers on ABCs with respiratory support and oxygenation, IV access, ECG monitoring, and possible use of naloxone dependent on agent taken and advice of medical direction.

f. Cyanide pp. 438–439

Cyanide can enter the body by different routes dependent on the product in which it is found. It is present in household items such as rodenticides and silver polish, as well as in foods such as fruit pits and seeds. It can be liberated into inhalable form through burning of nitrogen-containing products such as plastics, silks, or synthetic carpets. Cyanide also forms in patients on long-term therapy with nitroprusside. Regardless of entry, cyanide acts extremely quickly as a cellular asphyxiant, inhibiting the vital process of cellular respiration. Signs and symptoms include a burning sensation in mouth and throat, headache, confusion, combative behavior, hypertension, and tachycardia, followed by hypotension and further dysrhythmias, seizures and coma, and pulmonary edema. Management relies on removal from the source, immediate supportive measures, and treatment with a cyanide antidote kit containing amyl nitrite ampules, a sodium nitrite, and a sodium thiosulfate solution. Adding nitrites to blood converts some hemoglobin to methemoglobin, which binds cyanide, removing it from its free form in the blood. Thiosulfate binds with cyanide to form a soluble nontoxic compound. Note: Cyanide is rapidly toxic, so it is crucial you be familiar with a cyanide antidote kit if your unit carries one.

g. Narcotics/opiates p. 464

The narcotics can be taken orally or by injection. Pertinent assessment findings include CNS depression, constricted pupils, respiratory depression, hypotension, bradycardia, pulmonary edema, and coma. General management centers on ABCs with respiratory support and oxygenation, IV access, and ECG monitoring. You may use the antidote naloxone, which can be titrated to relieve symptoms of toxicity without provoking withdrawal symptoms in addicts. General instructions involve use of 1–2 mg naloxone IV or endotracheally per medical direction until respiration improves. Larger doses (2–5 mg) may be required in the management of Darvon overdose and alcoholic coma.

h. Cardiac medications
pp. 442–443

The number of available cardiac medications grows continually, and many classes exist, including antidysrhythmics, beta blockers, calcium channel blockers, glycosides, ACE inhibitors, etc. General pharmacology includes regulation of heart function by reducing heart rate, suppressing automaticity, reducing vascular tone, or some combination of these. Although overdose can be intentional, it often is due to an error in dosage. At the level of overdose, signs and symptoms include (1) nausea and vomiting, (2) headache, dizziness, and confusion, (3) profound hypotension, (4) cardiac dysrhythmias (usually bradycardic), (5) cardiac conduction blocks, and (6) bronchospasm and pulmonary edema (especially with beta blockers). Management centers on initiating standard toxicological emergency assessment and treatment immediately. Severe bradycardia may not respond well to atropine, so you should have an external pacing device at hand. Some cardiac medications have antidotes; these include calcium for calcium channel blockers, glucagon for beta blockers, and digoxin-specific Fab (Digibind) for digoxin. Contact medical direction before giving any of these antidotes.

i. Caustics
pp. 443–444

Caustic substances can either be acids or alkalis, and such substances are common at home and in the industrial workplace. Strong caustics can cause severe burns at the site of contact; if ingested, they can cause tissue destruction at the lips, mouth, esophagus, and more distal regions of the GI tract. Strong acids by definition have a pH less than 2; they are found in plumbing solutions and bathroom cleaners. Contact usually produces immediate, severe pain due to tissue coagulation and necrosis. Often this type of burn produces an eschar over the site, which may act as a shield to protect deeper tissues from damage. Because the substance is in the stomach much longer than the esophagus, the stomach is the more likely to sustain damage. Immediate or delayed hemorrhage is possible, as is perforation. Absorption of acids into the bloodstream produces acidemia, which needs to be managed along with the local, direct effects. Strong alkaline agents by definition have a pH greater than 12.5; they are present in solid or liquid form in household products such as drain cleaners. These agents cause local injury through liquefaction necrosis. Because of a delay in pain sensation, these agents are often present longer at the site of contact, allowing for greater tissue damage and deeper tissue injury. Solid products can stick to the oropharynx or esophagus, causing bleeding, perforation, and inflammation of central chest structures. Liquid alkalis are more likely to injure the stomach because, like the liquid strong acids, they pass quickly through the esophagus. Within 1–2 days of exposure to a strong alkali, complete loss of mucosal tissue can occur, followed either by gradual healing or further bleeding, necrosis, and stricture formation. Assessment findings include facial burns, pain in the lips, tongue, throat and/or gums, drooling and trouble swallowing, hoarseness, stridor, or shortness of breath, and shock from bleeding and vomiting. Both assessment and initiation of management must be rapid and aggressive to avoid significant morbidity and mortality. As with other toxicological situations, protect yourself and initiate standard toxicological assessment and treatment: Pay particular attention to the airway. Injury to the oropharynx and/or larynx may make airway control and ventilation very difficult and may go so far as to require cricothyrotomy. Because caustic substances do not adhere to activated charcoal, there is no indication for it. It is controversial whether ingestion of milk or water acts effectively to coat the stomach lining or dilute the caustic. It is clear that rapid transport is essential. Hydrofluoric acid, which is used to clean glass in laboratory settings and in etching glass in art work, is a specific example of a strong acid that can be lethal in even small exposure doses. Management specific to this agent is immersion of the exposed limb in iced water with magnesium sulfate, calcium salts, or benzethonium chloride (see textbook p. 444).

j. Common household substances
pp. 443–444

Many of these substances contain caustic agents (either strong acids or strong alkalis) as major ingredients; see objective i above for details.

k. Drugs abused for sexual purposes/sexual gratification
p. 463

This group includes a number of miscellaneous agents that are used to stimulate and enhance sexual experience but do not have medically approved indications for such use. MDMA, popularly known as Ecstasy, is an example. Ecstasy is a modified form of methamphetamine and has similar, although milder, effects. Look for its use on college campuses and in nightclub settings. Initial signs and symptoms of use include anxiety, tachycardia, nausea, and hypertension, followed by relaxation, euphoria, and feelings of enhanced emotional insight. Studies indicate prolonged use may cause brain damage. Cases that can lead to death have the following assessment findings: confusion, agitation, tremor, high temperature, and diarrhea. No specific treatment exists, so supportive measures should be taken. Flunitrazepam, or Rohypnol, is illegal in the U.S. but has been used as a "date rape drug" when slipped into a woman's drink. The drug is a strong benzodiazepine that causes sedation and amnesia. When this drug is suspected, treat as for other benzodiazepines but remember to look for consequences of sexual assault and be sure to treat them as well.

l. Carbon monoxide   p. 439

Carbon monoxide is a tasteless, odorless gas that is often created by incomplete combustion. Because of its chemical structure, it has an affinity for hemoglobin over 200 times greater than that of oxygen. Once carbon monoxide has bound to hemoglobin, it is very difficult to displace and it causes an effective hypoxia. Because of the variability of signs and symptoms (depending on dose and duration of exposure), many people ignore poisoning until toxic levels are in the blood. Early symptoms resemble those of the flu. Combining likely causes of carbon monoxide generation with early symptoms raises this red flag: Beware carbon monoxide poisoning in multiple patients living together in a poorly heated and ventilated space who have "flu-like" symptoms. Specific signs and symptoms include headache, nausea and vomiting, confusion or other manifestation of altered mental status, and tachypnea. Because of the difficulty of displacing carbon monoxide from hemoglobin, definitive treatment may require use of a hyperbaric chamber (in which oxygen is present at greater than atmospheric pressure). In the field, take these steps: Ensure safety of rescuing personnel, remove the patient(s) from contaminated area, begin immediate ventilation of affected area, and initiate supportive measures including high-flow oxygen via nonrebreather device (this last is critical).

m. Alcohols   pp. 463–468

Ethyl alcohol is the form of alcohol in beverages, and it is the single most common substance of abuse among Americans. Alcoholism, dependence on alcohol, progresses in much the same way as drug dependence discussed earlier in the chapter. The early symptoms of alcohol use, especially at low doses, include loss of inhibitions and emotionally excitatory effects, which can cause some of the aberrant behaviors associated with alcohol intoxication. Once ingested, alcohol is completely absorbed from the stomach and intestinal tract within approximately 30–120 minutes. After absorption, it is widely distributed in blood to all body tissues, and concentrations of alcohol in the brain rapidly approach the level in the blood. Alcohol's major physiologic effects are as a CNS depressant: toxicity, can include stupor, coma, and death. Because the liver is the major site of detoxification within the body, compromise of liver function increases the course and severity of alcohol intoxication. Another significant health effect is peripheral vasodilation, which results in flushing of the skin and a feeling of warmth. In cold conditions, this can increase loss of body heat and help to produce hypothermia. Alcohol-related diuresis is due to inhibition of vasopressin, a hormone responsible for homeostasis of water balance. The dry mouth associated with hangovers may in part be due to the alcohol-induced dehydration. Methanol, wood alcohol, is so toxic it is not safe for human consumption. However, methanol toxicity can occur either as an accident or because an alcoholic individual could not obtain ethyl alcohol. Methanol causes visual disturbances, abdominal pain, and nausea and vomiting even at low doses. Occasionally, methanol toxic patients complain of headache or dizziness or present with seizures and obtundation. Ethylene glycol, a related compound, can also be involved in toxic emergencies. It produces similar symptoms, but its CNS effects, including hallucinations, coma, and seizures, present at even earlier stages.

Assessment findings in an individual with chronic alcoholism include poor nutrition, alcoholic hepatitis, liver cirrhosis with subsequent esophageal varices, loss of sensation in hands and feet, loss of cerebellar function shown as poor balance and coordination, pancreatitis, upper GI hemorrhage (which is often fatal), hypoglycemia, subdural hematoma secondary to falls, and rib and extremity fractures, also secondary to falls. When you are in the field, keep in mind that conditions such as a subdural hematoma, sepsis, and diabetic ketoacidosis can, along with other conditions, mimic alcohol intoxication. For instance, the breath odor of ketoacidosis can resemble that of alcohol.

Abrupt discontinuance of alcohol by a dependent individual may provoke a withdrawal syndrome that can prove to be potentially lethal. Withdrawal symptoms can occur several hours after sudden abstinence and last up to 5–7 days. Common signs and symptoms include a coarse tremor of hands, tongue, and eyelids, nausea and vomiting, general weakness, increased sympathetic tone, tachycardia, sweating, hypertension, orthostatic hypotension, anxiety, irritability or depressed mood, and poor sleep. Seizures may occur, as can delirium tremens (DTs). DTs usually develop on the second or third day of withdrawal and are characterized by a decreased level of consciousness associated with hallucinations and misinterpretation of nearby events. Both seizures and delirium tremens are ominous signs.

Alcohol intoxication, whether acute or chronic, should not be underestimated as a toxic emergency. In cases of suspected alcohol abuse, manage as follows: (1) Establish and maintain the airway, (2) determine if other drugs or substances are involved, (3) start an IV with lactated Ringer's solution or normal saline, (4) use a Chemstrip and give 25 g $D_{50}W$ if the patient is hypoglycemic, (5) administer 100 mg thiamine IV or IM, (6) maintain a sympathetic and supportive attitude with the patient, and (7) transport to emergency department for further care. Note: Medical direction may suggest diazepam in severe cases of seizure or hallucination.

n. Hydrocarbons   pp. 444–445
Numerous household substances contain hydrocarbons, organic compounds composed primarily of carbon and hydrogen. Hydrocarbons include kerosene, naphtha, turpentine, mineral oil, chloroform, toluene, and benzene, and they are found in lighter fluid, paint, glue, lubricants, solvents, and aerosol propellants. Exposure can be via ingestion, inhalation, or surface absorption. Signs and symptoms of hydrocarbon exposure vary according to agent, dose, and route of exposure, but common problems include burns due to local contact, respiratory signs (wheezing, dyspnea, hypoxia, or pneumonitis from aspiration or inhalation), CNS signs (headache, dizziness, slurred speech, ataxia, and obtundation), foot and wrist drop with numbness and tingling, and cardiac dysrhythmias. Research has shown that fewer than 1% of hydrocarbon poisonings require physician care. In cases where you know the agent in question and in which the patient is asymptomatic, medical direction may permit the patient to stay at home. On the other hand, hydrocarbon poisonings can be very serious. If the patient is symptomatic, does not know the causative agent, or has taken a specific agent (such as halogenated or aromatic hydrocarbon compounds) that requires GI decontamination, standard toxicological emergency procedures and prompt transport are indicated.

o. Psychiatric medications   pp. 445–448
The tricyclic antidepressants were standard therapy for depression for years, despite concerns that their generally narrow therapeutic window made accidental toxic-level exposure, as well as intentional overdose, potentially common. Despite the introduction of newer, safer antidepressants, a number of tricyclics are still in use for depression, as well as chronic pain syndromes and migraine prophylaxis. Agents still in use include amitriptyline (Elavil), amoxapine, clomipramine, doxepin, imipramine, and nortriptyline. Signs and symptoms on assessment include dry mouth, blurred vision, urinary retention, and constipation. Late into overdose, you may find confusion and hallucinations, hyperthermia, respiratory depression, seizures, tachycardia and hypotension, and cardiac dysrhythmias (such as heart block, wide QRS complex, and *torsade de pointes*.) In addition to standard toxicological procedures, cardiac monitoring is critical because dysrhythmias are the most common cause of death. If you suspect a mixed overdose with a benzodiazepine, DO NOT use Flumazenil because it might precipitate a seizure. If significant cardiac toxicity is evident, sodium bicarbonate may be used as an additional therapy; contact Medical Control as needed.

p. Newer anti-depressants and serotonin syndromes   p. 447
In the recent past, a number of new antidepressants that are not related to the tricyclics have been introduced. Because of their high safety profile in both therapeutic and overdose amounts, these drugs have virtually replaced the tricyclics in clinical practice. This group includes trazodone (Desyrel), bupropion (Wellbutrin), and the large group of drugs known as selective serotonin reuptake inhibitors (SSRIs). Drugs in this group include Prozac, Luvox,

Paxil, and Zoloft. Their pharmacology, as indicated by group name, centers on prevention of reuptake of serotonin from neural synapses in the brain, theoretically raising the amount of serotonin available to modulate brain function. The usual signs and symptoms in overdose cases are generally mild, including drowsiness, tremor, nausea and vomiting, and sinus tachycardia. Occasionally trazodone and bupropion cause CNS depression and seizures, but deaths are rare, and they have been reported in situations with mixed overdoses and multiple ingestions. You should know that the SSRIs have been associated with serotonin syndrome, a constellation of signs/symptoms correlated with increased serotonin level and triggered by increasing the dose of SSRI or adding a second drug such as a narcotic or another antidepressant. Serotonin syndrome is marked by the following: (1) agitation, anxiety, confusion, and insomnia, (2) headache, drowsiness, and coma, (3) nausea, salivation, diarrhea, and abdominal cramps, (4) cutaneous piloerection and flushed skin, (5) hyperthermia and tachycardia, and (6) rigidity, shivering, incoordination, and myoclonic jerks. Because of the lower morbidity and mortality in these drugs compared with overdoses with the older antidepressants, standard toxicological emergency procedures suffice. The patient should discontinue all serotonergic drugs and you should institute supportive measures. Benzodiazepines or beta blockers are occasionally used to improve patient comfort, but they are rarely given in the field.

q. Lithium   pp. 447–448
Lithium is the most effective drug used in the treatment of bipolar disorder (a psychiatric disorder also known as manic depression). Pharmacology is unclear. However, it is known that lithium has a narrow therapeutic index, making toxicity relatively common during normal use and in overdose situations. Assessment findings of toxicity include thirst and dry mouth, tremor, muscle twitching, increased reflexes, confusion, stupor, seizures, coma, nausea, vomiting, diarrhea, and bradycardia and dysrhythmias. Lithium overdose should be treated primarily with supportive measures. Use standard toxicological procedures but remember that activated charcoal does not bind lithium and should not be used. Alkalinization of the urine with sodium bicarbonate and diuresis with mannitol may increase elimination of lithium, but severe toxicity requires hemodialysis.

r. MAO inhibitors   p. 446
Monoamine oxidase inhibitors (MAO inhibitors) have been used historically as psychiatric agents, primarily as antidepressants. Recently they have found limited use as treatment for obsessive-compulsive disorder. These drugs have always had relatively limited usage for several reasons: They have a narrow therapeutic index, multiple drug interactions, potentially serious interactions with foods rich in tyramine (for instance, red wine and cheese), and high morbidity and mortality in overdose incidents. The pharmacology of MAO inhibitors directly affects CNS neurotransmitters: The drugs inhibit the breakdown of norepinephrine and dopamine while increasing the molecular components necessary to produce more. Remember that overdose with this group of drugs is very serious, even though symptoms may not appear for up to 6 hours. Assessment findings include headache, agitation, restlessness, tremor, nausea, palpitations, tachycardia, severe hypertension, hyperthermia, and eventually bradycardia, hypotension, coma, and death. Newer MAO inhibitors have been introduced into the marketplace; they appear to be less toxic and avoid the food interactions that involved the older generation of MAO inhibitors. They are reversible in effect; however, overdose outcome data are not yet available for these drugs. Management includes reversal if the drug is in the newer class of reversible MAO inhibitors, prompt institution of standard toxicological procedures, and, if needed, symptomatic support for seizures and hyperthermia with use of benzodiazepines. If a vasopressor is needed, use norepinephrine.

s. Non-prescription pain medications: (1) nonsteroidal anti-inflammatory agents (2) salicylates (3) acetaminophen   pp. 448–450
(1) Nonsteroidal anti-inflammatory agents (called NSAIDs) are a large, commonly used group of drugs such as naproxen sodium, indomethacin, ibuprofen, and ketorolac (Toradol). Overdose is common, and assessment findings include headache, ringing in the ears (tinnitus), nausea, vomiting, abdominal pain, swelling of the extremities, mild drowsiness, dyspnea, wheezing, pulmonary edema, and rash and itching. There is no specific antidote for NSAID

toxicity, so use general overdose procedures including supportive care and transport to the emergency department for evaluation and any necessary symptomatic treatment.

(2) Salicylates are some of the most common over-the-counter drugs taken and among the most common taken in overdose. They include aspirin, oil of wintergreen, and some prescription combination medications. About 300 mg/kg aspirin can cause toxicity. In these amounts, the salicylate inhibits normal energy production and acid buffering in the body, resulting in metabolic acidosis that further injures other organ systems. Assessment findings include tachypnea, hyperthermia, confusion, lethargy and coma, cardiac failure and dysrhythmias, abdominal pain and vomiting, and non-cardiogenic (inflammatory) pulmonary edema and adult respiratory distress syndrome. The findings of chronic overdose are somewhat less severe and tend not to include abdominal complaints. It is thus difficult to distinguish chronic overdose from early acute overdose or acute overdose that has progressed past the initial abdominal irritation stage. In all cases, management of salicylate poisoning should be treated with use of standard toxicological emergency procedures. Activated charcoal definitely reduces drug absorption and should be used. If possible, learn the time of ingestion because blood levels measured at the right interval can be indicative of the expected degree of injury. Most symptomatic patients require generous IV fluids and may need urine alkalinization with sodium bicarbonate. Severe cases may require dialysis.

(3) Acetaminophen (paracetamol, Tylenol) has few side effects in normal dosage, and it is one of the most commonly used drugs in America for fever/pain. It is also a common ingredient in combination medications and is found in some prescription combination medications. In large doses, acetaminophen can be very dangerous: A dose of 150 mg/kg is considered toxic and may result in death secondary to liver damage. A highly reactive metabolite is responsible for most adverse effects, but this is avoided in most cases by detoxification. When large amounts enter the body in overdose, this detoxification system is overloaded and gradually depleted, leaving the metabolite in the circulation to cause liver necrosis. It is important for you to learn and remember that the signs and symptoms of toxicity appear in four stages: Stage 1—0.5 to 24 hours after ingestion, marked by nausea, vomiting, weakness, and fatigue; Stage 2—24 to 48 hours, marked by abdominal pain, decreased urine, elevated liver enzymes; Stage 3—72 to 96 hours, marked by liver function disruption; and Stage 4—4 to 14 days, marked by gradual recovery or progressive liver failure. Field management relies on standard toxicological procedures. Again, it is important to find time of ingestion because this may allow blood levels to be drawn at a time appropriate to predict potential injury. An antidote (N-acetylcysteine, or NAC, Mucomyst) is available and highly effective. However, NAC is usually given based on clinical and lab studies and in the hospital setting.

t. Theophylline p. 450
Theophylline is a member of the group of drugs called xanthines. It is generally used by patients with asthma or COPD because it has moderate bronchodilation and mild anti-inflammatory effects. It has a narrow therapeutic index and high toxicity, so it has been used less frequently recently. Thus, it is not a factor as often as it once was in overdose injuries. Assessment findings include agitation, tremors, seizures, cardiac dysrhythmias, and nausea and vomiting. Theophylline can cause significant morbidity and mortality. In an overdose setting, you must start toxicological emergency procedures immediately. Theophylline is on a short list of drugs that have significant entero-hepatic circulation. Thus, activated charcoal in multiple doses over time will continuously remove more and more theophylline from the body. Dysrhythmias should be treated according to ACLS procedures.

u. Metals pp. 450–451
With the exception of iron, heavy metal overdose is rare. Metals that can cause toxicity include lead, arsenic, and mercury, all of which affect numerous enzyme systems in the body and thus cause a variety of symptoms. Some also have direct local effects when ingested and they accumulate in various organs.

- *Iron:* The body needs only small daily amounts of iron; excess amounts are easily obtained through non-prescription supplements and multivitamins. Children have the tendency to overdose on iron by taking too many candy-flavored chewable vitamins containing iron.

Symptoms occur when more than 20 mg/kg of elemental iron are ingested. Excess iron causes GI injury and possible hemorrhagic shock, especially if it forms concretions (lumps formed when tablets fuse together). Patients with significant iron ingestions may have visible tablets or concretions in the stomach or small intestine on X-ray. Other signs and symptoms include vomiting (often hematemesis) and diarrhea, abdominal pain, shock, liver failure, metabolic acidosis with tachypnea, and eventual bowel scarring and possible obstruction. It is essential to start standard toxicological procedures promptly. Because iron inhibits GI motility, tablets remain in the stomach for a long time and may possibly be easier to remove via gastric lavage (especially if concretions are not present). Because activated charcoal does not bind metals, it should not be used for iron overdose or for any other metal overdose. Deferoxamine, a chelating agent, may be used in iron overdose as an antidote because it binds iron such that less enters cells to cause damage.

- *Lead and mercury:* Both metals are found in varying amounts in the environment. Lead was often used in glazes and paints before its toxic potential was realized. Mercury is a contaminant from industrial processing and is also found in some thermometers and temperature-control switches in homes. Both acute and chronic overdose are possible with both metals. Signs and symptoms of heavy metal toxicity include headache, irritability, confusion, coma, memory disturbance, tremor, weakness, agitation, and abdominal pain. Chronic poisoning can result in permanent neurological injury, which makes it crucial that heavy metal levels be monitored in the environment of a patient with toxicity. You need to remember the signs and symptoms of heavy metal poisoning and promptly institute standard procedures. Although activated charcoal is not helpful, various chelating agents (such as DMSA, BAL, and CDE) are available and may be used in definitive management in the hospital.

v. Plants and mushrooms pp. 452–453

Plants, trees, and mushrooms are common contributors to accidental toxic ingestions. You should know that many decorative home plants can present a toxic danger to children. Most Poison Control Centers distribute pamphlets that list relevant household plants. In nature, it is impossible to identify all toxic plants and mushrooms. A general approach for you to take is to obtain a sample of the offending plant if possible, trying to find a complete leaf, stem, or flower. Mushrooms are very difficult to identify from small pieces. Because many ornamental plants contain irritating material, be sure to examine the patient's mouth and throat for redness, blistering, or edema. Identify other findings during the focused physical exam. Mushroom poisonings generally involve a mistake in identification of edible mushrooms or accidental ingestion by children. Mushrooms in the class *Amanita* account for over 90% of deaths; they produce a poison that is extremely toxic to the liver and carry a mortality rate of about 50%. Signs and symptoms of poisonous plant ingestion include excessive salivation, lacrimation, diaphoresis, abdominal cramps, nausea, vomiting, and diarrhea, as well as decreasing levels of consciousness, eventually progressing to coma. Contact Poison Control if at all possible for guidance on management. If contact isn't possible, follow the procedures outlined under food poisoning (text pages 451–452).

12. Discuss common causative agents or offending organisms, pharmacology, assessment findings, and management for a patient with food poisoning, a bite, or a sting. pp. 451–461

Food poisoning can be due to a variety of causes including bacteria, viruses, and bacterial-associated chemical toxins. All notoriously produce varying degrees of gastrointestinal distress. Bacterial food poisonings range in severity. Bacterial exotoxins (secreted by bacteria) and enterotoxins (exotoxins associated with GI diseases) cause nausea, vomiting, diarrhea, and abdominal pain. Food contaminated with the bacteria *Shigella, Salmonella,* or *E. coli* can produce more severe reactions, often leading to electrolyte imbalance and hypovolemia. The world's most toxic poison is produced by *Clostridium botulinum,* and exposure presents as severe respiratory distress or even arrest. Fortunately, botulism rarely occurs except in cases of improper food storage procedures such as canning. A variety of seafood poisonings result from toxins produced by dinoflagellate-contaminated shellfish such as clams, mussels, oysters, and scallops. This exposure syndrome is called paralytic shellfish poisoning and can lead to respiratory arrest in addition to the GI symptoms. Toxicological emergencies can also arise from toxins found within commonly eaten fish. Bony fish poisoning (Ciguatera poisoning) is most frequent in fish caught in the Pacific Ocean or along the tropical reefs of Florida and the West Indies. Ciguatera may have an incubation period of 2–6 hours before producing myalgia and paresthesia. Scombroid (histamine) poisoning results from bacterial contamination of mackerel, tuna, bonitos, and albacore. Both Ciguatera and scombroid poisoning cause the standard GI symptoms; scombroid poisoning also produces immediate facial flushing due to histamine-induced vasodilation.

Except for botulism, food poisoning is rarely life threatening and treatment is largely supportive. In cases of suspected food poisoning, contact Poison Control and medical direction, and take the following steps: (1) perform necessary assessment, (2) collect samples of suspected food source, (3) support ABCs with airway maintenance, high-flow oxygen, intubation or assisted ventilation as needed, and establish IV access. In addition, consider administration of antihistamines (especially in seafood poisonings) and antiemetics.

Spider and snake bites can be common and significant toxicological emergencies in certain parts of the country. The brown recluse spider lives in southern and midwestern states. It is found in large numbers in Tennessee, Arkansas, Oklahoma, and Texas. It has also been reported in Hawaii and California. The brown recluse is about 15 mm in length, generally lives in dark, dry locations, and can often be found in or around a house. The bites themselves are usually painless, and bites often occur at night while the victim is asleep. The initial, local reaction occurs within minutes and consists of a small erythematous macule surrounded by a white ring. Over the next 8 hours or so localized pain, redness, and swelling develop. Tissue necrosis develops over days to weeks. Other symptoms include fever, chills, nausea, vomiting, joint pain, and in severe cases, bleeding disorders (namely, disseminated intravascular coagulation, DIC). Treatment is largely supportive, and there is no antivenin. Antihistamines may reduce systemic reactions and surgical excision may be required for necrotic tissue. Black widow spiders live in all parts of the continental U.S. and are often found in woodpiles or brush. The female spider bites, and the venom is very potent, causing excessive neurotransmitter release at the synaptic junctions. Immediate, local reaction includes pain, redness, and swelling. Progressive muscle spasms of all large muscles can develop and are usually associated with severe pain. Other systemic symptoms are nausea, vomiting, sweating, seizures, paralysis, and decreased level of consciousness. Field treatment is largely supportive, with reassurance an important factor. IV muscle relaxants may be needed for severe spasms. If medical direction orders it, you may use diazepam or calcium gluconate. Calcium chloride is ineffective and should not be used. Because hypertensive crisis is possible, monitor BP carefully. Transport as rapidly as possible so antivenin can be given in the hospital.

There are several thousand snake bites annually in the U.S., but few deaths. The assessment findings depend on snake, location of the bite, and the type and amount of venom injected. Two families of poisonous snakes are native to the U.S.: the pit vipers (cottonmouths, rattlesnakes, and copperheads) and the coral snake, a distant relative of the cobra. Pit viper venom contains hydrolytic enzymes capable of destroying most tissue components. They can produce hemolysis, destroy of other tissue elements, and may affect the clotting ability of the blood. They produce tissue infarction and necrosis, especially at the site of the bite. A severe pit viper bite can produce death within 30 minutes. However, most fatalities occur from 6 to 30 hours after the bite, with 90% within the first 48 hours. Assessment findings for pit viper bites include fang marks (often little more than a scratch or abrasion), swelling and pain at wound site, continued oozing from wound, weakness, dizziness, or faintness, sweating and/or chills, thirst, nausea and vomiting, diarrhea, tachycardia and hypotension, bloody urine and GI hemorrhage (these are late), ecchymosis, necrosis, shallow respirations progressing to respiratory failure, and numbness and tingling around face and head. The first goal in treatment is to slow absorption of venom; remember that about 25% of bites are dry, that is, no venom is injected. Antivenin is available but should only be considered for severe cases as evidence by marked systemic signs and symptoms. Routine treatment involves keeping the patient supine, immobilizing the affected limb with a splint, maintaining the extremity in a neutral position without any constricting bands, and giving supportive care with high-flow oxygen, IV with crystalloid fluid, and rapid transport. Note: DO NOT apply ice, cold pack, or freon spray to wound, DO NOT apply an arterial tourniquet, and DO NOT apply electrical stimulation from any source in an attempt to retard or reverse venom spread.

Coral snakes, which are small and with small fangs, are primarily found in the southwest. A mnemonic that you should remember is "Red touch yellow, kill a fellow; red touch black, venom lack." This indicates the stripe pattern of the coral snake: red-yellow-black-yellow-red. Coral snake venom contains some of the same enzymes as pit viper venom, but it additionally has a neurotoxin that will result in respiratory and skeletal muscle paralysis. Assessment findings include the following (noting that there may be no local or systemic effects for as long as 12–24 hours): localized numbness, weakness, and drowsiness, ataxia, slurred speech and excessive salivation, paralysis of tongue and larynx producing difficulty in swallowing and breathing, drooping of eyelids, double vision, dilated pupils, abdominal pain, nausea and vomiting, loss of consciousness, seizures, respiratory failure, and hypotension. Treatment includes the following steps: (1) wash the wound with lots of water, (2) apply a compression bandage and keep extremity at the level of the heart, (3) immobilize the limb with a splint, (4) start an IV with crystalloid fluid, and (5) transport to the emergency department for antivenin. Note: DO NOT apply ice, cold pack, or freon spray to the wound; DO NOT incise the wound; and DO NOT apply electrical stimulation from any device in an attempt to retard or reverse venom spread.

Stings (injection injuries) can come from insects and marine animals. Many people die from allergic reactions to insect stings, particularly wasps, bees, hornets, and fire ants. Only the common honeybee leaves a stinger. Wasps, hornets, yellow jackets, and fire ants sting repeatedly until removed from contact. Assessment findings include localized pain, redness, swelling, and a skin wheal. Idiosyncratic reactions are not considered allergic if they respond well to antihistamines. Signs and symptoms of an allergic reaction include localized pain, swelling, redness, and skin wheal, itching or flushing of skin or rash, tachycardia, hypotension, bronchospasm, or laryngeal edema, facial edema, and uvular swelling. General management includes washing of the sting area, gentle removal of stinger, if present (scrape, do not squeeze), application of cool compresses, and observation for allergic reaction or anaphylactic shock. Marine animal injection injuries are a threat in some coastal areas, especially in warmer, tropical waters. Toxin injection can be from jellyfish or coral stings or from punctures by the bony spines of animals such as sea urchins and stingrays. All marine venoms contain substances that produce pain that is disproportionate to the size of the injury. These toxins are unstable and heat sensitive, and heat will relieve the pain and inactivate the venom. Signs and symptoms of marine animal injection include intense local pain and swelling, weakness, nausea and vomiting, dyspnea, tachycardia, and hypotension or shock (in severe cases). In any case of suspected injection, treat by establishing and maintaining airway, application of a constriction bandage between the wound and the heart no tighter than a watchband (to occlude lymphatic flow only), application of heat or hot water, and inactivation or removal or any stingers. Because both fresh and salt water contain considerable bacterial and viral pollution, you should always be alert to possible secondary infection of a wound. In cases of marine-acquired infections, be sure to consider *Vibrio* species.

13. **Given several scenarios of poisoning or overdose, provide the appropriate assessment, treatment, and transport.** pp. 428–468

Remember that the basic assessment of a patient with a toxicological emergency includes careful scene size-up, protection of rescue personnel, and rapid response to any needs to support the ABCs. Treatment includes decontamination and use of antidotes, where available. Rapid transport is standard. Detailed specifics for many drugs, toxic substances, and animal bites and stings are given in other objectives for this chapter.

CASE STUDY REVIEW

Reread the case study on pages 427 and 428 in Paramedic Care: Medical Emergencies *before reading the discussion below.*

This case study demonstrates how paramedics react to a stressful emergency involving an unconscious person who proves to be someone familiar to them as a former patient. It demonstrates many of the general challenges involved in recognition and response to a life-threatening toxicological emergency.

Kevin, Charles, and David receive one of the briefest of calls, "unconscious person." Even before the team reaches the address, they realize that the address seems familiar to them; as they see the location, they remember that they have been called here before to care for a woman with a history of chronic depression and difficulty coping with stressful situations. The study does not state how David knows that a team had been called here as recently as four days previously; it is possible that the team called for log information after realizing that the patient was well known in their service sector.

Initial scene size-up does not reveal any sign of toxicological threat to the team. The woman's boyfriend, who placed the 911 call, is apparently unharmed by any gas or other potentially invisible threat. There are a number of clues obvious to the team that indicate that the woman's unconsciousness is tied to an intentional toxicological emergency: They see an empty bottle of Tylenol (acetaminophen) and an empty bottle of nortriptyline, a tricyclic antidepressant. The nearby pharmacy receipt has the current day's date on it. In addition, the team can smell alcohol in the air and can see several empty bottles of wine. Even as one team member begins an initial assessment of the patient, the others can conclude that a multiple-ingestion overdose has occurred that involves acetaminophen, a tricyclic antidepressant, and alcohol. This is substantiated by the only history, a statement by the boyfriend that the patient had called him and said she "just couldn't take it anymore." The timing of the ingestion is unclear. Certainly the woman was able to make a telephone call and speak coherently two hours or so before the 911 call was made.

Initial assessment reveals that the woman is alive but in extremis: She is unresponsive, has slow, shallow respirations indicative of respiratory depression, and tachycardia with weak pulses. The team begins with the ABCs, intubating the patient and beginning mechanical ventilation. Although the study does not state that they are also giving supplemental oxygen, you should assume that they are doing so with high-flow oxygen. They quickly establish IV access and place essential monitors; again, details are not given, but ECG monitoring and pulse oximetry would be indicated. Continuous assessment of vitals is essential in this type of unstable situation.

The team checks for signs of trauma or other coexisting conditions and finds evidence of previous suicidal intent: multiple shallow scars across both wrists. Rapid transport is initiated, and the team remembers to bring all bottles of medicine found at the scene. Despite their intensive supportive care, the patient does not improve en route and has a generalized, grand mal seizure in the emergency department. Further care and transfer to the ICU are insufficient, and the patient dies in the ICU roughly 48 hours after admission due to cardiac dysrhythmias and liver failure. An autopsy, the results of which are pending, may provide further information on the details of her ingestion and her progressive organ failure.

This vignette contains many of the elements of common toxicological emergencies: a severely ill patient, little history of the immediate event besides clues apparent at the scene, and a struggle for the paramedic team to support the woman's vital functions while transporting her to the hospital for more definitive treatment. This case study also points out something else you will see with some toxicological emergencies: It isn't possible to save every patient. Whether the emergency is accidental or intentional, some patients cannot be saved, even when everything is done correctly and promptly by the paramedic team.

CONTENT SELF-EVALUATION

MULTIPLE CHOICE

_____ 1. Which of the following statements about the epidemiology of toxicological emergencies is NOT true?
   A. The frequency of toxicological emergencies continues to increase both in number and severity.
   B. About 70% of accidental poisonings occur among children aged 6 years or younger.
   C. Toxicological emergencies account for about 5% of emergency department visits and EMS responses.
   D. More serious poisonings, especially in older children, may represent intentional poisoning by a parent or caregiver.
   E. Adult poisonings and overdoses account for 95% of the fatalities in this category.

_____ 2. Immediate effects of toxins are often localized to the site of entry, whereas delayed effects are often systemic in nature.
   A. True
   B. False

_____ 3. Many inhalation exposures are accidental, and leading agents include the following:
   A. carbon dioxide, carbon tetrachloride, and ammonia.
   B. toxic vapors, plants, and chlorine.
   C. carbon monoxide, nitrous oxide, and petroleum-based products such as gasoline.
   D. carbon monoxide, ammonia, and toxic vapors.
   E. chlorine, cleaners (soaps and alkalis), and carbon monoxide.

_____ 4. All of the following are guidelines to follow in cases of toxicological emergencies EXCEPT:
   A. maintaining a high index of suspicion for possible poisonings.
   B. recording everything you see or smell at the scene that might help determine cause.
   C. taking appropriate measures to protect all rescue personnel and any bystanders.
   D. centering general management on support of ABCs, decontamination of patient, and use of antidote, if there is one.
   E. removing the patient from a toxic environment as promptly as possible.

_____ 5. Never delay supportive measures or transport due to a delay in contacting Poison Control Center.
   A. True
   B. False

_____ 6. The most common route of entry for toxic substances is:
   A. inhalation.   D. injection.
   B. ingestion.   E. adsorption.
   C. surface absorption.

_____ 7. The three principles of decontamination are:
   A. removal of patient from toxic environment, reduction in intake of toxin, and increase in elimination of toxin from body.
   B. removal of patient from toxic environment, removal of patient's clothing and washing of patient's body, increase in elimination of toxin from body.
   C. removal of patient from toxic environment, reduction in intake of toxin, and use of antidote, if one.
   D. removal of patient's clothing and washing of body, reduction in intake of toxin, and reduction in absorption of toxin already in body.
   E. reduction in intake of toxin into the body, reduction of absorption of toxin already in the body, and increase in elimination of toxin from the body.

_____ 8. The most widely used means of reducing absorption of toxins in the body is:
   A. gastric lavage (stomach pumping).   D. whole bowel irrigation.
   B. activated charcoal.   E. chelating agents.
   C. syrup of ipecac.

_____ 9. Do not involve law enforcement in a possible suicide case until it is clear that suicide was intended.
   A. True
   B. False

_____ 10. Which of the following is not a question commonly asked of a poisoning patient during the focused history?
   A. How much of the agent(s) did you ingest?
   B. How long ago did you ingest the agent(s)?
   C. Were any people with you when you ingested the agent(s)?
   D. What is your weight?
   E. Have you attempted to treat yourself in any way?

_____ 11. The physical exam is crucial in toxicological emergencies, and it has two purposes: (1) documenting physical evidence of intoxication and (2) detecting any underlying illness or condition that might affect either patient's symptoms or outcome of exposure.
A. True
B. False

_____ 12. All of the following statements are correct when treating ingestion emergencies EXCEPT:
A. Maintaining the ABCs is the top priority along with monitoring of all vitals.
B. Prevention of aspiration is a major objective, and intubation may be necessary.
C. An IV at keep-vein-open rate is recommended for all potentially dangerous ingestion incidents.
D. Induce vomiting unless it is against local protocol or you are told not to do so by Poison Control.
E. Follow general treatment guidelines with decontamination procedures.

_____ 13. The first priorities, in proper order, with surface-absorption exposures are to remove the patient from the toxic environment, perform the initial assessment, and then ensure your safety.
A. True
B. False

_____ 14. The typical signs and symptoms of carbon monoxide poisoning include:
A. a burning sensation in mouth and throat, headache, and confusion.
B. headache, seizure or coma, tachypnea.
C. tachypnea, pulmonary edema, a burning sensation in mouth and throat.
D. tachypnea, tachycardia, headache, and confusion.
E. headache, nausea and vomiting, confusion or other altered mental status.

_____ 15. The narcotic toxidrome is characterized by CNS depression, whereas the sympathomimetic toxidrome is characterized by CNS excitation.
A. True
B. False

_____ 16. Response to poisoning with one of the cardiac medications often involves bradycardia, which may require use of:
A. atropine.   D. digoxin.
B. an external pacing device.   E. calcium.
C. a beta blocker.

_____ 17. Common assessment findings for ingestion with a caustic include all of the following EXCEPT:
A. chest and abdominal pain.   D. hoarseness and/or stridor.
B. drooling and trouble swallowing. E. pain in the lips, tongue, throat, or gums.
C. facial burns.

_____ 18. Drugs with narrow therapeutic indexes are more likely to be involved in accidental toxicological emergencies. Two such drugs are:
A. lithium and the selective serotonin reuptake inhibitors (SSRIs).
B. tricyclic antidepressants and salicylates.
C. tricyclic antidepressants and lithium.
D. tricyclic antidepressants and SSRIs.
E. salicylates and lithium.

_____ 19. It is particularly important to know time of ingestion when a blood test (timed properly) can predict degree of damage. Two drugs to which this statement especially applies are:
A. acetaminophen and tricyclics.
B. SSRIs and tricyclics.
C. acetaminophen and non-steroidal anti-inflammatory drugs.
D. salicylates and non-steroidal anti-inflammatory drugs.
E. salicylates and acetaminophen.

_____ 20. If you suspect mixed ingestion with tricyclics and benzodiazepines, do NOT use Flumazenil because it may precipitate seizures.
   A. True
   B. False

_____ 21. Serotonin syndrome includes all of the following signs and symptoms EXCEPT:
   A. nausea, diarrhea, abdominal cramps.
   B. hypotension.
   C. agitation and confusion.
   D. hyperthermia.
   E. rigidity, incoordination, myoclonic jerks.

_____ 22. Chelating agents are often useful in cases of toxicity due to:
   A. lithium.   D. heavy metals.
   B. theophylline.   E. salicylates.
   C. some cardiac medications.

_____ 23. All of the following statements are true about MAO inhibitors EXCEPT:
   A. Overdose cases may be very serious, even though initial signs/symptoms may appear hours after ingestion.
   B. MAO inhibitors have been used to treat depression and obsessive-compulsive disorder.
   C. MAO inhibitors as a group have a narrow therapeutic index.
   D. MAO inhibitors may interact negatively with foods containing tyramine, such as cheese and wine.
   E. In overdose, death usually follows the eventual signs of tachycardia, hypertension, and coma.

_____ 24. In cases of suspected food poisoning or poisoning involving plants and mushrooms, it is important to bring samples along with the patient if possible.
   A. True
   B. False

_____ 25. In cases involving bites or stings, fatalities are most likely among patients who have an allergic reaction or anaphylaxis to insect stings.
   A. True
   B. False

_____ 26. In common toxic drug ingestions, the use of benzodiazepines is frequently recommended with:
   A. alcohol, narcotics, and barbiturates.
   B. alcohol, hallucinogens, and barbiturates.
   C. cocaine, amphetamines, and hallucinogens.
   D. cocaine, alcohol, and amphetamines.
   E. cocaine, amphetamines, and barbiturates.

_____ 27. Which of the following statements about delirium tremens is NOT true?
   A. They usually develop 2–3 days after withdrawal of alcohol.
   B. They can occur in individuals who have experienced recent binge drinking.
   C. DTs are marked by decreased level of consciousness with hallucinations.
   D. Seizures and delirium tremens are ominous signs.
   E. DTs are associated with a significant mortality rate.

MATCHING

Write the letter of the definition in the space provided next to the term to which it applies.

_____ 28. injection

_____ 29. tolerance

_____ 30. toxin

_____ 31. inhalation

_____ 32. poisoning

_____ 33. substance abuse

_____ 34. therapeutic index (or window)

_____ 35. ingestion

_____ 36. delirium tremens (DTs)

_____ 37. enterotoxin

_____ 38. decontamination

_____ 39. surface absorption

_____ 40. overdose

_____ 41. toxidrome

_____ 42. withdrawal

_____ 43. addiction

A. an exposure to a nonpharmacological toxic substance
B. entry of a substance into the body via a break in the skin
C. result of drug discontinuance in which body reacts severely to absence of drug
D. group of clinical signs and symptoms consistently associated with exposure to a particular type of toxin
E. dependence on a drug, physiological, psychological, or both
F. potentially lethal syndrome found when alcohol withdrawn from chronic abusers
G. dosage range between effective and toxic dosages
H. need to progressively increase dosage to achieve same effect
I. process of minimizing toxicity by reducing amount of toxin absorbed into the body
J. entry of a substance into the body via the skin or mucous membranes
K. exposure to an amount of pharmacological substance greater than normally tolerated
L. bacterial exotoxin that produces GI symptoms and diseases such as food poisoning
M. entry of a substance into the body via the respiratory tract
N. any chemical that causes adverse effects on an organism exposed to it
O. use of pharmacological product for purposes other than those medically defined for it
P. entry of a substance into the body via the GI tract

FILL-IN-THE-BLANKS

Write the answers to the following questions in the spaces provided.

44. The four routes of entry into the body for toxins are _____ , _____ , _____ , and _____ .

45. The _____ are a chemical group often used as pesticides and frequently involved in surface-absorption emergencies.

SPECIAL PROJECT

Analyzing an Emergency Scene

Use your experience and what you have learned in this chapter to answer the questions about the following scenario.

You are called to the apartment of an elderly gentleman after his son phoned 911 to report that when he telephoned his father for a nightly check, his father had slurred speech and sounded confused. The son told dispatch that his father had felt "under the weather" with a cold recently but had otherwise been in his usual, somewhat fragile, state of health. No specifics were given.

You find the patient alone in his apartment. He is an unkempt, confused gentleman who repeatedly introduces himself and asks your names. He looks moderately uncomfortable, has nasal congestion and a mild cough, and says he has been "a bit ill" for several days. He states that he took a long nap, and then got up and took his pills. He says he doesn't need any help, he just needs to sit a bit to clear his head. When asked what pills he took, and how long ago, he says he "thinks" he just took the bedtime pills, but he may also have taken the afternoon ones because he might have slept through the normal time to take them. He doesn't know where the pharmacy bottles are because his visiting nurse makes up his pill case once a week. You note on the nightstand next to the bed a pill case, one of those that has the days of the week and several times per day marked on it with a compartment for each dosing time. You observe that several compartments for each day have tablets or capsules, often multiple.

1. What kind of toxicological emergency might this situation represent, and would you suspect accidental or intentional circumstances?

As you start your physical assessment, the patient says, "Oh, my, I'm dizzy," and sits awkwardly on the floor. His pulse is difficult to determine, but it is weak, slow, and possibly irregular.

2. What are your initial interventions?

3. What priorities do you give to calling the Poison Control Center, medical direction, and initiating transport?

4. What, if anything, do you take with you from the apartment?

CHAPTER 9
✳ Hematology

Review of Chapter Objectives

After reading this chapter, you should be able to:

1. **Identify the anatomy and physiology of the hematopoietic system.**   pp. 473–486

The components of the hematopoietic system include the blood, bone marrow, liver, spleen, and kidneys. The process of hematopoiesis forms the cellular components of blood. In the fetus, this first takes place outside the bone marrow in the liver, spleen, lymph nodes, and thymus. By the fourth month of gestation, the bone marrow begins to produce blood cells. After birth and across the span of life, bone marrow continues to fulfill this critical function barring the development of some pathological process.

In hematopoiesis, the stem cell reproduces to maintain a constant population of cells. Some stem cells further differentiate into myeloid multipotent stem cells that, in turn, differentiate into unipotent progenitors, which ultimately mature into the formed elements of blood: red blood cells, white blood cells, and platelets. Pluripotent stem cells may also differentiate into common lymphoid stem cells, ultimately becoming lymphocytes. Erythropoietin, the hormone responsible for red blood cell production, is produced by the kidneys and, to a lesser extent, the liver. The liver also removes toxins from the blood and produces many of the clotting factors and proteins in plasma. The spleen plays an important role in the immune system with its cells that scavenge abnormal blood cells and bacteria.

2. **Describe normal red blood cell (RBC) production, function, and destruction.**   pp. 474–476

Erythropoiesis, the process of RBC production, is stimulated by erythropoietin that is secreted by the kidneys when the renal cells sense hypoxia. In turn, this stimulates the bone marrow to increase red cell production resulting in increased RBC mass and thus effectively, albeit slowly, increases the oxygen carrying capacity of the blood.

The life span of a red blood cell is approximately 4 months, although hemorrhage, hemolysis (RBC destruction), or sequestration by the liver or spleen may significantly reduce its life span. The spleen and liver contain macrophages (a specialized type of scavenger white blood cell) that can remove damaged or abnormal cells from circulation.

3. **Explain the significance of the hematocrit with respect to red cell size and number.**   p. 476

Hematocrit is the packed cell volume of red blood cells per unit of blood. This measurement is obtained by spinning a sample of blood in a centrifuge to separate the cellular elements from the plasma. Red cells are by far the heaviest component of the blood, due to their carrying the iron-containing hemoglobin, and settle to the bottom of the tube. Immediately above the RBCs are the white blood cells and on top is the plasma layer. The height of the RBCs in the column is divided by the total height of the tube's contents (cellular component + plasma) and is reported as a percentage. The normal range is from 40 to 52 percent, although women tend to have slightly lower levels.

4. **Explain the correlation of the RBC count, hematocrit, and hemoglobin values.** p. 476

There are two ways that red blood cells are quantified and recorded: RBC count and hematocrit. Red blood cell count, reported in millions per cubic millimeter (mm^3), reflects the total number of RBCs. While normal values vary with age and gender, the typical range is 4.2 to 6.0 million/mm^3. The hematocrit reflects the packed cell volume of red cells, stated as a percentage of RBCs in a centrifuge-spun sample of blood. The normal range is from 40 to 52 percent, although women tend to have slightly lower levels.

Learning the concentration of hemoglobin is another means of determining the status of red blood cells. This concentration is expressed as the number of grams of hemoglobin present per deciliter of whole blood. There are two ways that the hemoglobin concentration can decrease. When the number of RBCs present is below normal, the hemoglobin will always be below normal. In some cases, the RBC count will be normal, but the amount of hemoglobin may be decreased. The standard of care measures both hemoglobin and hematocrit as they both indicate RBC volume and capability. Normal hemoglobin for a man is 12.0 to 15.0 g/dL and for a woman is 10.5 to 14.0 g/dL.

5. **Identify the characteristics of the inflammatory process.** p. 480

The inflammatory process is a nonspecific defense mechanism that wards off damage from microorganisms or trauma. It attempts to localize the damage while destroying the source, as it simultaneously facilitates repair. Causes of the process may be an infectious agent, trauma, or chemical or immunologic agents. Following local tissue injury, chemical messengers are released that attract white blood cells, increase capillary permeability, and cause vasodilation. This results in the redness, swelling, warmth, and pain associated with inflammation. Systemic inflammation is another type of inflammatory process occurring as a result of bacterial infection. Fever, which commonly accompanies systemic inflammation, is thought to occur as a response to chemical mediators released by macrophages in response to the causative infectious agent. These same mediators act on the brain, triggering sympathetic nervous system stimulation and causing heat conservation, vasoconstriction, and fever.

6. **Identify the difference between cellular and humoral immunity.** pp. 479–480

Lymphocytes, the primary cells of the immune system, are of two types: T cells and B cells. T cells, maturing in the thymus, are responsible for developing mediated or cellular immunity. In humoral immunity B cells produce antibodies to combat infection. Cellular immunity is responsible for antigen triggered release of effector cells and causes delayed hypersensitivity reactions, transplant rejection, and defense against intracellular organisms. Humoral immunity occurs when an antigen triggers the development and release of specific antibodies necessary for the body's defense.

7. **Identify alterations in immunologic response.** p. 480

A variety of factors such as drugs, disease, genetics, and infection can trigger alterations in the body's immunologic response. Genetics and viral infection can trigger the immune system to develop antibodies against the body's own tissues, causing a variety of localized or systemic diseases. Immunosuppressive drugs, like those used to prevent transplant rejection, and cancer chemotherapy agents, as well as the cancer itself, can also cause alterations, the most significant of which is a reduced ability to fight infections. Alterations in immunity may also be acquired through infection with the human immunodeficiency virus (HIV) which has an affinity for T lymphocytes, rendering the body at great risk for opportunistic infections. Regardless of the cause, alterations in immunologic response and the resultant risk of infection require that the EMS provider make every effort to protect patients from exposure to infection by good hand washing, correct IV techniques, and proper wound care.

8. **Describe the number, normal function, types, and life span of leukocytes (white blood cells), platelets, and red blood cells.** pp. 473–481

White blood cells originate in the bone marrow from undifferentiated stem cells. Leukopoiesis is the process by which stem cells differentiate into the various immature forms of the white blood cell (leukocyte). These immature forms known as -blasts mature to become granulocytes, monocytes, or lymphocytes. While leukocytes provide protection from foreign invasion, each type of white blood cell has its own unique function. Healthy people have between 5,000 and 9,000 white blood cells per milliliter of blood, but the presence of an infection can cause that number to rise to greater than 16,000.

Granulocytic white blood cells are of three types: basophils, eosinophils, and neutrophils. The basophils' primary function is in allergic reactions as they are storage sites for all of the body's circulating histamine. When stimulated, they degranulate and release histamine. Eosinophils can inactivate the chemical mediators of acute allergic response, thus modulating the anaphylactic response. The neutrophils' primary function is to fight infection.

Monocytes, another of the specialized WBCs, serve as the body's trash collectors, moving throughout the body to engulf both foreign invaders and dead neutrophils. Some monocytes remain in circulation, while others migrate to other sites to further mature into macrophages. Monocytes and macrophages also secrete growth factors to stimulate the formation of red blood cells and granulocytes. Some macrophages become fixed within tissues of the liver, spleen, lungs, and lymphatic system, becoming part of the reticuloendothelial system and having the capability to stimulate lymphocyte production in an immune response.

Lymphocytes, the primary cells of the body's immune response, can be found in the circulating blood, as well as in the lymph fluid and nodes, bone marrow, spleen, liver, lungs, skin, and intestine. These highly specialized cells contain surface receptor sites specific to a single antigen and initiate an immune response in order to rid the body of such agents.

Platelets or thrombocytes function to form a plug at an initial bleeding site and secrete several factors important to clotting. The normal number of platelets ranges from 150,000 to 450,000 per milliliter. Derived from megakaryocytes that arise from an undifferentiated stem cell in the bone marrow, platelets survive from 7 to 10 days and are removed from circulation by the spleen.

Erythropoiesis, the process of RBC production, is stimulated by erythropoietin that is secreted by the kidneys when the renal cells sense hypoxia. In turn, this stimulates the bone marrow to increase red cell production resulting in increased RBC mass and thus effectively, albeit slowly, increasing the oxygen carrying capacity of the blood.

The life span of a red blood cell is approximately 4 months, although hemorrhage, hemolysis (RBC destruction), or sequestration by the liver or spleen may significantly reduce its life span. The spleen and liver contain macrophages (a specialized type of scavenger white blood cell) that can remove damaged or abnormal cells from circulation.

9. List the leukocyte disorders. pp. 495–496

Disorders or problems of the white blood cells (leukocytes) have a significant impact on the body's defense system. These problems include leukopenia (too few white blood cells) or leukocytosis (too many white blood cells). A variation of leukopenia is neutropenia in which there are too few neutrophils; this is potentially dangerous, as the absolute count for neutrophils is an excellent indicator of the immune system's status. Improper white cell formation may also cause disorders such as leukemia (cancer of the hematopoietic cells) or lymphoma (cancer of the lymphatic system).

10. Describe the components of the hemostatic mechanism. pp. 481–483

Hemostasis involves three mechanisms that work to prevent or control blood loss, including vascular spasms that reduce the size of a vascular tear, platelet plugs (an aggregate of platelets that adheres to collagen), and lastly the formation of stable fibrin clots (coagulation).

11. Describe the intrinsic and extrinsic clotting systems and the function of coagulation factors, platelets, and blood vessels necessary for normal coagulation. pp. 481–483

Damage to cells or to the tunica intima (innermost lining of the blood vessels) triggers the clotting or coagulation cascade. This sequence of events (cascade) can be activated by either an intrinsic pathway (trauma to blood cells from turbulence) or an extrinsic pathway (damage to vessels).

Following the intrinsic pathway: platelets release substances that lead to the formation of prothrombin activator, which in the presence of calcium converts prothrombin to thrombin.

Thrombin converts fibrinogen to stable fibrin, again in the presence of calcium, which then traps blood cells and more platelets to form a clot.

The extrinsic pathway is triggered with the development of a tear in a blood vessel. When this occurs, the smooth muscle fibers in the tunica media (middle lining of the blood vessels) contract and the resultant vasoconstriction reduces the size of the injury. This action reduces blood flow through the area, effectively limiting blood loss and allowing platelet aggregation (formation of a platelet plug) and the subsequent conversion of prothrombin activator.

Clotting factors or proteins are primarily produced in the liver and circulate in an inactive state. Prothrombin and fibrinogen are the best known of these factors. Damaged cells send out a chemical message that activates a specific clotting factor. This activates each protein in sequence until a stable clot is formed.

An enzyme on the surface of the platelet membrane makes it sticky. It is this stickiness that allows platelet aggregation to occur.

12. Identify blood groups. pp. 484–485

The presence of certain antigens (proteins) on the surface of a donor's red blood cells allows the patient's body to recognize it as "self" or "not self." Following transfusion, antibodies in the patient's own blood attack the foreign antigens present in the transfused blood resulting in a transfusion reaction if the transfused blood contains opposing antigens. The presence or absence of such antigens and antibodies provides us with the blood typing system in use today.

For instance, someone with A antigen on his red cells would have anti-B antibodies. His blood type would be A. Conversely, someone with B antigen on his red cells would have anti-A antibodies. His blood type would be B. Others have both antigens present on their surface but neither antibody; their blood type would be type AB. With regard to transfusions, these individuals are known as universal recipients because they lack any antibodies to attack foreign cells. Some individuals have neither antigen but have both antibodies so their blood type is O. People with type O blood are known as universal donors in that their blood has no antigens and thus would not trigger a reaction.

In addition to the presence of A and B antigens, another factor to consider with regard to blood typing involves an antigen known as Rh found on red blood cells. If a person has the Rh factor, he is considered to be Rh positive; if not, he is Rh negative. When identifying an individual on the basis of blood type, all of these elements are taken into account. For example, one person may be O positive while another is AB negative.

13. Describe how acquired factor deficiencies may occur. pp. 483, 497–498

People who lack clotting factors can have bleeding disorders, which can occur as a result of genetics or medications. Some medications such as aspirin, dipyridamole (Persantine) and ticlopidine (Ticlid) decrease the stickiness of platelets by altering the surface enzyme that allows platelet aggregation. Others such as heparin and warfarin (Coumadin) cause changes within the clotting cascade to prevent clot formation. Heparin working together with antithrombin III (a naturally occurring thrombin inactivator) inactivates thrombin to prevent formation of the fibrin clot. Coumadin blocks the activity of vitamin K, which is necessary to generate the activated forms of clotting factors II, VII, IX, and X, thus effectively interrupting the clotting cascade.

14. Define fibrinolysis. p. 482

Fibrinolysis is the process through which plasmin dismantles a clot. Clot formation does not signal the end of the coagulation cascade. Once a fibrin clot is formed, it releases a chemical called plasminogen, which is subsequently converted to plasmin. Plasmin is capable of dismantling or lysing a clot through the process of fibrinolysis. This process takes place over a period of hours to days, by which time scarring has begun.

15. Identify the components of physical assessment as they relate to the hematology system. pp. 486–491

Many times hematological disorders are discovered and diagnosed when the patient seeks assistance for another medical condition, as the signs and symptoms associated with hematological problems may be quite varied. Fever often accompanies infection, white blood cell abnormalities (immunocompromised and prone to infection), and transfusion reactions. Acute hemodynamic compromise can be found in patients with anemia secondary to acute blood loss, coagulation disorders, or autoimmune disease. Confirmation of hematological disorders is usually dependent on laboratory analysis, but a complete history will go a long way toward developing an accurate diagnosis.

Additional specific considerations include mental status, dizziness, vertigo, or syncope, all of which may be indicative of anemia. Visual problems should alert you to the possibility of autoimmune disorders or sickle cell disease.

Skin color may be another indicator of hematological problems. Jaundice may indicate liver disease or hemolysis of red blood cells, while polycythemia is often associated with a florid (reddish) appearance, as pallor is with anemia. Observe for petechiae or purpura and bruising. Itching is commonly associated with hematological problems because of an excess of bilirubin as a result of liver disease or hemoglobin breakdown. Many patients report itching over a bruise. Look for evidence of prolonged bleeding, such as multiple bandages over a relatively minor wound.

Palpate the lymph nodes of the neck, clavicle, axilla, and groin. Enlarged lymph nodes are commonly seen in conjunction with hematopoietic disorders.

Gastrointestinal effects may be quite varied. Patients with clotting disorders may report epistaxis, bleeding gums, or melena. Many patients with clotting disorders report atraumatic bleeding of the gums. Ulcerations of the gums and oral mucosa as well as thrush (viral infection of the mouth) are often seen with immunocompromised patients. Abdominal pain is often seen in patients with hematological disorders. You may also be able to discern hepatic or splenic enlargement on your abdominal exam.

You should always ask about joint pain and examine the major joints closely in any patient in whom you suspect hematological problems. Minor trauma can cause significant hemarthrosis in patients with clotting disorders such as hemophilia. Many patients with autoimmune disorders frequently complain of arthralgia (joint pain) in all of their major joints.

You may see a variety of cardiorespiratory presentations that are linked to hematological disorders. Signs of hypoxia, such as tachypnea, tachycardia, and even chest pain, may be indicative of anemia. Occasionally, patients with bleeding disorders may develop hemoptysis. As always you should be alert to signs and symptoms of shock and be prepared to initiate prompt therapy.

Genitourinary signs and symptoms associated with hematological problems may include hematuria, bleeding into the scrotal sac, excessive menstrual bleeding, and infection. Sickle cell disease is the most common cause for priapism seen in the emergency setting. Recognize that a detailed physical exam of the genitourinary system is not appropriate in the prehospital setting.

16. Describe the pathology and clinical manifestations and prognosis associated with:

Anemia   **pp. 492–493**

The most common disease associated with red blood cells is defined as a hematocrit of less than 37 percent in women and less than 40 percent in men. The majority of patients remain asymptomatic until their hematocrit drops below 30 percent. Anemia is either due to a reduction in the total number of RBCs or quality of hemoglobin; it may also be due to acute or chronic blood loss. Anemia is a sign of an underlying disease process that is either destroying RBCs and hemoglobin or decreasing their production. Anemias may be hereditary or acquired.

The signs and symptoms associated with anemia are related to the associated hypoxia that results from the decrease in RBCs or hemoglobin. Depending on the rapidity of onset, signs and symptoms may be subtle or dramatic depending in some degree on the patient's age and underlying state of health. Signs and symptoms may include fatigue, dizziness, headache, pallor, and tachycardia, or dyspnea with exertion. If the anemia develops rapidly it may overwhelm the body's compensatory mechanisms, in which case you may observe postural or frank hypotension, tachycardia, peripheral vasoconstriction, and decreased mental status.

Anemia may be self-limited or can be a lifelong illness requiring transfusions on a recurring and periodic basis. Confirmation of the illness and determination of its cause will be predictive of its prognosis.

Leukemia pp. 495–496

Cancers of the hematopoietic cells occur when the precursors of white blood cells in the bone marrow begin to replicate abnormally. Initially the proliferation of WBCs is confined to the bone marrow but then spreads to the peripheral circulation. Leukemia is classified by the type of cell involved and may be either acute or chronic. Examples include acute or chronic lymphocytic leukemia, acute or chronic myelogenous leukemia, or hairy cell leukemia. Although leukemias may occur across the life span, some are more commonly associated with specific age groups. For instance, acute lymphocytic leukemia (ALL) is seen predominately in children and young adults, while chronic lymphocytic leukemia (CLL) is most common in the sixth and seventh decades of life.

The signs and symptoms of leukemia are variable, although anemia and thrombocytopenia (decreased number of platelets) are common. These patients often appear acutely ill, complain of fatigue, and are febrile due to secondary infection. Lymph nodes will be enlarged. The history often includes weight loss and anorexia, as well as a feeling of abdominal fullness or pain that occurs as a result of liver and spleen enlargement.

The management of leukemia is a marvel of modern medicine as treatments such as chemotherapy, radiation therapy, and bone marrow transplantation have resulted in cures of specific types. Where ALL was once a virtual death sentence, now more than 50 percent of the pediatric patients live a normal life with the disease cured or in remission.

Lymphomas p. 496

Lymphomas are cancers of the lymphatic system. Malignant lymphoma is classified by the cell type involved, which indicates the stem cell from which the malignancy arises, are either Hodgkin's or non-Hodgkin's lymphoma. In the United States each year, approximately 40,000 people are diagnosed with non-Hodgkin's lymphoma, while 7,500 are diagnosed with Hodgkin's lymphoma.

The most common presenting sign of non-Hodgkin's lymphoma is painless swelling of the lymph nodes, while those with Hodgkin's lymphoma typically have no related symptoms. Some patients report fever, night sweats, anorexia, weight loss, and pruritis.

The long-term survival rate is much better with Hodgkin's lymphoma. Many people with this disease who were treated with radiation, chemotherapy, or both are considered cured.

Polycythemia p. 494

Polycythemia is an abnormally high hematocrit occurring due to excess production of red blood cells. A relatively rare disorder, it typically occurs in people over the age of 50. It can occur secondary to dehydration. The increased red blood cell load increases the patient's risk of thrombosis. Most deaths from polycythemia are due to thrombosis.

The signs and symptoms of polycythemia vary. The primary finding is a hematocrit of 50 percent or greater, which is usually accompanied by an increased number of white blood cells and platelets. The large number of RBCs may cause platelet dysfunction resulting in bleeding abnormalities such as epistaxis, spontaneous bruising, and gastrointestinal bleeding. Other complaints may include headache, dizziness, blurred vision, and itching. Severe cases can result in congestive heart failure.

Disseminated intravascular coagulopathy p. 499

Disseminated intravascular coagulopathy (DIC), also called consumption coagulopathy, is a disorder of coagulation caused by the systemic activation of the coagulation cascade. Normally, inhibitory mechanisms localize coagulation to the affected area through a combination of rapid blood flow and absorption of the fibrin clot. In DIC, circulating thrombin cleaves fibrinogen to form fibrin clots throughout the circulation, causing widespread thrombosis and occasionally end-organ ischemia.

Bleeding, the most frequent sign of DIC, occurs due to the reduced fibrinogen level, consumption of coagulation factors, and thrombocytopenia. It most commonly results from sepsis, hypotension, obstetrical complications, severe tissue injury, brain injury, cancer, and major hemolytic transfusion reactions. The patient may exhibit a purpuric rash, often over the chest and abdomen. The disease is quite grave and has a poor prognosis.

Hemophilia   pp. 497–498

Hemophilia is a disorder in which one of the proteins necessary for blood clotting is missing or defective. A deficiency of factor VIII is called hemophilia A, which is the most common inherited disorder of hemostasis. The severity of the disease is related to the amount of available circulating factor VIII, and patients are classified as mild, moderate, or severe on that basis. A deficiency of factor IX is known as hemophilia B or Christmas disease, which is more rare but also more severe than hemophilia A.

Hemophilia is a sex-linked inherited bleeding disorder. The gene with the defective encoding is carried on the X chromosome; this means that if the mother is a carrier, her son will inherit this disorder. Conversely, female offspring who inherit the defective gene from their mother will be carriers, but will not exhibit the clotting defect. In order for a female to exhibit the defect, she must inherit the defect from both parents, that is, a mother who is a carrier and a father who has hemophilia. Hemophilia A affects 1 in 10,000 males.

The signs and symptoms of hemophilia include prolonged bleeding, numerous bruises, deep muscle bleeding characterized as pain or a "pulled muscle," and bleeding in the joints known as hemarthrosis.

Sickle cell disease   pp. 493–494

This disease is an inherited disorder of RBC production that causes hemoglobin to be produced in a "C" or sickle shape during low oxygen states. These patients also have a hemolytic anemia as a result of destruction of abnormal red blood cells. The average life span of sickled cells is about 1/6 that of a normal red cell, approximately 10 to 20 days versus 120 days. Additionally, the sickled shape increases the blood's viscosity, leading to sludging and obstruction of capillaries and small vessels. Blockage of blood flow to various tissues and organs is common usually following periods of stress. The process, called a vasoocclusive crisis, is characteristic of the disease and over time leads to organ damage, particularly in the cardiovascular, renal, and neurologic systems.

Sickle cell disease primarily affects African Americans, although other ethnic groups may also be affected, such as Puerto Ricans and people of Spanish, French, Italian, Greek, or Turkish heritage. If both parents carry the sickle cell gene, the chances are 1 in 4 that their child will have normal hemoglobin.

Patients will develop three types of problems. Vasoocclusive crisis causes severe abdominal and joint pain, priapism, and renal or cerebrovascular infarcts. Hematological crises present with a drop in hemoglobin, sequestration of RBCs in the spleen, and problems with bone marrow function. Infectious crises mark the third type of problem as the patients are functionally immunosuppressed and the loss of splenic function makes them vulnerable to infection. Infections become increasingly common and often are the cause of death.

Multiple myeloma   p. 499

Multiple myeloma is a cancerous disorder of plasma cells, the type of B cell responsible for producing immunoglobulins (antibodies). Rarely seen in patients under the age of 40, approximately 14,000 new cases are diagnosed each year.

Usually, multiple myeloma begins with a change or mutation in a plasma cell in the bone marrow. These cancerous cells crowd out the normal healthy cells and lead to a reduction in blood cell production. The patient then becomes anemic and prone to infection. The first sign is often a pain in the back or ribs as the diseased marrow weakens the bones and as a result, pathological fractures may occur. The resulting anemia leads to fatigue, and reduced platelet production places the patient at risk of bleeding. Calcium levels rise as a result of the bone destruction, and this often leads to renal failure.

17. **Given several preprogrammed patients with hematological problems,
    provide the appropriate assessment, management, and transport.**   pp. 472–499

Throughout your classroom, clinical, and field training, you will encounter a variety of real and simulated patients with hematological problems. Use the information provided in this chapter of your text, as well as the application of this information as demonstrated by your instructors, preceptors, and mentors to enhance your ability to assess, manage, and transport these patients.

CASE STUDY REVIEW

Reread the case study on pages 471 and 472 in Paramedic Care: Medical Emergencies *before reading the discussion below.*

This case study draws attention to the assessment, management, and transport of a patient with a hematologic disorder. Further, it also underscores the fact that the "nature of the call" as based on dispatch information may not in fact be the primary problem for the patient. In this case, for example, Christian and Victoria are dispatched for what seems to be a minor fall in a shopping mall, but instead turns out to be a potentially life-threatening event for their patient.

Medic 102 is dispatched for what appears to be a minor fall on a short flight of stairs at a shopping mall. As you'll recall, while it is important to treat the injuries caused by accidental falls, it is equally important to determine what caused the fall; so as always, scene size-up is an important part of the call. In addition to gauging the situation in terms of your personal safety and that of your patient and other people who may be present, you should be observant for possible contributing factors for the fall such as spills or poorly maintained or broken steps.

The initial impression of this patient escalates the gravity of the situation beyond that of a "minor fall." Although C.J. is conscious and able to localize his pain, it is readily apparent that he is unstable as evidenced by his confusion, tachypnea, and tachycardia, with a weakly palpable radial pulse and obvious profuse diaphoresis. Recognizing the severity of the situation, Christian and Victoria move quickly to expedite C.J.'s transport to the hospital; however, in doing so, they take appropriate concern for the potential for spinal injury by logrolling him onto a backboard and quickly initiating oxygen therapy and establishing vascular access.

Once en route to the hospital, Victoria performs a more complete assessment. In addition to the already noted large ecchymotic area on the right flank, she finds a large effusion of the right knee and, equally important, finds a Medic-Alert tag indicating that C.J. has hemophilia A. Victoria recalls from her training that hemophilia is a clotting deficiency disorder that requires the administration of clotting factors to formulate clots and makes even seemingly minor trauma a potential life threat. Although Victoria has observed an improvement in C.J.'s mental status since the administration of oxygen and fluids, she completes her assessment by obtaining vital signs. With a blood pressure of 90/60, pulse of 120, and respirations of 24, C.J. is currently stable but needs continued monitoring. Victoria applies a splint to C.J.'s right knee knowing that immobilization will help alleviate some of his pain as well preventing further injury.

She contacts the emergency department knowing that C.J.'s condition, injuries, and hemophilia will require more than a "routine trauma" response. On the basis of her radio report, the ED physician orders the needed clotting factor from the pharmacy and alerts the trauma team. Complete and concise reporting to the receiving facility allows them to adequately prepare and, ultimately, best meet the patient's physiologic needs.

CONTENT SELF-EVALUATION

MULTIPLE CHOICE

_____ 1. All of the following are components of the adult hematopoietic system EXCEPT the:
  A. blood.
  B. bone marrow.
  C. thymus.
  D. liver.
  E. spleen.

_____ 2. The major determinants of blood volume are red cell mass and:
  A. erythropoietin levels.
  B. plasma volume.
  C. total body water.
  D. stem cell percentage.
  E. bone marrow volume.

_____ 3. The component of the red blood cell that is responsible for transporting oxygen is the:
  A. basophil.
  B. granulocyte.
  C. hemoglobin.
  D. neutrophil.
  E. lymphocyte.

_____ 4. The Bohr effect describes the relationship between pH and oxygen delivery in that the more acidic the blood, the more readily oxygen is released to the tissues.
A. True
B. False

_____ 5. All of the following will cause a right shift of the oxyhemoglobin dissociation curve and thus increase the rate that oxygen is released to the tissues EXCEPT:
A. increased carbon dioxide.
B. increased temperature.
C. decreased pH.
D. decreased activity.
E. increased activity.

_____ 6. The term for the packed cell volume of red cells per unit of blood volume is:
A. hematocrit.
B. hemoglobin.
C. red blood cell count.
D. blood type.
E. white blood count.

_____ 7. White blood cells that primarily function in allergic reactions to release histamine are called:
A. lymphocytes.
B. neutrophils.
C. eosinophils.
D. monocytes.
E. basophils.

_____ 8. White blood cells that primarily function to fight infection are called:
A. lymphocytes.
B. neutrophils.
C. eosinophils.
D. monocytes.
E. basophils.

_____ 9. T cells and B cells, which play critical roles in immunity, are types of white cells called:
A. lymphocytes.
B. neutrophils.
C. eosinophils.
D. monocytes.
E. basophils.

_____ 10. The condition that occurs when the body develops antibodies against itself is called:
A. acquired immunodeficiency.
B. autoimmune disease.
C. rejection.
D. chemotaxis.
E. inherited immunodeficiency.

_____ 11. Causes of the inflammatory process include all of the following EXCEPT:
A. infectious agents.
B. chemical agents.
C. trauma.
D. immunologic agents.
E. genetics.

_____ 12. The formed blood cell components responsible for blood clotting are:
A. red blood cells.
B. white blood cells.
C. lymphocytes.
D. platelets.
E. monocytes.

_____ 13. The protein that on the surface of a blood cell that allows blood to be typed is known as a(n):
A. antibody.
B. antigen.
C. thrombocyte.
D. granulocyte.
E. monocyte.

_____ 14. The process of red blood cell destruction is known as:
A. sequestration.
B. fibrinolysis.
C. hemolysis.
D. hematopoiesis.
E. phagocytosis.

_____ 15. Tiny red dots found on the skin that may be indicative of hematological disorders are called:
A. purpura.
B. jaundice.
C. ecchymosis.
D. petechiae.
E. bruises.

_____ 16. An excess of bilirubin, either from liver disease or the breakdown of hemoglobin, can cause:
   A. gingivitis.
   B. generalized sepsis.
   C. arthralgia.
   D. priapism.
   E. pruritis.

_____ 17. Often, one of the earliest indications of hematological problems is:
   A. gingivitis.
   B. generalized sepsis.
   C. arthralgia.
   D. priapism.
   E. pruritis.

_____ 18. A hematocrit of 50 percent or greater is the principal finding in:
   A. anemia.
   B. leukopenia.
   C. polycythemia.
   D. thrombocytopenia.
   E. non-Hodgkin's lymphoma.

_____ 19. Painless swelling of lymph nodes is the most common presenting sign of:
   A. anemia.
   B. leukopenia.
   C. polycythemia.
   D. thrombocytopenia.
   E. non-Hodgkin's lymphoma.

_____ 20. An abnormal decrease in the number of platelets, which can be induced by many drugs, is:
   A. anemia.
   B. leukopenia.
   C. polycythemia.
   D. thrombocytopenia.
   E. non-Hodgkin's lymphoma.

MATCHING

Write the letter of the term in the space provided next to the most appropriate description of it.

A. erythropoietin
B. leukopoiesis
C. hematocrit
D. polycythemia
E. anemia
F. hemostasis
G. sickle cell disease
H. fibrinolysis
I. bilirubin
J. thrombosis
K. leukemia
L. antigen
M. thrombocytopenia
N. purpura
O. multiple myeloma

_____ 21. The packed cell volume of red blood cells per unit of blood

_____ 22. Clot formation

_____ 23. Protein on the surface of a donor's red blood cells that the patient's body recognizes as "not self"

_____ 24. Reddish-purple blotches related to multiple hemorrhages into the skin

_____ 25. An abnormally high hematocrit due to an excess production of red blood cells

_____ 26. An inherited disorder of red blood cell production

_____ 27. Byproduct of the breakdown of hemoglobin that is converted from porphyrin

_____ 28. An inadequate number of red blood cells or inadequate hemoglobin within the red blood cells

_____ 29. Hormone responsible for red blood cell production

_____ 30. Cancer of the hematopoietic cells

_____ 31. The process through which stem cells differentiate into the white blood cells' immature forms

_____ 32. The process through which plasmin dismantles a blood clot

_____ 33. An abnormal decrease in the number of platelets

_____ 34. A cancerous disorder of plasma cells

_____ 35. The combined three mechanisms that work to prevent or control blood loss

SPECIAL PROJECT

Completing a Table

Complete the table below by filling in the boxes.

Hematological Disorder	Common Signs and Symptoms	Prehospital Management
Anemia		
Hemophilia		
Leukemia		
Lymphoma		
Sickle Cell Anemia		

Chapter 10

Environmental Emergencies

Review of Chapter Objectives

After reading this chapter, you should be able to:

1. Define "environmental emergency." **p. 505**

An environmental emergency is a medical condition caused by or exacerbated by environmental factors such as weather, terrain, atmospheric pressure, or other local factors.

2. Describe the incidence, morbidity, and mortality associated with environmental emergencies. **p. 525**

The types of environmental emergencies most associated with any EMS provider's service sector are specific to that region: mountainous, coastal, desert, etc. In general, though, environmental emergencies are very common, and most paramedics will see such emergencies in their practice. It is vital that paramedics learn which types of emergencies are most likely in their locales and that they know the special rescue techniques and resources needed and available for such emergencies.

Specifics on morbidity and mortality: About 4,500 persons die annually from drowning in the U.S., making drowning the third most common cause of accidental death across age groups. Approximately 40 percent of these deaths are among children under age 5 years. There is a second peak among teenagers and a third among the elderly (the last due to bathtub incidents). Many more people each year sustain serious injury from near-drowning. Roughly 85 percent of near-drowning victims are male, and two-thirds of them do not know how to swim. Commonly, these situations are associated with fresh-water settings, especially swimming pools.

3. Identify risk factors most predisposing to environmental emergencies. **p. 505**

General risk factors that place an individual at greater risk for an environmental emergency include age (very young and very old), poor general health, fatigue, predisposing medical conditions, and certain prescription or over-the-counter medications. Among drowning and near-drowning cases, alcohol use by an adult victim or the supervising adult is common.

4. Identify environmental factors that may cause illness or exacerbate a pre-existing illness or complicate treatment or transport decisions. **p. 505**

Environments with certain characteristics are more likely to have emergencies: For instance, deserts may have tremendous variation in temperature between the hottest part of the day and overnight. Other such factors include current season, local weather patterns, atmospheric (high altitude) or hydrostatic (underwater) pressure, and the type of terrain. Rough or isolated terrain may significantly increase time for EMS response and for transport to the appropriate treating facility.

5. Define "homeostasis" and relate the concept to environmental influences. **pp. 505–506**

Homeostasis is the body's ability to maintain a steady and normal internal environment despite changing external conditions. In this chapter, external conditions that are explored in the context of environmental emergency are (1) extremes in temperature, (2) drowning (fresh-water or salt-water), (3) atmospheric (high altitude) or hydrostatic (underwater diving) pressure, and (4) nuclear radiation.

6. Identify normal, critically high, and critically low body temperatures. p. 509

In the core of the body, temperature usually varies within 1° of 98.6°F (37°C). Heat exhaustion occurs at core temperatures above 100°F (37.8°C), and heatstroke can occur at 105°F (40.6°C) and higher. In contrast, mild hypothermia is associated with core temperatures of roughly 90–95°F (32–35°C). Severe hypothermia develops when core temperature drops below 90°F (32°C). The upper and lower core-body temperatures compatible with survival are roughly 114°F and 86°F, respectively.

7. Describe several methods of temperature monitoring. p. 508

Core body temperature can be monitored with a tympanic or rectal thermometer. Peripheral body temperature, which is usually a little bit lower, can be measured with use of an oral thermometer or a thermometer placed under the armpit (an axillary temperature). Approximate peripheral temperature or change in peripheral temperature can often be discerned by touch.

8. Describe human thermal regulation, including system components, substances used, and wastes generated. pp. 506–510, 517

The human body does not generate "cold," it generates heat, and this process is called thermogenesis. There are three types of thermogenesis: The most basic and vital type is thermoregulatory thermogenesis, in which the nervous system and endocrine system work together to control the rate of cellular metabolism, which directly changes the rate of internal heat production. In work-induced thermogenesis, heat is produced through the work of skeletal muscles during exercise. In a cool or cold environment, muscles will produce some additional heat through shivering. The last type of heat generation is diet-induced thermogenesis, and it reflects the heat generated by cells as they process food and nutrients and eventually metabolize the breakdown products.

The body's thermal regulation is achieved through coordination of the nervous and endocrine systems. This is intuitively logical because these two systems are the control systems for all major body functions. Cells in the hypothalamus, a structure at the base of the brain, have the ability to act as a thermostat. As nerve cells, they sense the temperature of the core blood passing by them and they can receive messages from temperature sensors located in other parts of the body. Additional sensor cells for core temperature are located in the spinal cord, abdomen, and around the great veins in the chest. Peripheral sensors are in the skin and subcutaneous tissue.

On a cool day, peripheral temperature may drop. When the hypothalamic cells get the message, the cells act as endocrine cells, producing and secreting a hormone into the blood that acts to increase work-induced thermogenesis. Heat is produced through shivering. Also piloerection, or "goose bumps," the standing of small hairs, results in decreased air flow over the skin surface. If the environment is so cold that both peripheral and core temperature drop, the hypothalamic cells secrete hormones that increase heat production through all three means: thermoregulatory, work-induced, and diet-induced thermogenesis. (In the last, body cells burn fats and thus produce more heat.) In addition, core temperature, which is critical for survival, is maintained in part by reducing blood flow (and thus, heat) to the most peripheral tissues, the skin and subcutaneous tissues. In contrast, when the thermostat cells sense peripheral temperature is too high (as when you exercise vigorously), they stop releasing the hormone that stimulates thermogenesis. Not only is heat production slowed, but mechanisms to dissipate heat into the external environment are also activated. These include dilation of blood vessels in the skin and subcutaneous tissue (why people flush in the heat) and sweating.

This method of control, in which the production of a substance (in this case, heat) is turned off by the presence of that substance, is called negative feedback. Heat feeds back on the thermostat cells to turn off production of more heat. Think about the thermostat and furnace in a house. They work in a very similar fashion.

Thermogenesis consumes nutrient fuel for cells—fats, proteins, and carbohydrates—and it results in waste products such as carbon dioxide and water (from cellular respiration and fat breakdown) and urea (from protein breakdown). Extensive skeletal muscle use may also result in lactic acid accumulation. Heat dissipation through sweating consumes water, urea, and salts that are lost onto the skin surface.

9. **List the common forms of heat and cold disorders.** pp. 510–516

The common heat disorders are variants of hyperthermia, elevated core body temperature: In terms of increasing severity, these conditions are heat (muscle) cramps, heat exhaustion, and heat-stroke. Cold disorders are frostbite, trench foot, and hypothermia.

10. **List the common predisposing factors and preventive measures associated with heat and cold disorders.** pp. 510–511, 517–518

Important predisposing factors for hyperthermia include age, general health, and medications. Both the very young and the very old have less responsive heat regulating systems and can tolerate less variation in their core body temperature. Persons who have diabetes with autonomic neuropathy are at higher risk for hyperthermia because damage to the autonomic nervous system may interfere with proper messaging to the CNS about temperature and may interfere with the heat-dissipating processes of vasodilation and sweating. Several groups of medications can affect body temperature. Diuretics predispose to dehydration, which impairs ability to sweat. Beta blockers interfere with vasodilation, impair ability to increase heart rate in response to volume loss, and may interfere with temperature messages to the CNS. Psychotropics and antihistamines interfere with thermoregulation within the CNS. Additional factors include acclimatization to local conditions, length and intensity of heat exposure, and environmental factors such as humidity and wind. Preventive measures for heat disorders include three major elements. First, maintenance of adequate fluid intake is vital, and remember that thirst alone is an inadequate indicator for dehydration. Second, you should allow yourself time for acclimatization to the hot environment, which results in more perspiration with lower salt concentration, thus conserving body-fluid volume. Last, it is important to limit exposure to hot environments.

Important predisposing factors for hypothermia are the same: age, general health, and medications. Both the very young and the very old have less responsive heat generating systems to combat cold exposure and cannot tolerate cold environments. The elderly may become hypothermic in environments that are only somewhat cool to others. Persons with inadequately treated hypothyroidism have suppressed metabolisms, which prevents proper responsiveness to cold. In addition, malnutrition, hypoglycemia, Parkinson's disease, fatigue, and other medical conditions can interfere with the body's ability to combat cold exposure. Drugs that interfere with heat-generating mechanisms include narcotics, alcohol, phenothiazines, barbiturates, antiseizure medications, antihistamines and other allergy medications, antipsychotics, sedatives, antidepressants, and various analgesics such as aspirin, acetaminophen, and NSAIDs. Additional factors include prolonged or intense exposure, which directly affects both morbidity and mortality, and coexisting weather conditions (such as high humidity, brisk winds, or accompanying rain, all of which magnify the effect of cold). Preventive measures can decrease the morbidity of cold-related injury, and these include dressing warmly, being rested, which maximizes the ability of the heat-generating mechanisms to replenish energy reserves, appropriate eating at proper intervals to support metabolism, and limitation of exposure to cold environments.

11. **Define heat illness, hypothermia, frostbite, near-drowning, decompression illness, and altitude illness.** pp. 510, 517, 523, 525, 531, 536

- *Heat illness* is increased core body temperature (CBT) due to inadequate thermolysis (heat dissipation).
- *Hypothermia* is a state of low body temperature, particularly low core body temperature. Frostbite is environmentally induced freezing of body tissues causing destruction of cells.
- *Near-drowning* is an incident of potentially fatal submersion in liquid which did not result in death or in which death occurred more than 24 hours after submersion.
- *Decompression illness* is the development of nitrogen bubbles within body tissues due to a rapid reduction of air pressure when a diver returns to the surface; this is commonly called "the bends."

- *High altitude illness* is caused by a decrease in ambient pressure causing a low-oxygen environment and resultant hypoxia.

12. Describe the pathophysiology, signs and symptoms, and predisposing factors, preventive actions, and treatment for heat cramps, heat exhaustion, heatstroke, and fever. pp. 511–516

Heat cramps are caused by overexertion and dehydration in a hot environment. They occur when the temperature- and exercise-induced sweating (which consumes water and electrolytes including sodium) depletes the body of so much water and electrolytes that the actively exercising skeletal muscle fibers cramp. Signs and symptoms include cramping in fingers, arms, legs, or abdominal muscles. Patients are generally mentally alert with a feeling of weakness, but they may be dizzy or faint. Vital signs are stable, although temperature may be normal or slightly elevated. Skin is likely to be moist and warm. Note that heat cramps may be painful but they are NOT considered to be an actual heat illness. The general predisposing factors and preventive measures for all heat-related disorders are discussed with objective 10. Treatment for heat cramps is usually easily accomplished. First, remove the patient from the hot environment to a cooler one such as a shady area or an air-conditioned ambulance. For severe cramps, you can administer an oral saline solution (approximately 4 tsp salt/gallon water) or a sports electrolyte drink. Do NOT use salt tablets, which are not absorbed readily and can irritate the stomach causing ulceration or hypernatremia. If the patient cannot take liquids readily, an IV of normal saline may be needed. Palliative care may include muscle massage or moist towels over patient's head and the cramping muscles.

Heat exhaustion, which is considered a mild heat illness, is an acute reaction to heat exposure, and it is the most common heat-related illness seen by EMS providers. The loss of water and electrolytes (notably sodium) from working in a hot environment, combined with general vasodilation as a heat-dissipating mechanism, leads to a decreased circulating blood volume, venous pooling, and reduced cardiac output. The presenting symptoms are due to dehydration and sodium loss secondary to sweating. Because the symptoms are not unique to heat exhaustion, diagnosis requires presentation in the appropriate environmental setting. Remember that untreated heat exhaustion can progress to heatstroke. The signs and symptoms of heat exhaustion include increased body temperature (over 100°F, 37.8°C), cool clammy skin with heavy perspiration, rapid, shallow breathing, and a weak pulse. Signs of active thermolysis may include diarrhea and muscle cramps. The patient will feel weak and, in some cases, may lose consciousness. There also may be CNS symptoms such as headache, anxiety, paresthesia, and impaired judgment or even psychosis. The general predisposing factors and preventive measures for all heat-related disorders are discussed with objective 10. Treatment includes removal of the patient from the hot environment and placement in a supine position. For severe cramps, you can administer an oral saline solution (approximately 4 tsp salt/gallon water) or a sports electrolyte drink. Do NOT use salt tablets, as discussed above. If the patient cannot take liquids readily, an IV of normal saline may be needed. Remove some clothing and fan the patient to increase heat dissipation. Be careful not to cool the patient to the point of chilling him or her. Stop fanning if shivering develops, and consider covering the patient lightly. If shock is suspected, treat accordingly. If symptoms do not resolve, consider the possibility of increased core body temperature and evolution of heatstroke.

Heatstroke is a true environmental emergency, one in which the body's hypothalamic temperature regulation is lost and there is uncompensated hyperthermia resulting in cell death and damage to the brain, liver, and kidneys. Generally, heatstroke is characterized by body temperature above 105°F (40.6°C), CNS disturbances, and (usually) cessation of perspiration. It is thought that sweating stops either because of destruction of sweat glands or because of sensory overload resulting in their temporary dysfunction. Patients may present with signs and symptoms including cessation of sweating, hot skin that is either moist or dry (depending on whether sweat has dried), very high core temperatures, deep respirations that become shallow and rapid respirations that may later slow, a rapid, full pulse that may slow later, hypotension with low or absent diastolic reading, confusion or disorientation or unconsciousness, and possible seizures. Field management centers on immediate cooling of the patient's body and replacement of fluids. First, remove the patient from the environment; if this is not done, other measures will be only minimally useful. Initiate rapid active body cooling to a target temperature of 102°F (39°C). This can be accomplished en route to the hospital. Remove the patient's clothing and cover with sheets soaked in tepid water. If necessary, either fanning or misting may be used. Be sure you avoid over-cooling because this can trigger reflex hypothermia. Tepid water avoids the risk of producing reflex peripheral vasoconstriction and shivering that can be produced by exposure to cold water. In addition, use high-flow oxygen and assist respirations if they are shallow. Use pulse oximetry if available. Administer fluid therapy orally (if possible) or IV. In many cases, orally will suffice. Remember in this setting that electrolyte replacement is not nearly as necessary as water/volume replacement. If IVs are needed, start one or two and make the initial infusion with the line(s) wide open. Be sure to monitor the ECG because dysrhythmias can develop at any time. Avoid vaso-pressors and anticholinergic drugs because they may inhibit sweating and can contribute to devel-opment of a hyperthermic state in high-humidity, high-temperature environments. Lastly, monitor body temperature for trends toward target temperature or for other shift. If you work in a hot climate, try to make sure your thermometers measure above 106°F and below 95°F.

Fever (or pyrexia) is defined simply as elevation of body temperature above the normal for the individual. The body develops fever when pathogens cause infection, in turn stimulating produc-tions of pyrogens, substances produced either by the pathogen or by cells involved in an inflamma-tory or immune response to the pathogen. Pyrogens produce fever by resetting the hypothalamic thermostat to a high level. The increase in temperature is largely due to increased metabolic activ-ity. When production of pyrogen stops (or pathogen attack stops), the thermostat resets to normal and fever ends. Although fever typically presents in a setting of infectious disease, it may be difficult to distinguish from heatstroke, particularly if there is no history available and CNS signs are appar-ent. If you are unsure of diagnosis, treat for heatstroke. Treatment for fever should be undertaken when the patient is uncomfortable or when a child has a history of febrile seizures. Remove extra layers of clothing or bedclothes to allow body cooling. Consider use of an antipyretic agent such as acetaminophen or ibuprofen. Acetaminophen is available in rectal suppository form if vomiting is a concern. Note that sponge baths and cool-water immersion should not be used because they can cause a rapid drop in temperature with reflex shivering and increase in body temperature.

13. Describe the contribution of dehydration to the development of heat disorders. p. 515

Dehydration often accompanies heat disorders because it inhibits vasodilation and heat dissipa-tion (thermolysis). Dehydration leads to orthostatic hypotension and the following symptoms: nausea, vomiting, abdominal distress, vision disturbances, decreased urine output, poor skin tur-gor, and signs of hypovolemic shock. These may present along with the signs and symptoms of heatstroke. When assessment suggests dehydration, rehydration is critical. IV fluids may be needed, especially when the patient has altered mental status or is nauseated. An adult with mod-erate to severe dehydration may require 2–3 liters of IV fluids or more.

14. Describe the differences between classical and exertional heatstroke. p. 514

Heatstroke is often divided into two types: classic and exertional. In classic heatstroke, the patient probably has chronic disorders, and increased core body temperature is due to deficient ther-moregulatory function. Predisposing conditions include age, diabetes, and other medical condi-tions. In classic heatstroke, hot, red, dry skin is common. In contrast, exertional heatstroke often occurs in persons in good general health, and the increased core body temperature is due to over-whelming heat stress. Contextually, there is excessive ambient temperature, excessive exertion, prolonged exposure, and poor acclimatization. In exertional heatstroke, skin may well be moist from prior sweat. If heatstroke is tied to exertion, you may find severe metabolic acidosis caused by lactic acid accumulation. Hyperkalemia may also develop due to release of potassium from injured muscle cells, renal failure, or metabolic acidosis.

15. Identify the fundamental thermoregulatory difference between fever and heatstroke. p. 516

The fundamental difference is that the trigger for temperature disruption is endogenous (inter-nal) in fever and exogenous (external) in heatstroke. In fever, the hypothalamic thermostat is actually reset to a high level by pyrogens, substances associated with infection and the body's responses to it. The thermostat resets to the normal level when pyrogens disappear from the body. In heatstroke, exposure to high ambient temperatures depletes the body of the materials necessary for compensation (such as water and electrolytes for perspiration) and then causes the hypothalamic thermoregulatory processes to be lost. The ensuing uncompensated hyperthermia, with very high core body temperatures, begins the process of organ damage (if untreated) with potential for death.

16. Discuss the role of fluid therapy in the treatment of heat disorders. **p. 515**

Objective 13 discusses the role of dehydration in heat disorders. Because dehydration plays an increasingly significant role in heat cramps, heat exhaustion, and heatstroke, rehydration becomes increasingly pivotal to treatment success. Remember in milder forms of heat disorders, such as heat cramps, that the patient's perception of thirst is a poor indication of the degree of dehydration present. Fluid, whether it is administered orally or IV, is important in restoring the body's thermolytic abilities. In heat exhaustion and heatstroke, replacement of fluid (often by IV due to patient nausea, inability to swallow, or inability to take in fluids orally fast enough to be successful) is critical. Remember that an adult with moderate to severe dehydration can require 2–3 liters or more of replacement fluid.

17. Describe the pathophysiology, predisposing factors, signs, symptoms, and management of the following:

a. hypothermia **pp. 517–523**

Hypothermia is defined as a state of low core body temperature, which can be due to inadequate heat generation, excessive cold stress, or a combination of both. Hypothermia can be discussed in several contexts. First, it can be mild (core temperature greater than 90°F or 32°C) or severe (core temperature less than 90°F). In both forms signs and symptoms of hypothermia are present. Onset of symptoms can be acute (falling through ice into a lake), subacute (hikers trapped on a mountain during a winter snowstorm), or chronic (homeless individuals living outdoors during the winter). In many cases of acute and subacute hypothermia, the individual may not have any underlying predisposing factors for hypothermia: The pathophysiology of hypothermia rests on exposure to unsurvivable cold (as in the example of falling in the lake) or extended exposure to very cold conditions (the hiking example). In both settings, the body's ability for thermogenesis is simply overwhelmed. In other cases, an individual with impaired capacity for compensation is exposed to normal or cool conditions and develops hypothermia when a healthy individual would not or develops hypothermia before a healthy person would do so. Medical conditions that predispose to hypothermia include inadequately treated hypothyroidism, which depresses the body's metabolic rate, brain tumors or head trauma, which may impair hypothalamic function, as well as myocardial infarction, diabetes, hypoglycemia, drugs, poor nutrition, sepsis, or very young or old age.

Signs and symptoms of hypothermia are given in Table 10-2 (text page 520). Your assessment of an individual with mild hypothermia will likely reveal lethargy, shivering, lack of coordination, pale, cold, dry skin, and an early rise in blood pressure, heart rate, and respiratory rates. In severe hypothermia, you may find no shivering, loss of voluntary muscle control, hypotension, and an unpredictable pulse and respiration. On the ECG, you may find dysrhythmias. The most common presenting dysrhythmia is atrial fibrillation. With progressive cooling of the body core, a variety of dysrhythmias may appear, with eventual bradycardia or asystole. Note: The severely hypothermic patient requires assessment of pulse and respirations for at least 30 seconds every 1–2 minutes. Management includes: (1) removal of wet garments; (2) protection against further heat loss and wind chill (calling for passive external warming with blankets, moisture barriers, etc.); (3) maintenance of patient in horizontal position; (4) avoidance of rough handling, which can trigger dysrhythmias; (5) monitoring of core temperature; and (6) monitoring of cardiac rhythm. Persons with mild hypothermia may be rewarmed with active external techniques such as warmed blankets or heat packs. In contrast, active rewarming of the severely hypothermic patient is best carried out in the hospital because of the possibility of complications such as ventricular fibrillation. If transport to the hospital will require more than 15 minutes, you may need to begin active rewarming in the field. Beware of rewarming shock and cold diuresis, both of which are discussed on text page

522. As a final aid in putting the pieces of hypothermia care together, review the algorithm on text page 521.

b. superficial and deep frostbite   pp. 523-524

Frostbite is an environmentally induced freezing of body tissues. As tissues freeze due to the excessive cold, ice crystals form within cells and water is drawn from cells into the extracellular space. As the ice crystals expand, cells are destroyed. Damage to blood vessels from ice-crystal formation causes loss of vascular integrity, which results in further tissue swelling and loss of distal blood flow. Peripheral tissues are more exposed to cold and thus more likely to be involved in frostbite. Thus, frostbite is largely seen in the extremities and in areas of the head and face. Predisposing factors are the same as those for hypothermia, and they are discussed with objective 10. The role of predisposing factors is often straightforward in terms of pathophysiology. A patient with diabetes, for instance, may have impaired peripheral circulation, and this relatively low flow of warm blood may make the extremities more vulnerable to frostbite. Two types of frostbite are defined based on the extent of tissue freezing: superficial and deep frostbite. Superficial frostbite (also called frostnip) involves some freezing of epidermal tissue, resulting in initial redness followed by blanching and diminished sensation. Deep frostbite involves both the epidermal and subcutaneous layers; there is a white, hardened appearance. Sensation is lost. Subfreezing temperatures are necessary for frostbite (otherwise, cellular water wouldn't freeze) but are not necessary for hypothermia. You will find that many patients with frostbite also do have hypothermia. You will also find that there is tremendous variation in presentation of frostbite. Some patients will feel little pain at the outset, whereas other will complain of bitter pain. Physical exam is a better indicator of the extent of frostbite. In superficial frostbite, there will be some degree of compliance felt beneath the frozen layer upon palpation; in deep frostbite, the frozen part will be hard and noncompliant. Treatment involves the following steps. First, do not thaw the affected area if there is any possibility of refreezing and do not massage the frozen area or rub with snow. Both may result in more extensive damage. Do administer analgesia prior to thawing, and do transport to the hospital for rewarming by immersion. If transport will be delayed, thaw the frozen part in a 102–104°F water bath. Water will need to be changed frequently as it cools. Do cover the thawed part with loosely applied, dry, sterile dressings and elevate and immobilize the thawed part. Do not puncture or drain blisters, and do not rewarm frozen feet if they are required for walking out of a hazardous situation.

c. near-drowning   pp. 525–528

Near-drowning is defined as submersion that is survived for at least 24 hours. The pathophysiology parallels that of drowning. Following submersion, a conscious person will have complete apnea for up to three minutes as an involuntary reflex as he struggles to keep his head above water, and during this period blood is shunted to the heart and brain. During apnea, $PaCO_2$ will rise to greater than 50 mmHg while PaO_2 falls to less than 50 mmHg. The hypoxic stimulus eventually overrides the sedative effects of the hypercarbia, resulting in CNS stimulation. While conscious, the panicky victim typically swallows a lot of water into the stomach, stimulating severe laryngospasm and bronchospasm. Especially in near-drowning victims, this effect prevents significant influx of water into the lungs (and is thus termed a dry drowning or near-drowning). Another effect of laryngospasm is worsening hypoxia, which causes a deepening coma. Morbidity or delayed mortality in near-drowning is primarily due to asphyxia from airway obstruction secondary to water in the airways (if a wet event) or laryngospasm and bronchospasm (if a dry near-drowning). Water in the lungs of a near-drowning survivor may cause lower-airway disease. A number of factors affect survival, and these include the cleanliness of the water, the duration of submersion, and the age and general health of the victim. Children have a longer survival time and a greater probability of successful resuscitation. Most significant is water temperature. In general, the colder the water, the greater the chance for survival. Usually, you expect brain death after 4–6 minutes without oxygen. However, some patients in cold water (below 68°F) may be resuscitated after 30 minutes or more in cardiac arrest. A possible physiologic factor in this phenomenon is the mammalian diving reflex. When a person dives into cold water, the submersion of the face inhibits breathing, drops heart rate, and causes vasoconstriction in tissues relatively resistant to asphyxia even as blood flow to the heart and brain continue. The colder the water, the greater the shunting of blood to brain and heart. This is the origin of the saying "the cold water drowning victim is not dead until he is warm and dead."

Field treatment for near-drownings in either saltwater or fresh water is similar: The first goal is to correct the profound hypoxia. Treatment includes the following steps: Remove the patient from the water. If possible, initiate ventilation while the victim is still in the water. Note that both steps require a trained, equipped rescue swimmer. Suspect head and neck injury if there was a fall or a dive involved; rapidly place victim on long backboard and use C-spine precautions. Then, protect from heat loss by removing wet clothing, laying the patient on a warm surface, and covering the body to the extent possible. The remaining steps are familiar to all resuscitations: Examine for airway patency, breathing, and pulse. If needed, begin CPR and defibrillation. Manage the airway as needed with suctioning and airway adjuncts. Administer 100% oxygen. Use respiratory rewarming, if available and if transport time will exceed 15 minutes. Establish an IV of lactated Ringer's or normal saline for venous access and run at 75 mL/hr. Follow ACLS protocols if the patient is normothermic. If hypothermic, the patient should be treated for hypothermia as discussed in the text. Note: Resuscitation is NOT indicated if immersion is known to have been extremely prolonged (unless hypothermia IS present) or if there is evidence of decomposition. All near-drowning victims should be admitted for observation for possible late complications including adult respiratory distress syndrome (ARDS).

d. decompression illness   **pp. 531, 532–534**

Decompression illness, or the bends, is due to nitrogen bubbles coming out of solution in the blood and tissues, causing increased pressure on various body structures and occluding circulation in small blood vessels. This occurs in joints, tendons, the spinal cord, skin, brain, and inner ear. The trigger is a rapid ascent after exposure to a depth of 33 feet or more for a time sufficient to allow body tissues to become saturated with nitrogen. Predisposing factors for the individual include older age, obesity, fatigue, alcohol consumption before or after dive, and a history of medical problems. General factors are cold water diving, diving in rough water, strenuous diving conditions, history of previous decompression incident, overstaying time at a given dive depth, diving at 80 feet or more, too rapid an ascent, heavy exercise before or after dive, flying after diving (within 24 hours), or driving to high altitude after dive. Signs and symptoms include joint and abdominal pain, fatigue, paresthesia, and CNS disturbances. If the nitrogen bubbles occlude blood flow such that areas of local ischemia develop, tissue damage may occur.

Patients with decompression illness usually seek treatment within 12 hours of ascent, but some may not seek help until 24 hours afterward. Early oxygen therapy may reduce symptoms substantially, and divers who are given high-concentration oxygen have a significantly better treatment outcome. Prehospital management includes a number of steps. First, assess ABCs and administer CPR, if needed. Administer oxygen at 100% concentration with a non-rebreather mask. Intubate if the patient is unconscious. Keep the patient in a supine position and protect him or her from excessive heat or cold, wetness, or noxious fumes. If the patient is conscious and alert, give nonalcoholic liquids such as fruit juice or oral balanced salt solutions. Evaluate and stabilize the patient at the nearest emergency department prior to transfer to a recompression chamber for definitive therapy. Begin IV fluid replacement with electrolyte solutions if the patient is unconscious or seriously injured, otherwise, use lactated Ringer's solution. DO NOT use 5% dextrose in water. If there is evidence of CNS involvement, give dexamethasone, heparin, or diazepam as instructed by medical direction. If air evacuation is used, cabin pressure must be maintained at sea level to avoid worsening of the illness. Be sure to send the diving equipment for examination, if possible.

e. diving emergency   **pp. 530–536**

The underlying physiology of diving emergencies is based on dissolution of gases in water, specifically, oxygen, carbon dioxide, and other gases dissolved in a diver's blood and body tissues. Pressure increases during descent, causing more gas to dissolve. During ascent, decreasing pressure allows gases to come out of solution, and they are eliminated gradually through respiration. If ascent is too rapid, however, dissolved gases, primarily nitrogen, come out of solution and expand in volume quickly, forming bubbles in the blood, brain, spinal cord, inner ear, muscles, and joints. Scuba diving injuries are due to barotrauma (changes in pressure), pulmonary over-pressure, arterial gas embolism, decompression illness, cold, panic, or a combination. Accidents generally occur at one of four phases of the dive: on the surface, during descent, at the bottom, or during ascent. Risk factors at the surface include presence of lines or kelp in which a diver can become entangled, cold water, which might induce shivering or even blackout, and boats or other large objects in the area. Barotrauma during descent is a factor in emergencies occurring during that period. If the diver cannot equilibrate the pressure between the nasopharynx and middle ear, he or she can experience severe pain, ringing in the ears, dizziness, and hearing loss, any of which can cause disorientation or panic, leading to an emergency. A similar problem of disequilibration can occur in the sinuses, producing frontal headache or pain below the eyes. Emergencies at the bottom often involve nitrogen narcosis, a state of stupor commonly called "rapture of the deep." Other emergencies occur when a diver begins to run out of oxygen and panics. Injury during ascent can involve barotrauma or decompression illness. The most serious form of barotrauma is pulmonary over-pressure, a condition in which expansion of air within the alveoli is greater than the tissue can handle and rupture of alveoli occur. If this occurs, the lung sustains structural damage and air entering the circulatory system can cause an arterial gas embolism. Pneumomediastinum (air in the mediastinum) and pneumothorax can also occur.

In a diving emergency, gather all evidence of air embolism and decompression illness together. Specific questions center on the timing and nature of the phases of the dive, as well as the diver's experience and state of equipment. Signs and symptoms of pulmonary over-pressure include substernal chest pain, respiratory distress, and diminished breath sounds. Treatment is the same as for pneumothorax of any other origin (see Chapter 1, "Pulmonology"). The signs and symptoms of arterial gas embolism (AGE) begin within 2–10 minutes of ascent with a rapid, dramatic onset of sharp tearing pain and other symptoms related to the specific organ system affected by lack of blood flow. The most common presentation resembles that of a stroke, with confusion, vertigo, visual disturbances, and loss of consciousness. Presentation may include hemiplegia as well as cardiopulmonary collapse. The key to diagnosis is the history of the dive. Treatment after assessment of ABCs includes use of 100% oxygen via nonrebreather mask, placement of patient in supine position, frequent monitoring of vitals, IV fluids at keep-vein-open rate, and use of a corticosteroid if ordered by medical direction. Transport to a recompression chamber as rapidly as possible under conditions that keep air pressure at that of sea level. Pneumomediastinum produces substernal chest pain, irregular pulse, abnormal heart sounds, reduced blood pressure and narrow pulse pressure, and change in voice. Cyanosis may or may not be present. Field management includes use of high-concentration oxygen via nonrebreather mask, IV with lactated Ringer's or normal saline per medical direction, and transport to an emergency department. Nitrogen narcosis causes the same concerns regarding mental and physical function as present with any other type of intoxication, with the addition of a person's functioning underwater during a dive. Altered level of consciousness and impaired judgment are key in assessment. Treatment involves return to shallow depth as this produces self-resolution.

Less frequent diving problems include oxygen toxicity due to prolonged exposure to high partial pressures of oxygen, hyperventilation, and hypercapnia due to inadequate clearance of carbon dioxide through the breathing equipment. Oxygen toxicity can lead to lung damage or even seizures. Hyperventilation due to excitement or panic may lead to muscle cramps or even decreased level of consciousness. Hypercapnia may also lead to unconsciousness. Finally, poorly prepared air tanks may be contaminated with other gases, which can increase the risk of hypoxia, narcosis, and accidental injury.

f. altitude illness   pp. 536–539
In contrast to diving emergencies, high altitude illnesses are due to decreased ambient pressure creating a low-oxygen environment. As barometric pressure decreases at higher altitudes, lower oxygen availability can both trigger related disorders and aggravate existing medical conditions such as angina, congestive heart failure, COPD, and hypertension. Even in very healthy individuals, rapid ascent to high altitudes without time for acclimatization can cause illness. It is difficult to predict who will be affected by altitude illness: The predictor is hypoxic ventilatory response. There are two medications that may act to prevent altitude illness: acetazolamide and nifedipine. High altitude illness begins to be manifest at approximately 8,000 ft

(2,400 m) above sea level. Aspen, Colorado is located at 2,438 m, and it has 26% less oxygen per volume of air than at sea level. The range considered high altitude is 4,900–11,500 ft. Here, the hypoxic environment causes decreased exercise tolerance, although without major disruption of normal oxygen transport in the blood. The range for very high altitude is 11,500–18,000 ft, and this causes extreme hypoxia during exercise or sleep. Extreme altitude (greater than 18,000 ft) will cause severe illness in virtually everyone. Some signs and symptoms of altitude illness include malaise, anorexia, headache, sleep disturbance, and respiratory distress that worsens with exertion. Specific disorders include acute mountain sickness, high altitude pulmonary edema, and high altitude cerebral edema.

Acute mountain sickness (AMS) usually manifests in an unacclimatized person who ascends rapidly to an altitude of 2,000 m (6,600 ft) or higher. Signs and symptoms include lightheadedness, breathlessness, weakness, headache, and nausea and vomiting. More serious signs can develop, especially if the person continues to ascend: weakness to the point of requiring assistance to dress and eat, severe vomiting, decreased urine output, shortness of breath, and altered level of consciousness. Mild AMS is self-limiting and often improves in 1–2 days if no further ascent occurs. Treatment for AMS consists of halting ascent or possibly lowering altitude, use of acetazolamide and anti-nauseants as needed. Supplemental oxygen will relieve symptoms but is typically used only in severe cases. Definitive treatment for all high altitude illnesses is descent.

High altitude pulmonary edema (HAPE) results from increased pulmonary pressure and hypertension caused by changed blood flow in higher altitude. Children are most susceptible, and men are more susceptible than women. Initial symptoms include dry cough, mild shortness of breath on exertion, and slight crackles in the lungs. Symptoms of progression include severe dyspnea and cyanosis, coughing productive of frothy sputum, and weakness that may progress to coma and death. In its early stages, HAPE is completely reversed by descent and use of oxygen. If immediate descent isn't possible, oxygen can completely reverse HAPE but requires 36–72 hours to do so. Such a supply is rarely available to mountain climbers. An alternative is a portable hyperbaric bag, the use of which simulates a descent of roughly 5,000 ft. Acetazolamide may decrease symptoms. Other medications such as morphine, nifedipine, and furosemide may be useful but carry risk for complications such as hypotension and dehydration.

The exact cause of high altitude cerebral edema (HACE) is unknown. It usually presents as deteriorating neurological status in a patient with AMS or HAPE. The increased fluid in the brain tissue causes increased intracranial pressure. Symptoms include altered mental status, ataxia, decreased level of consciousness, and coma. If descent isn't possible, oxygen and steroids and a hyperbaric bag may help. If coma develops, it may persist for days after descent to sea level, but it usually resolves, although it may leave residual disability.

18. Identify differences between mild, severe, chronic, and acute hypothermia.   **p. 518**

As discussed with objective 17a, mild hypothermia is defined by a core temperature greater than 90°F (32°C) in the presence of signs/symptoms of hypothermia, whereas severe hypothermia is defined as core temperature less than 90°F in the presence of signs/symptoms of hypothermia. Acute hypothermia involves sudden exposure to a cold environment as can happen when someone falls through the ice on a frozen lake. Chronic hypothermia may occur in predisposed persons in ambient temperatures inadequately cold to produce hypothermia in a healthy, appropriately dressed individual. In the U.S., look for it among homeless persons who have endured frequent and prolonged cold stress outdoors.

19. Discuss the impact of severe hypothermia on standard BCLS and ACLS algorithms and transport considerations.   **pp. 520–523**

Severe hypothermia (core temperature less than 86°F or 30°C) mandates a switch from passive rewarming and some degree of active external rewarming to active internal rewarming, which may include use of warm IV fluids, warm, humid oxygen, peritoneal lavage, extracorporeal rewarming, and esophageal rewarming tubes. If pulse or breathing is absent, severe hypothermia mandates continuance of CPR but withholding of IV fluids and limitation of electrical conversion to three times maximum. There are also specific considerations for resuscitation when core temperature is 86°F or less (discussed on text pages 522–523). Drug metabolism in the severely hypothermic patient is significantly decreased, and levels may accumulate that will become toxic when the patient is rewarmed. In addition, it may not be possible to electrically defibrillate a heart that is at a temperature less than 86°F.

20. Differentiate between fresh-water and saltwater immersion as they relate to near-drowning. pp. 526–527

There are differences between fresh-water and saltwater near-drowning because of the difference in the salt content of the water. You should know, however, that although the pathophysiology is different, there is no difference in the end result or in field management. In fresh-water settings, a massive amount of hypotonic water diffuses across the alveolar/capillary interface, resulting in hemodilution, an expansion in blood plasma volume with relative reduction in erythrocyte concentration. Hemodilution produces a thickening of the alveolar walls with inflammatory cells, hemorrhagic pneumonitis, and destruction of surfactant. Surfactant is the lipid substance secreted by lung cells that regulates surface tension on the fluid lining the alveoli, helping to keep them open. Loss of surfactant leads to fluid buildup in the small airways with atelectasis. Because some blood flowing through the lungs is now not oxygenated, hypoxemia results. Saltwater settings are different because the ambient water is hypertonic to that in the body. Thus, water is drawn from the bloodstream into the alveoli, producing pulmonary edema and profound shunting. Hypoxemia again results. In addition, saltwater near-drownings feature respiratory and metabolic acidosis due to retention of carbon dioxide and the development of anaerobic metabolism.

21. Discuss the incidence of "wet" versus "dry" drownings and the differences in their management. p. 525–526

While conscious, the panicky victim typically swallows a lot of water into the stomach, stimulating severe laryngospasm and bronchospasm. Especially in near-drowning victims, this effect prevents significant influx of water into the lungs (and is thus termed a dry drowning or near-drowning). Another effect of laryngospasm is worsening hypoxia, which causes a deepening coma. Morbidity or delayed mortality in near-drowning is primarily due to asphyxia from airway obstruction secondary to water in the airways (if a wet event) or laryngospasm and bronchospasm (if a dry near-drowning). Water in the lungs of a near-drowning survivor may cause lower-airway disease. Dry drownings occur in about 10 percent of drowning victims, which means wet drownings are by far more common.

22. Discuss the complications and protective role of hypothermia in the context of near-drowning. pp. 525, 527–528

In general, the colder the water, the greater the patient's chance for survival. Usually, you expect brain death after 4–6 minutes without oxygen. However, some patients in cold water (below 68°F) may be resuscitated after 30 minutes or more in cardiac arrest. A possible physiologic factor in this phenomenon is the mammalian diving reflex. When a person dives into cold water, the submersion of the face inhibits breathing, drops heart rate, and causes vasoconstriction in tissues relatively resistant to asphyxia even as blood flow to the heart and brain continues. The colder the water, the greater the shunting of blood to brain and heart. This is the origin of the saying "the cold water drowning victim is not dead until he is warm and dead."

23. Define self-contained underwater breathing apparatus (scuba). p. 528

Scuba is the commonly known abbreviation for self-contained underwater breathing apparatus, a portable system that contains compressed air that is delivered to a diver so he or she can breathe underwater.

24. Describe the laws of gases and relate them to diving emergencies and altitude illness. pp. 528–529

Three laws pertaining to the behavior of gases under different physical conditions relate to environmental emergencies.
- *Boyle's law* states that a volume of gas is inversely proportional to its pressure when temperature remains constant. As you increase pressure (as happens during a dive), gas is compressed

into increasingly smaller volumes. One liter of air at the surface fills 500 mL at 33 feet of water depth, and the same one liter fills only 250 mL at 66 feet. As a diver ascends, pressure decreases toward that at the surface and the gas present in tissues and in the blood expands to occupy ever greater volumes. The reason controlled ascent is so important is that the sudden dissolution of gas into bubble form associated with rapid assent causes occlusion of small blood vessels by bubbles, the disorder known as decompression illness. With increasing altitudes, the problem is the reverse. The gas molecules in air expand to occupy an increasingly larger volume, and thus a lungful of air contains ever less gas (including oxygen) at higher altitudes, and hypoxemia and tissue hypoxia can result.

- *Dalton's law* states that the total pressure of a mixture of gases (such as air) is equal to the sum of the partial pressures of each individual gas. Air is roughly 78% nitrogen, 21% oxygen, and 1% carbon dioxide and other trace gases. As altitude changes (upward or downward), those proportions remain the same. The fraction of oxygen in air does not change.
- *Henry's law* states that the amount of a gas dissolved in a given volume of fluid is proportional to the pressure of the gas above it. This law is most relevant to diving. As a person descends to greater depths, oxygen is increasingly used up in cellular metabolism, whereas nitrogen, which is inert, does not change in quantity. Instead, it dissolves into body water. As the person ascends, those gases (particularly nitrogen, because it is present in the greatest amount) come out of the blood and tissues and form bubbles. The correct rate of ascent allows the gas to form bubbles at a rate for which the body can compensate.

25. Differentiate between the various diving emergencies. pp. 530–531

See the discussion with objective 17e. Briefly, one disorder, nitrogen narcosis, is unrelated to change in pressure (barotrauma). Instead, it reflects the sedative and intoxicating effect of nitrogen on the CNS. Disorders related to barotrauma include decompression illness during rapid ascent, in which nitrogen bubbles forming in blood and other body fluids cause severe pain and the possibility of areas of ischemia secondary to occlusion of small blood vessels by bubbles. Lung overinflation associated with rapid ascent can cause pulmonary over-pressure accidents, in which air expansion can rupture alveoli, resulting in hemorrhage and reduced oxygen and carbon dioxide transport, as well as complications due to air leakage.

26. Identify the various conditions that may result from pulmonary over-pressure accidents. pp. 531, 534

Lung overinflation associated with rapid ascent can cause pulmonary over-pressure accidents, in which air expansion can rupture alveoli, resulting in hemorrhage and reduced oxygen and carbon dioxide transport, as well as air leakage into the mediastinum, a condition termed pneumomediastinum. Another condition associated with pulmonary over-pressure is arterial gas embolism (AGE), in which a large bubble of free air can enter the circulation, travel through the left side of the heart, and eventually lodge at some point in the systemic circulation, setting up the possibility of cardiac, pulmonary, or cerebral compromise.

27. Describe the function of the Divers Alert Network (DAN) and how its members may aid in the management of diving-related illnesses. pp. 535–536

The Divers Alert Network (DAN) serves as a non-profit consultant for diving-related health concerns, and it can be contacted through Duke University Medical Center in North Carolina. There are both emergency (919-684-8111) and non-emergency (919-684-2948) telephone numbers.

28. Describe the specific function and benefit of hyperbaric oxygen therapy for the management of diving accidents. p. 533

Decompression illness may require recompression, which can be accomplished by placing the patient in a hyperbaric oxygen chamber (a chamber in which pressure of oxygen is maintained at greater-than-atmospheric levels). In this setting, nitrogen redissolves, relieving the illness. Controlled decompression then allows the nitrogen to come out of solution and be eliminated without forming bubbles. Arterial gas embolism also requires prompt treatment in a recompression chamber so the air embolism can dissolve, relieving the ischemia associated with its occlusion of a blood vessel. These are the only diving-related conditions for which hyperbaric oxygen is standard. In some cases, it may also be required for patients with pulmonary over-pressure.

29. Define acute mountain sickness (AMS), high altitude pulmonary edema (HAPE), and high altitude cerebral edema (HACE). pp. 538–539

- *Acute mountain sickness (AMS)* represents sudden-onset hypoxia in a person unacclimatized to the current altitude. Signs and symptoms are generally mild and the illness often resolves spontaneously within 1–2 days of living at the higher altitude. AMS usually develops after a rapid ascent to an altitude of 2,000 m (6,600 ft) or higher.
- *High altitude pulmonary edema (HAPE)* is a more serious condition caused by increased pulmonary pressure and hypertension due to altitude-induced changes in blood flow. Either immediate descent or 36–72 hours of supplemental oxygen usually relieves the condition.
- *High altitude cerebral edema (HACE)* reflects increased intracranial pressure due to increased fluid in the brain. The pathophysiologic mechanism is unclear. Even with proper treatment, residual disability may result if coma developed before definitive treatment (descent, oxygen, steroids) could improve the patient's condition.

30. Discuss the symptomatic variations presented in progressive altitude illnesses. pp. 538–539

The symptoms associated with AMS are so mild that the patient may never request treatment, and they resemble those associated with severe overexertion (in both cases because root cause is insufficient oxygen and stressed body systems). In HAPE, symptoms of similar severity (cough, shortness of breath on exertion) progress to those of a clearly serious illness: dyspnea, possibly with cyanosis, and coughing productive of frothy sputum. Weakness can progress to coma. The presentation of HACE may follow presentation of AMS or HAPE. The presentation of HACE itself reflects the progressive neurologic deterioration associated with increased intracranial pressure: altered mental status and decreasing level of consciousness, ataxia, and coma.

31. Discuss the pharmacology appropriate for the treatment of altitude illnesses. pp. 537–539

If AMS requires medication, treatment usually consists of acetazolamide and anti-nauseants such as prochlorperazine. Supplemental oxygen will relieve symptoms but is usually reserved for severe cases. HAPE in its early stages can be treated with rapid descent and supplemental oxygen. If descent is not an option, oxygen in combination with a portable hyperbaric bag is useful; pharmacological adjuncts include acetazolamide, morphine, nifedipine, and furosemide. Acetazolamide carries the least risk for complications. HACE is treated with descent, oxygen with a hyperbaric bag, and steroids to reduce intracranial swelling.

32. Given several preprogrammed simulated environmental emergency patients, provide the appropriate assessment, management, and transportation. pp. 505–544

Attention to the ABCs is always important, and this doesn't change with environmental emergencies. The need to move the patient from the harmful environment to one conducive to recovery is special, although not unique (as with inhalation toxicological emergencies). Among the heat disorders, heatstroke is the most serious, and rapid transport is always required.

Hypothermia always requires transport to a hospital setting. The urgency in rewarming varies with the degree of hypothermia, as do some potential complications on rewarming such as cardiac dysrhythmias. Superficial and deep frostbite differ in the depth of tissue affected by freezing; care while en route to the hospital is similar. Early recognition is important to the EMS provider, but prevention is the most important of all steps.

Near-drownings require immediate care and rapid transport to the hospital. Although more than 90% of near-drowning patients survive without sequelae, ARDS can occur as a potentially deadly late complication. Emergencies related to air pressure (diving and altitude) can vary in severity and setting, but immediate care and removal to an appropriate environment as soon as possible are key to treatment. Again, these emergencies are better prevented than treated. Knowing what resources are available in the area is important to treating any of these types of emergencies.

CASE STUDY REVIEW

Reread the case study on page 504 in Paramedic Care: Medical Emergencies *before reading the discussion below.*

This case study demonstrates how paramedics react to a relatively common wintertime emergency: a patient with apparent hypothermia. The case study demonstrates how assessment findings reveal diagnosis, and, as presentation changes, how diagnosis and treatment change as well. The case study also demonstrates how contraindications to certain management steps appear at different stages of hypothermia.

The EMS team is en route to work on a winter day described as "bitterly cold" when they hear a priority call for an unconscious man found lying in snow. As they respond, they do not know any particulars regarding age, possible medical conditions, or even how long the man has been exposed to the snow and cold air.

They find a young man who is huddled and shivering on ice-covered ground. Breathing is shallow and irregular; the approximate number of respirations per minute is not given. The man is conscious, and, although confused, gives a brief, plausible history. He had been out celebrating and passed out. (The case study does not state whether the man admitted to use of alcohol or other drugs during the celebration, substances that may increase vulnerability to hypothermia.) The patient adds he may have been exposed to the elements for a "couple of hours." Important assessment findings include bradycardia, mild hypotension, and a core temperature of 86°F.

At this point, the assessment contains a few elements suggesting mild hypothermia and others pointing to severe hypothermia. Findings consistent with mild hypothermia include the presence of shivering, detectable although irregular respirations, and a level of consciousness sufficient to give a brief history. In contrast, there are also more ominous signs of severe hypothermia: bradycardia and hypotension. The core temperature of 86°F defines the case as severe hypothermia (core temp. less than 90°F).

The team knows that the man has severe hypothermia, and they know they must act quickly as they can expect his condition to continue to deteriorate, perhaps precipitously, as long as he is in the cold environment. Indeed, before they can intervene, the patient's presentation does decline: Shivering stops and speech becomes unintelligible.

The partners quickly move the man into the warm ambulance, remove his wet clothing, apply cardiac and core temperature monitors, and then begin active external rewarming with water bottles at the head, neck, chest, and groin. (The study does not note if the patient was covered with blankets or other insulating material, but you can assume that he was because the other initial actions taken by the team comply with management guidelines.) During this period core temperature does continue to drop, to 85°F. Findings from the cardiac monitor are not given but presumably are stable, as no action is taken against dysrhythmia.

The temperature drop below 86°F signals a new level of urgency. At this temperature, active internal rewarming is mandated with measures such as warm IV fluid, warm humid oxygen, as well as the possible steps of peritoneal lavage, extracorporeal rewarming, and esophageal rewarming tubes. In the prehospital setting, the measures most likely to be available are the warm IV fluid and warm, humid oxygen. The team also knows that they have reached a critical temperature in terms of cardiac instability: Dysrhythmias or asystole are now very real possibilities, and, indeed, the rough handling associated with road construction triggers ventricular fibrillation. Cardioversion is unsuccessful (an expected finding as hearts are generally considered to be incapable of response to defibrillation at temperatures below 86°F).

The providers respond with traditional support for the ABCs: intubation, ventilation with warmed oxygen, and chest compressions. The team makes another correct decision for treatment at this low temperature: They refrain from giving medications via the IV because they know drug metabolism is significantly decreased at this low core body temperature. The drugs may not be useful in the short term and may accumulate to a toxic level once the body core is rewarmed.

At the emergency department, more resources are available to rewarm the patient, and, after core temperature comes rises over 86°F, the usual ACLS protocols are used to stabilize the patient, who eventually recovers fully.

CONTENT SELF-EVALUATION

MULTIPLE CHOICE

_____ 1. General risk factors that predispose a person to developing an environmental illness include all of the following EXCEPT:
   A. predisposing medical conditions such as diabetes.
   B. fatigue.
   C. high levels of fluid intake.
   D. use of certain over-the-counter or prescription medications.
   E. age: either very young or old persons.

_____ 2. Homeostasis is the body's ability to maintain a steady, normal internal environment in the face of changing external conditions.
   A. True
   B. False

_____ 3. Which process is NOT one that results in body heat loss into the environment?
   A. evaporation   D. radiation
   B. convection   E. diffusion
   C. respiration

_____ 4. Which group of medications does NOT predispose a person to hyperthermia?
   A. psychotropics   D. beta blockers
   B. antiepileptics   E. antihistamines
   C. diuretics

_____ 5. Thirst is an adequate indicator of dehydration.
   A. True
   B. False

_____ 6. Dehydration is often intimately associated with heat disorders because it inhibits peripheral vasodilation and limits sweating.
   A. True
   B. False

_____ 7. In situations where it is unclear whether the diagnosis is fever or heatstroke, always treat for both conditions.
   A. True
   B. False

_____ 8. Medical conditions that may predispose to hypothermia include all of the following EXCEPT:
   A. hypothyroidism.   D. thin body build.
   B. malnutrition.   E. hypoglycemia.
   C. Parkinson's disease.

_____ 9. Rewarming is not the mirror image of the cooling process.
   A. True
   B. False

_____ 10. Which is NOT appropriate as a rewarming measure for mild to moderate hypothermia?
   A. warmed blankets   D. heat packs
   B. warmed IV fluids   E. heat lamp
   C. peritoneal lavage

_____ 11. Management guidelines for frostbite include all of the following negatives EXCEPT:
   A. Do not thaw affected area if possibility of refreezing exists.
   B. Do not massage the frozen area or rub with snow.
   C. Do not puncture or drain any blisters.
   D. Do not warm frozen feet if patient will need to walk out of hostile environment.
   E. Do not give analgesia prior to thawing.

_____ 12. The physiology of fresh-water and saltwater drownings differs, and these differences contribute to differences in prognosis and field management.
A. True
B. False

_____ 13. Resuscitation of a drowning victim is not indicated when:
A. respirations have ceased.
B. cardiac asystole exists.
C. the patient has been pulled from freezing water and is very cold himself.
D. immersion is known to have been extremely long.
E. head or neck injury due to trauma is evident.

_____ 14. Which gas law is most applicable to decompression illness?
A. Boyle's law
B. Dalton's law
C. Henry's law
D. Ohm's law
E. Venturi's law

_____ 15. Which of the following might be administered IV to a near-drowning patient?
A. plasmanate
B. dextran
C. lactated Ringer's
D. D_5W
E. hetastarch

_____ 16. One of the most severe complications of near-downing is:
A. "the squeeze."
B. ARDS.
C. DAN.
D. barotrauma.
E. pneumomediastinum.

_____ 17. The condition whose chief signs and symptoms include altered levels of consciousness and impaired judgment is:
A. AGE.
B. "the squeeze."
C. "the bends."
D. pneumomediastinum.
E. nitrogen narcosis.

_____ 18. The condition whose signs and symptoms include substernal chest pain, irregular pulse, abnormal heart sounds, reduced blood pressure and narrow pulse pressure, and a change in voice is:
A. AGE.
B. "the squeeze."
C. "the bends."
D. pneumomediastinum.
E. nitrogen narcosis.

_____ 19. The condition whose signs and symptoms include altered mental status, ataxia, decreased level of consciousness, and coma is:
A. AGE.
B. DAN.
C. HACE.
D. HAPE.
E. AMS.

_____ 20. The unit of local tissue energy deposition in cases of radiation exposure is the:
A. Geiger.
B. RAD.
C. QF.
D. gamma.
E. radioisotope.

MATCHING

Write the letter of the definition in the space provided next to the term it describes.

_____ 21. basal metabolic rate

_____ 22. core temperature

_____ 23. acclimatization

_____ 24. thermolysis

_____ 25. thermoregulation

_____ 26. hypothalamus

_____ 27. negative feedback

_____ 28. heat disorder

A. the temperature of deep body tissues
B. maintenance of a particular body temperature
C. control mechanism through which a substance turns off its further production
D. regulatory structure that serves as part of neurological and endocrine systems
E. increased core body temperature due to inadequate heat dissipation
F. metabolism required simply to maintain body stability
G. loss of body heat to external environment
H. reversible changes in the body that compensate for environmental change

Write the letter of the physiologic or pathophysiologic state in the space provided next to the approximate core body temperature range with which it occurs.

_____ 29. 90°–95°F

_____ 30. 100°–105°F

_____ 31. 86°–90°F

_____ 32. 96°–100°F

_____ 33. 66°–86°F

_____ 34. 105°–114°F

A. severe hypothermia
B. heat exhaustion
C. severe hypothermia with poor prognosis for cardiac stability/resuscitation
D. potentially survivable heatstroke or high fever
E. mild hypothermia
F. normal range

Write the letter of the clinical characteristics in the space provided next to the appropriate disorder.

_____ 35. heat exhaustion

_____ 36. deep frostbite

_____ 37. high altitude cerebral edema

_____ 38. severe hypothermia

_____ 39. acute mountain sickness (early phase)

_____ 40. heatstroke

_____ 41. pulmonary over-pressure

_____ 42. nitrogen narcosis

_____ 43. mild hypothermia

_____ 44. decompression illness

_____ 45. high altitude pulmonary edema

A. moderately decreased core temperature, shivering, lethargy, early rise in heart and respiratory rates
B. dry cough and dyspnea progressing to cough productive of frothy sputum and severe dyspnea
C. severe pain and CNS disturbances that develop during a rapid ascent from a dive to depth below 40 feet
D. environmentally induced freezing of skin and subcutaneous tissues with hardness on palpation, no sensation
E. altered mental status and decreasing level of consciousness, ataxia
F. substernal chest pain that develops during ascent, often from shallow depths, associated with respiratory distress and diminished breath sounds
G. lightheadedness, shortness of breath, nausea after rapid ascent to altitude of 6,600 feet or more
H. stuporous state that develops during deep dives rather than during descent or ascent
I. severely increased core temperature, loss of sweating, hypotension, possible seizures
J. somewhat increased core temperature, rapid, shallow respirations, weak pulses
K. severely decreased core temperature, no shivering, hypotension, dysrhythmias, undetectable pulse and respirations

Write the letter of the key prevention measure in the space provided next to the disorder to which it applies.

_____ **46.** heat disorders (heat cramps, heat exhaustion, heatstroke)

_____ **47.** high altitude illness

_____ **48.** cold disorders (hypothermia)

A. maintain adequate fluid intake, limit exposure to hostile environment, and allow acclimatization

B. dress appropriately, get plenty of rest, eat appropriately, and limit exposure to hostile environment

C. limit exertion, eat properly, consider prophylactic medications, and allow acclimatization

LISTING

49. List the three forms of thermogenesis.

_____

_____

_____

50. List the two major mechanisms for heat dissipation.

_____

_____

51. List the two major mechanisms for heat conservation.

_____

_____

CHAPTER 11
Infectious Disease

Review of Chapter Objectives

After reading this chapter, you should be able to:

1. **Describe the specific anatomy and physiology pertinent to infectious and communicable diseases.** pp. 557–560

   The body's first line of defense against many infectious agents is the skin. Additionally, components of the respiratory system also assist in this endeavor by creating turbulent airflow, while nasal hairs trap pathogens and mucus in the lower airways also traps and kills pathogens. Cilia in the airways move the mucus to the mouth and nose for expulsion. Other bacteria are removed from the body via feces and urine. However, there are three body systems that specifically protect against disease; these are the immune system, the complement system, and the lymphatic system.

   The immune system fights disease by protecting the body from foreign invaders in a mechanism initiated by the inflammatory response and involving white blood cells. There are two types of immune system response: cell-mediated immunity that employs T lymphocytes and humoral immunity that depends on the B lymphocytes to form antibodies. The complement system recognizes surface proteins, providing alternative pathways to combat infection. The lymphatic system is a secondary circulatory system that collects overflow fluid from tissue spaces and filters it before returning it to the circulatory system. The spleen is an essential organ of the lymphatic system whose white pulp generates antibodies and produces B and T lymphocytes, while the red pulp removes unwanted particulate matter, such as old or damaged red blood cells.

2. **Define specific terminology identified with infectious/communicable diseases.** pp. 549–601

   Infectious diseases are illnesses caused by infestations of biological organisms, such as bacteria, viruses, fungi, protozoans, or helminths. Microorganisms that normally reside in our bodies without causing disease are referred to as normal flora and protect us from pathogens (disease-causing organisms). Opportunistic pathogens are ordinarily non-harmful bacteria that cause disease only under unusual circumstances, such as a weakened immune system.

3. **Discuss public health principles relevant to infectious/communicable diseases.** pp. 549–550

   The task of public health epidemiologists is to study how infectious diseases affect populations, as well as to predict and describe how disease moves from individuals to populations and determine what the impact of the disease is on the population. Paramedics must evaluate the host (patient), what they believe to be the infectious agent, and the environment. Based on that assessment, they may opt to use more aggressive personal protective equipment. They must also consider the patient, those in the patient's environment, and the environment where the patient is being transported all to be at risk for infection.

4. Identify public health agencies involved in the prevention and management of disease outbreaks. p. 550

Local agencies including hospitals, fire departments, and EMS agencies cooperate with state and local health departments to monitor and report the incidence and prevalence of disease. Additionally, there are numerous federal agencies involved in tracking the morbidity and mortality of infectious disease, as well as setting standards for workplace disease prevention and control standards. These include: the U.S. Department of Health and Human Services (DHHS) Centers for Disease Control and Prevention (CDC), the National Institute for Occupational Safety and Health (NIOSH), and the U.S. Department of Labor's Occupational Safety and Health Administration (OSHA).

5. List and describe the steps of an infectious process. pp. 555–557

The elements of disease transmission include the interactions of host, infectious agent, and environment. Infectious agents invade hosts by either direct or indirect transmission, and may be bloodborne, airborne, or transmitted by fecal-oral route. Factors that affect the likelihood that an exposed individual will become infected and then actually develop disease include correct mode of entry, virulence (strength), number of organisms transmitted, and host resistance.

6. Discuss the risks associated with infection. pp. 549, 551, 555–557

Infection is the presence of an agent within the host, without necessarily causing disease. Not all exposures result in transmission of microorganisms, nor are all infectious agents communicable. Risk of infection is considered theoretical if transmission is acknowledged to be possible but has not actually been reported. It is considered measurable if factors in the infectious agent's transmission and associated risks have been identified from reported data. Generally, the risk of disease transmission increases if a patient has open wounds, increased secretions, active coughing, or any ongoing invasive treatment where exposure to an infectious body fluid is likely.

7. List and describe the stages of infectious diseases. pp. 555–557

Exposure to an infectious agent may result in contamination or penetration. Penetration implies that infection has occurred, but infection should never be equated with disease. Once infected, the host goes through a latent period when he cannot transmit an infectious agent to someone else. This is followed by the communicable period when the host may exhibit signs of clinical disease and can transmit the infectious agent to another host. The time between exposure and the appearance of symptoms is known as the incubation period, which may range from a few days to months or years.

Most viruses and bacteria have antigens that stimulate the body to produce antibodies. The presence of these antibodies in the blood indicates exposure to the particular disease that they fight. This process is known as seroconversion. The window phase refers to the time between exposure and seroconversion. The disease period is the duration from the onset of signs and symptoms of disease until the resolution of symptoms or death.

8. List and describe infectious agents, including bacteria, viruses, fungi, protozoans, and helminths (worms). pp. 550–554

- *Bacteria:* microscopic single-celled organisms (1–20 micrometers in length) that can be differentiated by their reaction to a chemical staining process; classified by type as spheres (cocci), rods, spirals.
- *Viruses:* disease-causing organisms that are much smaller than bacteria and are only visible with an electron microscope; obligate intracellular parasites, they can grow and reproduce only within a host cell.
- *Fungi:* plant-like microorganisms, most of which are not pathogenic.
- *Protozoans:* single-celled parasitic organisms with flexible membranes and ability to move; rarely a cause of disease in humans, but commonly considered opportunistic pathogens in those patients with compromised immune function.

- *Helminths (worms):* parasitic organisms that live in or on another organism and are common causes of disease where sanitation is poor; various forms include pinworms, hookworms, trichinella.

9. Describe characteristics of the immune system, including the categories of white blood cells, the reticuloendothelial system (RES), and the complement system.
pp. 557–560

The immune system is the body's mechanism for defending against foreign invaders. The various cells involved in the immune response are sometimes collectively referred to as the reticuloendothelial system (RES) because their locations are so widely scattered throughout the body. Reticulo means network and endothelial refers to certain cells that line blood vessels, the heart, and various body cavities. Key to the immune system's response is the ability to differentiate "self" from "nonself." Once an invader is recognized as "nonself," a series of actions is initiated to eradicate the foreign material; this process is known as the inflammatory response. This response involves selected leukocytes (white blood cells) that attack the infectious agent in a process called phagocytosis. Neutrophils act first and then 12–24 hours later are followed by macrophages. The macrophages release chemotactic factors, which trigger additional immune system responses.

The complement system provides an alternative pathway to deal with foreign invaders more quickly than is accomplished through cell-mediated or humoral immunity. This system of at least 20 proteins works with antibody formation and the inflammatory reaction to combat infection by starting a cascade of biochemical events triggered by tissue injury.

10. Describe the processes of the immune system defenses, including humoral and cell-mediated immunity.
pp. 557–560

There are two types of immune system response: cell-mediated immunity, which generates various forms of T lymphocytes that react against specific antigens, and humoral-mediated immunity, which results from antibodies (immunoglobulins) formed from mature B lymphocytes in the lymph nodes and bone marrow. Humoral immunity is responsible for the immune system properties of memory and specificity. Other classes of white blood cells, monocytes, eosinophils, basophils, and natural killer (NK) cells, also participate in the general immune response. There are five classes of human antibodies: IgG—major class of immunoglobulin in the immune response; it crosses the placental barrier and thus plays an important role in producing immunity prior to birth; IgM—formed early in most immune responses; IgA—primary immunoglobulin in exocrine secretions; IgD—acts as an antigen receptor and is present on the surface of B lymphocytes; IgE—attaches itself to mast cells in the respiratory and intestinal tracts, playing a critical role in allergic reactions.

11. In specific diseases, identify and discuss the issues of personal isolation.
pp. 561–604

Understanding the mechanism for disease transmission, as well as the relationship between infectious agent, host, and environment, will allow the EMS provider to make appropriate decisions regarding personal protection against disease. To supplement the body's natural defenses against disease, EMS providers must protect themselves against infectious exposures. Prevention is the most effective approach to infectious disease. All body fluids are possibly infectious, and universal precautions should be followed at all times.

12. Describe and discuss the rationale for the various types of personal protection equipment.
pp. 561–567

Personal protective equipment provides an additional barrier to exposure, thus minimizing the risk of infection from bloodborne and airborne organisms. Isolating all body substances and avoiding contact with them further reduces risk of exposure. Using disposable items for patient care also decreases risk, as does exercising caution around "sharps." Thorough and vigorous hand washing also goes a long way to reduce inadvertent contamination. Dispose of biohazard wastes as proscribed by local laws and regulations. Decontaminate and disinfect infected equipment according to local SOPs and protocols.

13. **Discuss what constitutes a significant exposure to an infectious agent.**   pp. 567–568

All exposures to blood, blood products or any potentially infectious material should be immediately reported to the designated infectious disease control officer (IDCO). The nature of the exposure is assessed based on route (percutaneous, mucosal, or cutaneous), dose, and nature of the infectious agent. For instance, in the case of HIV, the highest risk exposure involves percutaneous exposure with a large volume of blood, a high antibody titer against a retrovirus in the source patient, deep percutaneous injury, or actual intramuscular injection.

14. **Describe the assessment of a patient suspected of, or identified as having, an infectious/communicable disease.**   pp. 568–569

When assessing any patient, you should maintain a high index of suspicion that an infectious agent may be involved. Evaluate every environment for its suitability to transmit infectious agents and always maintain appropriate BSI.

Be alert to clues about the potential for infectious disease based on the patient's past medical history and medication use, as well as his or her chief complaint and the history of present illness. Look for general indicators of infection, such as unusual skin signs or rashes, fever, weakness, profuse sweating, malaise, or dehydration. Follow the standard format for assessing medical patients.

15. **Discuss the proper disposal of contaminated supplies such as sharps, gauze, sponges, and tourniquets.**   pp. 561–565

Any patient care supplies (gauze, sponges, and tourniquets) that have been contaminated by blood or body fluids should be disposed of as biohazard waste in leak-proof biohazard bags and in accordance with local protocol. Dispose of all contaminated sharps in properly labeled puncture-resistant containers.

16. **Discuss disinfection of patient care equipment and areas where patient care occurred.**   pp. 566–567

Decontaminate infected equipment according to local protocols in the appropriate designated area. The decontamination process begins with the removal of surface dirt and debris using soap and water, then disinfect as appropriate, and finally sterilize if required. There are four levels of decontamination:
- *low-level disinfection*—appropriate for routine cleaning and removing visible body fluids
- *intermediate-level disinfection*—appropriate for cleaning equipment that has been in contact with intact skin
- *high-level disinfection*—required for all reusable devices that have come in contact with mucous membranes
- *sterilization*—required for all contaminated invasive instruments

17. **Discuss the seroconversion rate after direct significant HIV exposure.**   pp. 560, 570–571

HIV is detected through the presence of antibodies specific to HIV. When a person develops antibodies after exposure to a disease, his previously negative test will be positive indicating that seroconversion has taken place. The estimated probability of a health care worker becoming infected by a work-related exposure to virus-containing blood is 0.2 to 0.44%.

18. **Discuss the causative agent, body systems affected and potential secondary complications, routes of transmission, susceptibility and resistance, signs and symptoms, patient management and protective measures, and immunization for each of the following:**

- **Human immunodeficiency virus (HIV)** pp. 570–574
  —HIV is a retrovirus with affinity for human T lymphocytes with the CD4 marker.
  —Transmitted via blood, blood products, and body fluids, HIV enters the body through breaks in the skin, mucous membranes, eyes, or by placental transmission (13–30% transmission rate).
  —Destruction of the immune system leads to the development of opportunistic infections and cancers.
  —There is no vaccine or cure, although postexposure prophylaxis with triple therapy (two reverse transcriptase inhibitors and one protease inhibitor) may be helpful.
  —Practice BSI for all potential blood/body fluid exposures during patient care activities.

- **Hepatitis A (HAV)** pp. 574–575
  —Hepatitis A virus is transmitted by fecal-oral route. It has an incubation period of 3 to 5 weeks, with greatest probability of transmission in the latter half of that period.
  —The disease causes inflammation of the liver (also known as viral or infectious hepatitis) evidenced by general malaise, fever, anorexia, nausea and vomiting, and possibly jaundice, although many infections are asymptomatic.
  —Vaccines (Havrix and Vaqta) provide effective active immunization.
  —EMS workers should employ universal precautions against bloodborne or fecal-oral transmission.

- **Hepatitis B (HBV)** p. 575
  —Hepatitis B virus is transmitted by direct contact with contaminated blood or body fluids and is very highly infectious. There is a 1.9–40% transmission rate via cutaneous exposure and a rate of 5–35% via needle stick. The HBV incubation period is 8–24 weeks.
  —HBV causes inflammation of the liver (also known as serum hepatitis) evidenced by general malaise, fever, anorexia, nausea and vomiting, and possibly jaundice, cirrhosis, and malignancies. Some 60–80% of infections, however, are asymptomatic.
  —Vaccines (Recombivax HB, Engerix B) provide effective immunization after completion of series of three IM injections and follow-up antibody screening.
  —Employ universal precautions against bloodborne transmission.

- **Hepatitis C (HCV)** pp. 575–576
  —Hepatitis C virus is transmitted by direct contact with contaminated blood or body fluids.
  —A majority of patients have chronic hepatitis C, which has the ability to cause active disease years later.
  —HCV often causes liver fibrosis, which progresses over the years to cirrhosis.
  —Effective vaccines do not yet exist, although there has been some success in treating disease with alpha interferon, often in combination with ribavirin.
  —Employ universal precautions against bloodborne transmission.

- **Hepatitis D (HDV)** p. 576
  —Hepatitis D virus seems only to coexist with hepatitis B.
  —HDV virus is transmitted by direct contact with contaminated blood or body fluids.
  —HDV causes inflammation of the liver evidenced by general malaise, fever, anorexia, nausea and vomiting, and possibly jaundice, cirrhosis, and malignancies.
  —Immunization against HBV confers immunity to HDV.
  —Employ universal precautions against bloodborne transmission.

- **Hepatitis E** p. 576
  —Hepatitis E virus is transmitted, like hepatitis A, by the fecal-oral route; it is more commonly associated with contaminated drinking water.
  —Hepatitis E causes inflammation of the liver evidenced by general malaise, fever, anorexia, nausea, and vomiting. It occurs primarily in young adults, with highest rates among pregnant women.
  —Employ universal precautions against fecal-oral transmission.

- **Tuberculosis (TB)** pp. 576–579
  —The causative bacteria of the disease is *Mycobacterium tuberculosis*.
  —TB is commonly transmitted through airborne droplets but may also be contracted by direct inoculation through mucous membranes and broken skin or by drinking contaminated milk.
  —The communicability of TB is variable, with an incubation period of 4 to 12 weeks, although disease usually develops from 6 to 12 months after infection.
  —TB primarily affects the respiratory system, including a highly contagious form in the larynx, and may spread to other organ systems causing extrapulmonary TB.
  —No vaccine exists, although postexposure prophylaxis is helpful.
  —Protect against disease transmission by practicing universal precautions, plus donning an N95 (or HEPA) respirator, as well as employing appropriate respiratory precautions while performing CPR or intubation; masking the patient will also reduce exposure to droplet nuclei.

- **Meningococcal meningitis** pp. 582–583
  —The causative organism for meningococcal meningitis is *Neisseria meningitidis*.
  —The infection asymptomatically colonizes in the upper respiratory tract of healthy individuals and then is transmitted by respiratory droplets.
  —Presentation includes fever, chills, headache, nuchal rigidity with flexion, arthralgia, lethargy, malaise, altered mental status, vomiting and seizures; characteristic petechiae rash common in pediatric cases.
  —The incubation period from is from 2 to 4 days, but potentially as long as 10 days.
  —Meningococcal vaccines are available against some of the serotypes but are not routinely recommended for routine immunization of health care workers; postexposure drug prophylaxis is effective.
  —Practice universal precautions and using masks on self or patient.

- **Pneumonia** pp. 579–580
  —Pneumonia's causative organism may be bacterial, viral, or fungal, although the most common pathogen is *Streptococcus pneumoniae*.
  —It is transmitted by airborne droplet inhalation.
  —Acute lung infection is characterized by fever, chills, dyspnea, productive cough, pleuritic chest pain, and adventitious lung sounds indicative of consolidation.
  —An effective vaccine exists for at risk populations: children under 2 years of age, adults over age 65, and anyone without a spleen. Routine vaccination of EMS personnel is not required.
  —Use of respiratory precautions is advised.

- **Tetanus** pp. 594–595
  —*Clostridium tetani* bacillus is the causative organism.
  —Tetanus is transmitted by exposure to *C. tetani* spores, which are present in the soil, street dust, and feces. The condition is often associated with puncture wounds, deep lacerations, or injections.
  —Localized symptoms include rigidity of muscles in close proximity to wound. Generalized symptoms include pain and stiffness of the jaw that may progress to cause muscle spasm and rigidity of the entire body; respiratory arrest may result.
  —The incubation period is variable (usually 3 to 21 days, or 1 to 3 months); shorter periods are linked to more severe illness.
  —Universal precautions should afford sufficient protection, although respiratory protection and goggles are advised for intubation.
  —Vaccinations usually begin in childhood (DTP or diphtheria-tetanus toxoid, pertussis) and every 10 years thereafter; postexposure prophylaxis is often recommended.

- **Rabies** pp. 592–594
  —The causative organism is the rabies virus, a member of the *Rhabdovirus* family and *Lyssavirus* genus, which affects the nervous system
  —Rabies is transmitted in the saliva of an infected animal by bites, through an opening in the skin, or by direct contact with a mucous membrane. Once it enters the body, it then travels

along motor and sensory fibers to the spinal ganglia corresponding to the site of invasion and then to the brain, creating an encephalomyelitis that is almost always fatal.

—Rabies is characterized by a nonspecific prodrome that typically lasts 1 to 4 days (malaise, fever, chills, sore throat, myalgia, anorexia, nausea, vomiting, and diarrhea); this is followed by the encephalitic phase that begins with periods of excessive motor activity, followed by confusion, hallucinations, tetany, and seizures. Focal paralysis appears and if untreated causes death within 2 to 6 days. Attempts to drink water may produce laryngospasm, causing profuse drooling associated with hydrophobia.

—BSI precautions are appropriate and the use of masks may be prudent.

—Several options for rabies immunization are available and are recommended for animal care workers. Postexposure prophylaxis should be discussed on a case-by-case basis with a physician.

- **Hantavirus**   pp. 589–590
—This family of viruses is carried by rodents such as the deer mouse.

—Transmission is primarily by inhalation of aerosols caused by the stirring up of the dried urine, saliva, and fecal droppings of these rodents. Contamination of food and autoinoculation after handling objects tainted by rodent droppings may also cause transmission.

—Hantavirus causes hantavirus pulmonary syndrome (HPS) whose signs and symptoms include fatigue, fever, muscle aches, headaches, nausea, vomiting and diarrhea, and—after 4 to 10 days—pulmonary edema occurs. Hemodynamic compromise occurs approximately 5 days after onset.

—There is no vaccine available.

—Wear masks when in dusty, unoccupied buildings for extended periods of time.

- **Chickenpox**   pp. 581–582
—Chickenpox is caused by the varicella zoster virus (VZV) in the herpesvirus family.

—It is transmitted by airborne droplet inhalation plus direct contact with weeping lesions or contaminated linens.

—Respiratory symptoms include malaise and low-grade fever, followed by a rash that starts on the face and trunk and progresses to the rest of the body including the mucous membranes. The fluid-filled vesicles that form the rash rupture, leaving small ulcers that scab over within a week.

—The incubation period is from 10 to 21 days.

—An effective vaccine exists (Varivax) and is required in some states for admission to elementary school or day care; it is also recommended for susceptible health care workers.

—Employ universal precautions and place masks on patients. Extensive decontamination of the ambulance and any equipment used for patient with chickenpox is strongly recommended.

- **Mumps**   pp. 585–586
—The mumps virus is a member of the genus *Paramyxovirus*.

—It is transmitted through respiratory droplets and direct contact with saliva of infected patients.

—The infection is characterized by painful enlargement of the salivary glands. It presents as a feverish cold followed by swelling and stiffening of the parotid salivary gland in front of the ear, often bilaterally.

—The incubation period is 12 to 25 days.

—A mumps live-virus vaccine is available and should be administered with measles and rubella (MMR) to all children over 1 year of age.

—Standard BSI precautions are advised; EMS personnel should not work without an established MMR immunity.

- **Rubella**   p. 586
—The carrier is the rubella virus of the genus *Rubivirus*.

—It is transmitted by inhalation of infective droplets.

—Rubella is generally milder than measles. It is characterized by a low-grade fever and sore throat, and accompanied by a fine, pink rash on the face, trunk, and extremities that lasts about 3 days.

—The incubation period is 12 to 19 days.

—Immunization should be combined with mumps and measles (MMR) and, due to its devastating effects in a developing fetus, every woman should be immunized prior to becoming pregnant.

—Standard BSI precautions are advised; EMS personnel should not work without an established MMR immunity.

- **Measles**   p. 585

—The carrier is the measles virus of the genus *Morbilli*.

—It is transmitted by droplet inhalation and direct contact.

—Known also as rubeola or hard measles, it is characterized by fever, conjunctivitis, malaise, cough, and nasopharyngeal congestion. Koplik's spots (bluish-white specks with a red halo approximately 1 mm in diameter) appear on the oral mucosa, followed within 24 to 48 hours by a maculopapular rash lasting about 6 days, moving from head to toe.

—The incubation period is 7 to 14 days.

—Immunization is 97–99% percent effective and is usually administered in conjunction with mumps and rubella (MMR).

—Standard BSI precautions are advised, along with vigilant hand washing and masks; EMS personnel should not work without an established MMR immunity.

- **Pertussis (whooping cough)**   p. 587

—Pertussis is caused by the bacterium *Bordetella pertussis*.

—It is transmitted via respiratory secretions or in an aerosolized form and is highly contagious.

—The disease has a three-phase clinical presentation. The catarrhal phase of 1 to 2 weeks resembles a common cold and fever. In the paroxysmal phase of 1 month or longer, fever subsides and the patient develops a mild cough that quickly becomes severe and violent. Rapid consecutive coughs are accompanied by deep high-pitched inspiration, and coughing produces copious thick mucus and may lead to increased intracranial pressure and, potentially, intracerebral hemorrhage. Finally, in the convalescent phase, the frequency and severity of the coughs decrease, and the patient is no longer contagious.

—The incubation period is 6 to 20 days.

—Mask the patient and observe standard BSI precautions, including postexposure hand washing. Booster doses of DTP (diphtheria-tetanus toxoid, pertussis) should be considered.

- **Influenza**   pp. 584–585

—Influenza is caused by viruses designated types A, B, C.

—It is transmitted by airborne droplet inhalation, direct contact, or autoinoculation.

—The disease is characterized by sudden onset of chills, fever (usually of 3 to 5 days duration), malaise, muscle aches, nasal discharge, and cough that may be severe and of long duration.

—The incubation period is from 1 to 3 days.

—Immunization is available and recommended for the elderly, those who live in institutional settings, military recruits, and health care workers.

—Antiviral agents such as amantadine are available but are only effective against type A.

—Universal BSI precautions and good hand washing are recommended.

- **Mononucleosis**   p. 588

—The causative organism of mononucleosis is Epstein-Barr virus (EBV).

—It is transmitted by direct oropharyngeal contact with an infected person.

—Clinical presentation includes fatigue, fever, sore throat, oral discharges, and tender, enlarged lymph nodes. Splenomegaly is not uncommon.

—The incubation period is 4 to 6 weeks.

—No vaccine is available.

—Observe universal BSI precautions, and good hand washing practices are recommended.

- **Herpes Simplex 1 and 2**   pp. 587–588, 598

—There are two forms of herpes simplex, herpes simplex virus type 1 (HSV-1) and herpes simplex virus type 2 (HSV-2).

—HSV-1 is transmitted in the saliva of carriers.

—HSV-1 affects the oropharynx, face, lips, skin, fingers, and toes, although it can cause menin-goencephalitis in newborns and aseptic meningitis in adults. Following an incubation period of 2 to 12 days, fluid-filled vesicles form that soon deteriorate to small ulcers. Lesions may be accompanied by fever, malaise, and dehydration. Lesions usually disappear in 2 to 3 weeks but may recur throughout the patient's life.

—HSV-2 is sexually transmitted, although it may be transmitted during childbirth as the infant moves through the birth canal.

—Presentation of HSV-2 includes vesicular lesions on the genitals, rectum, anus, perineum, or mouth depending on the type of sexual activity. Females may be asymptomatic. Fever and enlarged lymph nodes often accompany initial infection. Lesions last up to several weeks and may recur throughout the patient's lifetime.

—Immunization is not available for either form.

—Universal precautions are absolutely essential, along with good hand washing.

- **Syphilis**   pp. 596–598
—Syphilis is caused by the spirochete *Treponema pallidum*.

—It is transmitted by direct contact with exudates from other syphilitic lesions of the skin and mucous membranes, semen, blood, saliva, and vaginal discharges.

—The disease has four stages: primary syphilis—painless lesion forms 3 to 6 weeks after expo-sure; secondary syphilis—bacteremic stage occurs 5 to 6 weeks after lesion heals; macu-lopapular rash on hands and feet, condyloma latum (painless wart-like lesions on warm, moist skin areas that are very infectious); latent stage—symptoms abate for months to years; tertiary syphilis—wide variety of presentations (cardiovascular, neurologic).

—The incubation period is 3 weeks.

—No immunization is available.

—Universal precautions are absolutely essential along with use of good hand washing practices.

- **Gonorrhea**   p. 596
—Gonorrhea is caused by a gram-negative bacterium, *Neisseria gonorrhoeae*.

—It is transmitted by direct contact with exudates of mucous membranes, primarily from direct sexual contact.

—Presentation varies: in men, it most commonly causes dysuria and purulent discharge, then epididymitis; in women, there is commonly no pain or discharge unless it develops into pelvic inflammatory disease.

—The incubation period is 10 to 14 days.

—Universal precautions are absolutely essential along with use of good hand washing practices.

- **Chlamydia**   pp. 598–599
—Chlamydia is caused by a genus of intracellular parasites most like gram-negative bacteria, *Chlamydia trachomatis*.

—It is transmitted by sexual activity and by hand-to-hand transfer of eye secretions; it often coexists with gonorrhea.

—Presentation varies with symptoms in a manner similar to gonorrhea, but less severe: in men, it most commonly causes dysuria and purulent discharge, then epididymitis; women may have no pain or discharge unless it develops into pelvic inflammatory disease.

—The incubation period is 10 to 14 days.

—Universal precautions are absolutely essential along with use of good hand washing practices.

- **Scabies**   p. 601
—Scabies is caused by infestation of a mite, *Sarcoptes scabiei*.

—The condition is contracted by exposure through close personal contact, from hand holding to sexual contact. Mites remain viable on clothing or bedding for up to 48 hours.

—Upon attaching to a new host, the female burrows into the epidermis to lay eggs within $2^{1}/_{2}$ minutes. Larvae hatch shortly and are full-grown adults in 10 to 20 days. Primary symptom of the condition is intense itching.

—The incubation period is 2 to 6 weeks after infestation. It remains communicable until all mites and eggs are destroyed.

—No immunization is available.

—Bag and remove all linens immediately. Decontaminate stretcher and patient compartment as for lice. Remove and decontaminate any clothing that may have contacted the patient.

- **Lice (Pediculosis)**   **p. 600**

—There are three varieties of infestation: *Pediculus humanus var. capitis* (head lice), *Pediculus humanus var. corporis* (body lice), and *Pthirus pubis* (pubic lice or crabs).

—Lice are transmitted by direct contact, which may or may not be associated with sexual activity.

—Eggs hatch within 7 to 10 days.

—Infestation results in parasitic infection of the skin of the scalp, trunk, or pubic area, which is primarily characterized by intense itching. Red macules, papules, and urticaria commonly appear on the shoulders, buttocks, abdomen, or genital areas.

—No immunization is available.

—Spray the ambulance interior close to the cot and the area by the patient's head with an insecticide, preferably one containing permethrin. Wipe and clean all surfaces to remove insecticide residues.

- **Lyme disease**   **pp. 595–596**

—Lyme disease is caused by the tick-borne spirochete *Borrelia burgdorferi*.

—It is transmitted by the bite of an infected tick.

—A flat, painless red lesion may appear at bite site (and may appear to resemble a bull's eye). This may be accompanied by malaise, headache, and muscle aches; then the spirochete spreads to the skin, nervous system, heart, and joints. Meningitis, cardiac conduction defects, and arthritis are common. Recurrence can appear months to years after initial exposure.

—The incubation period ranges from 3 to 32 days.

—Immunization is available (LYMErix) as a series of three vaccinations.

—Employ universal precautions. Also, when responding in wooded areas, check for ticks, and spray the ambulance compartment with an arthropod-effective insecticide.

- **Gastroenteritis**   **p. 590–591**

—Causative organisms for the condition may be viruses, bacteria, and parasites.

—It is highly contagious via the fecal-oral route, including the ingestion of contaminated food or water.

—Prolonged vomiting and diarrhea may cause dehydration and electrolyte disturbances.

—No immunization is available.

—Follow universal precautions and use aggressive hand washing.

19. **Discuss other infectious agents known to cause meningitis including streptococcus pneumonia, haemophilus influenza type B, and various varieties of viruses.**   **p. 582**

Meningitis is often caused by other infectious agents, particularly *Streptococcus pneumoniae* and *Haemophilus influenzae* type B. *Streptococcus* is the most common cause of adult pneumonia and the leading cause of otitis media in children. Vaccines have proven to be very effective, especially in children. *Haemophilus* was once the leading cause of meningitis in children from 6 months to 3 years of age but the development of a vaccine in the early 1980s has virtually eliminated its incidence. While a variety of viruses have also been known to cause meningitis, in otherwise healthy individuals viral meningitis is a self-limited disease that lasts 7 to 10 days.

20. **Identify common pediatric viral diseases.**   **pp. 581–582, 585–587**

The most common cause of viral illness in children is *respiratory syncytial virus* (RSV), most commonly causing pneumonia and bronchiolitis in infants and young children. Croup and pharyngitis have also been attributed to viruses, such as the parainfluenza virus and rhinovirus. All of these are transmitted by direct inhalation of infected droplets or through exposed mucosal surfaces, as well as autoinoculation from unwashed hands after handling contaminated surfaces.

21. **Discuss the characteristics of and organisms associated with febrile and afebrile diseases including bronchiolitis, bronchitis, laryngitis, croup, epiglottitis, and the common cold.** pp. 584–590

The common cold (viral rhinitis) is caused by the any of the more than 100 serotypes of rhinovirus. Transmission is caused by direct inhalation of infected droplets or through exposed mucosal surfaces, as well as autoinoculation from unwashed hands after handling contaminated surfaces. The incubation period is from 12 hours to 5 days, with an average of 48 hours. Generally, it is a mild illness characterized by nasal congestion, rhinitis, and cough.

Bronchiolitis, bronchitis, laryngitis, croup, and epiglottitis may have bacterial or viral origins, although epiglottitis is most commonly due to *Haemophilus influenzae, Streptococcus pneumoniae,* or *Staphylococcus aureus,* while croup is usual viral.

All of these are transmitted by direct inhalation of infected droplets or through exposed mucosal surfaces, as well as autoinoculation from unwashed hands after handling contaminated surfaces.

22. **Articulate the pathophysiological principles of an infectious process given a case study of a patient with an infectious/communicable disease.** pp. 550–601

As already discussed, the interactions between a host, an infectious agent, and the environment are the elements of disease transmission. Recognizing that infectious agents invade hosts through either direct or indirect transmission, you should generally be able to determine which is applicable given the patient presentation. Your role as an EMS provider is to interrupt disease transmission while providing safe and effective care for your patient, based on your recognition of signs and symptoms and your knowledge of the physiologic priorities for emergency care.

23. **Given several preprogrammed infectious disease patients, provide the appropriate body substance isolation procedure, assessment, management, and transport.** pp. 550–601

Throughout your training, you will encounter a variety of real and simulated patients with a variety of infectious diseases. Use the information provided in your text as well as the application of this information as demonstrated by your instructors, preceptors, and mentors to enhance your ability to assess, manage, and transport these patients. Remember that prevention is the best approach and, for that reason, you should presume that every patient is potentially infectious and take appropriate precautions to minimize your exposure. Your own personal accountability in the area of infection control is equally important: Do not go to work if you have any signs or symptoms of illness, keep your immunizations up to date, and always practice effective hand washing.

CASE STUDY REVIEW

Reread the case study on page 548 in Paramedic Care: Medical Emergencies *before reading the discussion below.*

This case study draws attention to the potential for EMS personnel to be exposed to infectious and communicable disease when in the course of routine delivery of emergency care.

Elizabeth and Stuart are dispatched on a routine call for a person complaining of difficulty breathing. The patient looks acutely ill and the observed signs and symptoms indicate a pulmonary infection. The report of prolonged respiratory problems, recent weight loss, night sweats, and hemoptysis should raise the index of suspicion for tuberculosis. Appropriately, they administer oxygen via nonrebreather mask and establish vascular access at a keep-open rate.

Although not specified in this scenario, it is hoped that Elizabeth and Stuart practiced universal precautions while caring for this patient, just as with any other. It is reasonable and appropriate to adopt a high-index-of-suspicion-driven response to potential exposures to any infectious agent. Fortunately, their exposure to this patient did not result in their becoming infected with tuberculosis.

CONTENT SELF-EVALUATION

MULTIPLE CHOICE

_____ 1. Microscopic single-celled organisms that can be differentiated by their reaction to a chemical staining process are called:
A. helminths.
B. bacteria.
C. viruses.
D. fungi.
E. protozoans.

_____ 2. Single-celled parasitic organisms that are a common cause of opportunistic infection are called:
A. helminths.
B. bacteria.
C. viruses.
D. fungi.
E. protozoans.

_____ 3. All microorganisms that reside in our bodies are pathogenic.
A. True
B. False

_____ 4. Visible only by electron microscope, obligate intracellular parasites that resist antibiotic treatment are called:
A. helminths.
B. bacteria.
C. viruses.
D. fungi.
E. protozoans.

_____ 5. All of the following are airborne diseases EXCEPT:
A. meningitis.
B. tuberculosis.
C. measles.
D. syphilis.
E. influenza.

_____ 6. The presence of an infectious agent within the host, without necessarily causing disease, is referred to as:
A. infection.
B. contamination.
C. communicable.
D. exposure.
E. virulence.

_____ 7. All of the following are factors that affect disease transmission EXCEPT:
A. mode of entry.
B. virulence.
C. dose of organism.
D. host resistance.
E. type of organism.

_____ 8. Surface proteins on viruses and bacteria that stimulate the production of antibodies are called:
A. pathogens.
B. prokaryotes.
C. antigens.
D. prions.
E. eukaryotes.

_____ 9. The creation of antibodies following an exposure to a disease is called:
A. incubation.
B. seroconversion.
C. latency.
D. infection.
E. contamination.

_____ 10. All of the following are agents for the body's general immune response EXCEPT:
A. neutrophils.
B. monocytes.
C. macrophages.
D. lymphocytes.
E. antigens.

_____ 11. Cellular-mediated immunity does not result in the formation of antibodies against foreign antigens.
A. True
B. False

_____ 12. The principle immunoglobulin in human serum and the major class of immunoglobulin in the immune response is:
  A. IgA.   D. IgG.
  B. IgD.   E. IgM.
  C. IgE.

_____ 13. The body's formation of antibodies against itself is known as:
  A. autoinoculation.   D. phagocytosis.
  B. contamination.   E. cellular-mediated immunity.
  C. autoimmunity.

_____ 14. Antibodies, B lymphocytes, and T lymphocytes are produced by the:
  A. thymus.   D. bone marrow.
  B. spleen.   E. lymph nodes.
  C. complement system.

_____ 15. Sterilization is the recommended level of decontamination for all equipment used by EMS personnel.
  A. True
  B. False

_____ 16. At the scene of a motor vehicle accident, all of the following are appropriate infection control measures EXCEPT:
  A. wearing gloves and changing them between patients.
  B. using protective eyewear or face shields to limit splash exposures.
  C. recapping needles to reduce risk of needlestick to others.
  D. decontaminating all reusable equipment.
  E. putting all contaminated dressings in a leak-proof biohazard bag.

_____ 17. Risk factors for developing infectious disease include:
  A. immunosuppression.   D. alcoholism.
  B. diabetes.   E. all of the above
  C. artificial heart valves.

_____ 18. Which of these infectious diseases poses the greatest risk to EMS personnel as a result of work-related exposures?
  A. AIDS   D. hepatitis B
  B. tuberculosis   E. hantavirus
  C. hepatitis A

_____ 19. The most significant problem associated with HIV is:
  A. opportunistic infection.   D. blindness.
  B. hemorrhage.   E. splenomegaly.
  C. dementia.

_____ 20. The most common form of hepatitis transmitted by the fecal-oral route is:
  A. hepatitis A.   D. hepatitis D.
  B. hepatitis B.   E. hepatitis E.
  C. hepatitis C.

_____ 21. Primarily a respiratory disorder, the most common preventable adult infectious disease in the world is:
  A. hepatitis A.   D. pneumonia.
  B. tuberculosis.   E. influenza.
  C. HIV.

_____ 22. Your 60-year-old patient reports an acute onset of high fever, chills, dyspnea, pleuritic chest pain, and a productive cough. You suspect:
  A. hantavirus.   D. pneumonia.
  B. tuberculosis.   E. influenza.
  C. HIV.

_____ 23. Your patient has a low-grade fever and malaise and is covered from head to toe with fluid-filled vesicles and small ulcers. You suspect:
   A. measles.   D. meningitis.
   B. rubella.   E. scabies.
   C. chickenpox.

_____ 24. Your patient reports an acute onset of high fever, stiff neck, and severe headache. You suspect:
   A. measles.   D. meningitis.
   B. rubella.   E. scabies.
   C. chickenpox.

_____ 25. All of the following are viral infections that may be contracted in the EMS setting EXCEPT:
   A. measles.   D. meningitis.
   B. rubella.   E. scabies.
   C. chickenpox.

_____ 26. The most important personal precaution against disease transmission is:
   A. effective hand washing.
   B. up-to-date immunizations.
   C. postexposure prophylaxis.
   D. disinfection of equipment.
   E. compliance with infection control policies.

_____ 27. Your partner reports a sudden onset of fever, chills, malaise, muscle aches, nasal discharge, and a cough. You suspect:
   A. hantavirus.   D. pneumonia.
   B. tuberculosis.   E. influenza.
   C. HIV.

_____ 28. All of the following are causative organisms for food poisoning EXCEPT:
   A. _Escherichia coli._   D. _Salmonella._
   B. _Haemophilus influenzae._   E. _Shigella._
   C. _Campylobacter._

_____ 29. The clinical presentation of encephalitis often mimics that of meningitis.
   A. True
   B. False

_____ 30. All of the following are sexually transmitted diseases EXCEPT:
   A. HSV-2.   D. HPV.
   B. chlamydia.   E. gonorrhea.
   C. HAV.

SPECIAL PROJECT

Decontamination Procedures

Complete the table below regarding decontamination procedures.

Method and Cleaning Agent	Indication	Effectiveness
Low-level disinfection *Agent:*		
Intermediate-level disinfection *Agent:*		
High-level disinfection *Agent:*		
Sterilization *Agent:*		

CHAPTER 12

✳

Psychiatric and Behavioral Disorders

Review of Chapter Objectives

After reading this chapter, you should be able to:

1. **Define behavior and distinguish among normal behavior, abnormal behavior, and the behavioral emergency.** pp. 608–609

   Behavior is a person's observable conduct and activity, while a behavioral emergency is a situation in which a patient's behavior becomes so unusual, bizarre, or threatening that it alarms the patient or another person and requires the intervention of EMS and/or mental health personnel. The differentiation between "normal" and "abnormal" behavior is largely subjective and widely variable based on culture, ethnic group, socioeconomic class, environment, and personal interpretation and opinion.

2. **Discuss the prevalence of behavioral and psychiatric disorders.** p. 609

   It is estimated that 20 percent of the population has some type of mental health problem and that as many as 1 in 7 will require treatment for an emotional disturbance.

3. **Discuss the pathophysiology of behavioral and psychiatric disorders.** pp. 609–610

   The general causes of behavioral and psychiatric disorders are biological (organic), psychosocial, and sociocultural. Biological (organic) causes are related to disease processes or structural changes in the brain. Psychosocial causes are related to the patient's personality, dynamics of unresolved conflict, or crisis management methods. Sociocultural causes are related to the patient's actions and interactions within society. It should be noted that many psychiatric disorders are due to altered brain chemistry.

4. **Discuss the factors that may alter the behavioral or emotional status of an ill or injured individual.** pp. 609–610

   Remember that you cannot be sure that a patient is suffering from a purely psychological condition until you have completely ruled out medical conditions, such as hypoglycemia, traumatic injury, and substance abuse. Failure to comply with the prescribed medication regimen may cause exacerbation of a patient's psychiatric condition and lead to the development of a behavioral emergency. Societal events (rape, assault, and acts of violence) may contribute to alterations in someone's emotional status, as can interpersonal events, such as death of a loved one or loss of a relationship.

5. **Describe the medical legal considerations for management of emotionally disturbed patients.** pp. 627–628

The laws of consent specify that any competent person has the right to refuse to consent to treatment. Further, no competent person may be transported against his/her will. Any person who is in imminent danger of harming him-/herself or others is not considered competent to refuse treatment and transport. Most states have laws that allow persons fitting this criterion to be transported against their will to a hospital or approved psychiatric facility for evaluation.

6. **Describe the overt behaviors associated with behavioral and psychiatric disorders.** pp. 614–625

Overt behaviors that may be associated with behavioral emergencies include hand gestures (clenched fists, wringing hands, etc.) or postures (cowering, visible tension, etc.) that you may observe in your patient. The patient may display strange or threatening facial expressions. The patient's speech may reveal disorientation, fixations, unrealistic judgments, or unusual thought processes. Other behaviors you may observe include pacing, picking at one's skin, or appearing to pull things from the air. There are many different kinds of such overt behaviors, and they can differ or overlap depending on the specific disorder.

7. **Define the following terms:**

- **Affect** p. 611
  Visible indicators of mood or the impression that someone else may have about one's mood based on one's appearance. For instance, a person with a flat affect gives the appearance of being disinterested and is often lacking facial expression.

- **Anger** p. 617
  This can be described as feelings of hostility or rage to compensate for an underlying feeling of anxiety.

- **Anxiety** pp. 616–617
  This is a state of uneasiness, discomfort, apprehension, and restlessness.

- **Confusion** p. 611
  This is a state of being unclear or unable to make a decision easily.

- **Depression** pp. 618–619
  This is a profound sadness or feeling of melancholy.

- **Fear** p. 611
  Fear is a feeling of alarm and discontent in the expectation of danger.

- **Mental status** p. 611
  This is defined as the state of the patient's cerebral functioning.

- **Open-ended question** p. 612
  This is the type of question that cannot be answered by "yes" or "no" and requires a longer response from the person being questioned.

- **Posture** p. 611
  This term refers to the position, attitude, or bearing of the body.

8. **Describe verbal techniques useful in managing the emotionally disturbed patient.** pp. 611–613

The key to dealing with the emotionally disturbed patient is to listen carefully. Place yourself at the patient's level, but keep a safe and proper distance, not invading the patient's personal space. Ask open-ended questions that require your patient to respond in detail. Be comfortable with silence and take whatever time is necessary to get the whole story of the situation. Do not lie to or make fun of the patient. Be nonjudgmental.

9. **List the appropriate measures to ensure the safety of the paramedic, the patient, and others.** pp. 610–612, 627–631

As with any call, determining scene safety is critical. Many behavioral emergencies, for which you are dispatched, will also warrant mutual response by law enforcement personnel. Gain control of the scene. Remove anyone who agitates the patient or adds confusion to the scene. Examine the environment for signs of violence and potential weapons. Approach every situation cautiously and when feasible observe the patient from a distance first before approaching. Avoid invading the patient's personal space. Watch for signs of aggression. If a patient becomes violent, use of restraint may become necessary; in such cases, carefully follow your service's protocols for such circumstances and be sure to document your actions thoroughly.

10. **Describe the circumstances when relatives, bystanders, and others should be removed from the scene.** p. 611

It is important to gain control of the scene as quickly as possible. Remove anyone who agitates the patient or adds to the confusion on the scene. Generally, it is a good idea to limit the number of people around the patient. You may even find it necessary to totally clear the room or to move the patient to a quiet area.

11. **Describe techniques to systematically gather information from the disturbed patient.** pp. 611–613, 627

Your interpersonal skills are crucial to your success as an EMS professional but never more so than when you are caring for a patient who is having a behavioral emergency. Limit environmental distractions at the scene. Introduce yourself and note how the patient responds to you, altering your approach if the patient becomes agitated. Establish eye contact. Place yourself at the patient's level. Listen carefully. Take your time. Do not physically threaten the patient. Ask open-ended questions. Be truthful with the patient and never play along with hallucinations or delusions. Focus your questioning and assessment on the immediate problem.

12. **Identify techniques for physical assessment in a patient with behavioral problems.** pp. 611–613, 627–631

All of the interpersonal skills discussed above that allow you to effectively interview patients will need to be incorporated into your physical assessment activities. Generally, the examination of a behavioral emergency patient is largely conversational. If you need to perform hands-on assessment activities, defer their completion until you have had the opportunity to establish rapport and, even then, do not make any sudden moves that may startle the patient. If a patient is restrained, be sure to monitor him or her frequently and carefully to assure that the airway is patent and that he or she is not experiencing positional asphyxia.

13. **List situations in which you are expected to transport a patient forcibly and against his will.** pp. 627–631

Any person who is in imminent danger of harming him-/herself or others is not considered competent to refuse treatment and transport. Patients who are suicidal or homicidal meet this criterion. Most states have laws that allow persons fitting this criterion to be transported against their will for evaluation. The authority to make this decision varies from state to state. Other situations are not so clear-cut and require you to use clinical judgment and follow your service's protocols.

14. **Describe restraint methods necessary in managing the emotionally disturbed patient.** pp. 628–631

The primary objective is to restrict the patient's movement to prevent him from harming himself or others. Your own agency's rules will dictate the appropriate technique and method for restraint. The following rules always apply: use minimum necessary force; use appropriate devices; remember that restraint is not punitive; and carefully monitor anyone who is restrained. Before initiating any restraint activities, make sure that you have sufficient help, as this minimizes the potential for injury to the patient or yourself.

15. List the risk factors and behaviors that indicate a patient is at risk for suicide.   **p. 624**

All of the following are considered to be risk factors for suicide: previously attempted suicide, depression, age (15 to 24 years of age or over 40), substance abuse, social isolation, major separation trauma, major physical stresses, loss of independence, suicide of a parent. Also significant is having possession of a mechanism for suicide and having a specific plan and/or expressing it.

16. Use the assessment and patient history to differentiate between the various behavioral and psychiatric disorders.   **pp. 610–625**

Most psychiatric disorders have two diagnostic elements: symptoms of the disease/disorder and indications that the disease/disorder has impaired major life functions or interfered with the activities of daily living. It is not the role of EMS personnel to diagnose behavioral disorders, as this can be a difficult task even for skilled mental health professionals. The overview of psychiatric disorders is intended to increase your general understanding of behavioral problems.

The most helpful thing you can do is to perform a mental status exam (MSE) as part of your routine assessment. The elements of an MSE include: general appearance, behavioral observations, orientation, memory, sensorium, perceptual processes, mood and affect, intelligence, thought processes, insight, judgment, psychomotor.

17. Given several preprogrammed behavioral emergency patients, provide the appropriate scene size-up, initial assessment, focused assessment, and detailed assessment, then provide the appropriate care and patient transport.   **pp. 608–631**

Throughout your training, you will encounter a variety of real and simulated patients with behavioral or psychiatric emergencies. Use the information in the text, as well as the application of this information as demonstrated by your instructors, preceptors, and mentors to enhance your ability to assess, manage, and transport patients with behavioral emergencies. Every emergency call has an element of behavioral emergency in it; your patience and professionalism will help minimize the emotional component for everyone involved.

CASE STUDY REVIEW

Reread the case study on pages 607 and 608 in Paramedic Care: Medical Emergencies *before reading the discussion below.*

This case study draws attention to the assessment and management of a commonly encountered patient presentation, in which an individual is exhibiting bizarre behavior in a public setting.

The paramedics arrive on-scene and obtain information about the situation from the store manager who has placed the 911 call. When the patient notices their arrival and becomes more agitated, they retreat to the ambulance and request assistance from law enforcement personnel.

As is often the case, the police officers recognize the patient from previous interactions with him. Before approaching the patient, the paramedics and police officers coordinate their plans and anticipate the potential need for restraint. Using a team approach to subdue and restrain the patient minimizes the risk of injury for all involved. Once the patient is safely restrained, a thorough assessment is performed to rule out possible medical or traumatic causes for the patient's altered mental status and agitation. En route to the hospital the patient is carefully monitored to insure his well-being.

CONTENT SELF-EVALUATION

MULTIPLE CHOICE

_____ 1. Organic causes for behavioral emergencies include all of the following EXCEPT:
    A. tumor.   D. infection.
    B. depression.   E. hypoglycemia.
    C. substance abuse.

_____ 2. It is always safe to assume that a patient exhibiting bizarre behavior is suffering from a psychological problem or disease.
   A. True
   B. False

_____ 3. The term that describes the state of a patient's cerebral functioning is:
   A. affect.
   B. mood.
   C. mental status.
   D. orientation.
   E. sensorium.

_____ 4. The best approach for gaining information from a behavioral emergency patient is to:
   A. ask questions requiring yes or no answers.
   B. talk loudly to establish control.
   C. ask open-ended questions.
   D. physically restrain the patient before questioning.
   E. move quickly to expedite transport and then question.

_____ 5. The structured exam designed to quickly evaluate a patient's level of mental functioning is the:
   A. neurologic exam.
   B. mental status exam.
   C. psychiatric evaluation.
   D. Glasgow Coma Score.
   E. stroke assessment scale.

_____ 6. The most likely way to provoke violence or aggression in a behavioral emergency patient is to:
   A. listen carefully to his responses.
   B. appear patient and unhurried.
   C. ask open-ended questions.
   D. invade his personal space.
   E. avoid rapid or sudden movements.

_____ 7. Panic attack, phobias, and posttraumatic stress syndrome are classified as:
   A. types of schizophrenia.
   B. personality disorders.
   C. variants of depression.
   D. bipolar disorders.
   E. anxiety disorders.

_____ 8. The most prevalent form of psychiatric problem is:
   A. schizophrenia.
   B. personality disorder.
   C. depression.
   D. bipolar disorder.
   E. anxiety disorder.

_____ 9. Profound sadness, diminished ability to concentrate, and feelings of worthlessness are commonly associated with:
   A. schizophrenia.
   B. personality disorders.
   C. depression.
   D. bipolar disorders.
   E. anxiety disorders.

_____ 10. Medications commonly used in the management of schizophrenia are:
   A. antipsychotics.
   B. sedatives.
   C. antihistamines.
   D. antipsychotics and sedatives.
   E. sedatives and antihistamines.

_____ 11. Common causes of dementia include all of the following EXCEPT:
   A. Alzheimer's disease.
   B. head trauma.
   C. cardiac seizure.
   D. Parkinson's disease.
   E. AIDS.

_____ 12. Hallucinations, delusions, and disorganized thought, speech, and behavior are commonly associated with:
   A. schizophrenia.
   B. personality disorders.
   C. depression.
   D. bipolar disorders.
   E. anxiety disorders.

_____ 13. The compelling desire to use a substance, inability to reduce use of a substance, and repeated unsuccessful efforts to quit using that substance are indicators of:
   A. psychological dependence.
   B. physical dependence.
   C. substance tolerance.
   D. factitious disorder.
   E. somatoform disorder.

_____ 14. The primary objective in patient restraint is to:
   A. initiate punitive response.
   B. stop dangerous behaviors.
   C. limit patient strength.
   D. reduce legal liability.
   E. encourage patient cooperation.

_____ 15. When a pediatric or geriatric patient is experiencing a behavioral emergency, the paramedic should always consider using chemical restraints.
   A. True
   B. False

MATCHING

Write the letter of the word or phrase in the space provided next to its definition.

A. delirium
B. dementia
C. schizophrenia
D. delusions
E. hallucinations
F. catatonia
G. paranoid
H. bipolar disorder
I. personality disorder
J. depersonalization

_____ 16. Feeling detached from oneself

_____ 17. Condition characterized by relatively rapid onset of widespread disorganized thought

_____ 18. Fixed false beliefs

_____ 19. Condition that results in persistently maladaptive behavior

_____ 20. Sensory perceptions with no basis in reality

_____ 21. Condition characterized by one or more manic episodes, with or without subsequent or alternating periods of depression

_____ 22. Condition characterized by immobility, rigidity, and stupor

_____ 23. Common disorder involving significant behavioral changes and disorganized thought

_____ 24. Preoccupation with feelings of persecution

_____ 25. Condition involving gradual development of memory impairment and cognitive disturbance

SPECIAL PROJECT

Crossword Puzzle

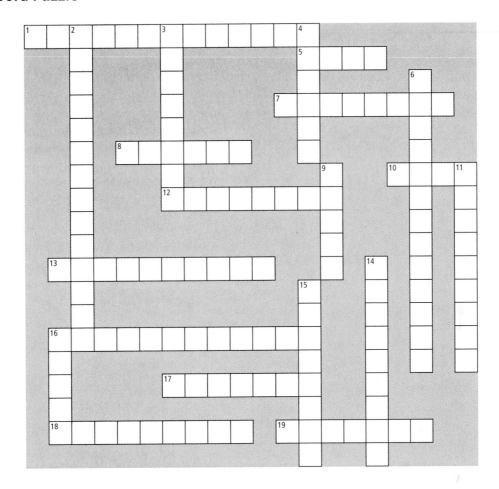

Across
1. Common mental health problem associated with significant behavioral change and a loss of contact with reality
5. Feeling of alarm in expectations of danger
7. Person's observable conduct and activity
8. Excessive fear that interferes with functioning
10. Pervasive emotion that colors a person's perception of the world
12. Condition involving gradual development of memory impairment and cognitive disturbance
13. One of the three general causes of behavioral emergencies, related to disease processes or structural changes
16. Another of the three general causes of behavioral emergencies, related to the person's personality style, unresolved conflicts, or crisis management methods
17. Sometimes known as a manic-depressive mood disorder
18. Displays of rigidity, immobility, and stupor often associated with schizophrenia
19. Intentional taking of one's own life commonly seen in association with depression

Down
2. Sensory perception with no basis in reality
3. Preoccupation with a feeling of persecution
4. Visible indicators of mood
6. Another of the three general causes of behavioral emergencies, related to the patient's actions and interactions with society
9. Excessive excitement or activity
11. Fixed false beliefs that are not widely held within the context of the individual's cultural or religious group
14. Extreme response to stress characterized by impaired ability to deal with reality
15. Condition characterized by a relatively rapid onset of widespread disorganized thought
16. Extreme anxiety resulting in great emotional distress

CHAPTER 13

Gynecology

Review of Chapter Objectives

After reading this chapter, you should be able to:

1. **Review the anatomic structures and physiology of the female reproductive system.** pp. 637–641

   The most important female reproductive structures are located within the pelvic cavity. Essential to reproduction, these structures include the ovaries, fallopian tubes, uterus, and vagina. The external genitalia have accessory functions, in that they protect body openings and play an important role in sexual functioning.

2. **Identify the normal events of the menstrual cycle.** pp. 641–643

   A monthly hormonal cycle prepares the uterus to receive a fertilized egg. The first 2 weeks of the cycle (known as the proliferative phase) are dominated by estrogen causing the uterine lining to thicken. In response to a surge of luteinizing hormone, ovulation takes place and an egg is released from the ovary. The secretory phase is the stage of the menstrual cycle immediately surrounding ovulation. If the egg is not fertilized, the woman's estrogen level drops sharply while the progesterone level dominates. Uterine vascularity increases in anticipation of implantation. If fertilization does not occur, estrogen and progesterone levels fall, triggering vascular changes leaving the endometrium ischemic. The ischemic endometrium is shed during the menstrual phase (menstruation), along with a discharge of blood, mucus, and cellular debris. Menstrual flow usually lasts 3 to 5 days, with an average blood loss of 50 ml.

3. **Describe how to assess a patient with a gynecological complaint.** pp. 643–646

   The most common gynecological complaints are abdominal pain and vaginal bleeding. Complete your initial assessment in the usual manner and then proceed with a focused history and physical exam. Specific questions will need to be asked that are pertinent to reproductive function and dysfunction. If pertinent, be sure to gather information about her obstetrical history, including pregnancies and deliveries. It is important to document the date of the patient's last menstrual period (LMP). You should also ask what form of birth control, if any, she uses and, if pertinent, whether she uses it regularly. Pay particular attention to the physical exam, which will be limited to assessment of the abdomen and potentially (in the presence of serious bleeding) inspection of the patient's perineum. Gently auscultate and palpate the abdomen. Be sure to note the color, character, and volume of any blood lost. An internal vaginal exam should never be performed in the prehospital setting.

4. **Explain how to recognize a gynecological emergency.** pp. 643–646

   As with any emergency situation, vital signs are useful clues as to your patient's status as well as its severity. Be alert for early signs of shock or a positive tilt test, both of which point to significant blood loss. If possible, estimate blood loss. The use of two sanitary pads per hour is considered significant bleeding.

5. Describe the general care for any patient experiencing a gynecological emergency.   **pp. 646–647, 649**

Management of gynecological emergencies is focused on supportive care. Rely on your initial assessment guidance in your decision making about oxygen therapy, ventilatory support, and vascular access. In the presence of shock, follow your local protocols for fluid resuscitation and use of the PASG. In cases of heavy bleeding, do not pack dressings in the vagina. Continue to monitor the patient's status and bleeding en route to definitive care. Equally important is the psychological support that you give your patient. Protect her modesty and privacy.

6. Describe the pathophysiology, assessment, and management of the following gynecological emergencies.

a. Pelvic inflammatory disease   pp. 647–648

Pelvic inflammatory disease (PID), the most common cause of nontraumatic abdominal pain in women in the childbearing years, is an infection of the female reproductive tract that is most commonly caused by gonorrhea or chlamydia. Predisposing factors include: multiple sexual partners, prior history of PID, recent gynecological procedure, or an IUD. The patient will look acutely ill and will often present with diffuse lower abdominal pain, and may also have fever, chills, nausea, vomiting, and possibly a foul-smelling vaginal discharge. The patient may also walk with a shuffling gait due to pain. Blood pressure may be normal, and fever may or may not be present. Palpation of the lower abdomen usually elicits moderate to severe pain. The primary management in the field is supportive care and a position of comfort during transport. If the patient appears septic, then administer oxygen and initiate IV therapy.

b. Ruptured ovarian cyst   p. 648

Cysts are fluid-filled pockets, and, when they develop in the ovary, they can rupture and be a source of abdominal pain. The rupture spills a small amount of blood into the abdomen, irritating the peritoneum and causing abdominal pain and rebound tenderness. Usually the patient complains of moderate to severe unilateral abdominal pain that may radiate to the back; it may be associated with vaginal bleeding. The patient may also report pain during intercourse or a delayed menstrual period. The primary management in the field is supportive care and a position of comfort during transport.

c. Cystitis   p. 648

A bacterial infection of the urinary bladder (cystitis) is a common cause of abdominal pain that may be accompanied by urinary frequency, dysuria, and a low-grade fever. The pain is generally located just above the symphysis pubis unless the infection has spread to the kidneys, in which case there is likely to be flank pain as well. The primary management in the field is supportive care and a position of comfort during transport.

d. Mittelschmerz   p. 648

Mid-cycle abdominal pain may accompany ovulation. The unilateral lower quadrant pain is usually self-limited and may be accompanied by mid-cycle spotting. Treatment is symptomatic.

e. Endometritis   p. 648

Endometritis, an infection of the uterine lining, is an occasional complication of miscarriage, childbirth, or gynecologic procedures. Commonly reported signs and symptoms include mild to severe lower abdominal pain, a bloody and foul-smelling discharge, and fever that may mimic PID. The primary management in the field is supportive care and a position of comfort during transport. If the patient appears septic, then administer oxygen and initiate IV therapy.

f. Endometriosis   pp. 648–649

Endometriosis is a condition in which endometrial tissue is found outside the uterus. Most commonly, it is found in the abdomen and pelvis. Regardless of the site, the tissue responds to the hormones of the menstrual cycle, thus bleeding in a cyclic manner. The condition is most common in women between 30 and 40 and is rare in postmenopausal women. The patient complains of dull, cramping pelvic pain, usually related to menstruation. The primary management in the field is supportive care and a position of comfort during transport.

g. Ectopic pregnancy p. 649

Ectopic pregnancy is the implantation of a fetus outside of the uterus, most commonly in the fallopian tubes. Patients usually report severe unilateral abdominal pain that may radiate to the shoulder on the affected side, a late or missed menstrual period, and sometimes vaginal bleeding. As the fetus develops, the tube can rupture, triggering a massive, life-threatening hemorrhage. Absorb the bleeding but do not pack the vagina. Ectopic pregnancy is a surgical emergency, and the primary management in the field is supportive care and a position of comfort during transport, as well as oxygen administration and IV therapy for fluid resuscitation.

h. Vaginal hemorrhage pp. 649–650

Nontraumatic vaginal hemorrhage is rarely encountered in the prehospital setting unless it is severe. Do not presume that such bleeding is due to normal menstrual flow. Most commonly, it is due to a spontaneous abortion (miscarriage) and is associated with cramping abdominal pain and the passage of clots and tissue. Other possible causes include cancerous lesions, PID, or the onset of labor. Absorb bleeding but do not pack the vagina. The primary management in the field is supportive care and a position of comfort for the patient, as well as oxygen administration and IV therapy for fluid resuscitation. If the bleeding is due to miscarriage, this will likely be a significant emotional event for your patient, so your kind and considerate care is important.

Traumatic vaginal bleeding may result from sexual assault, blunt-force injuries to the lower abdomen, seat-belt injuries, objects inserted into the vagina, self-attempts at abortion, and lacerations following childbirth. Bleeding in such cases should be managed by direct pressure over a laceration or a cold pack applied to a hematoma. Never pack the vagina. Provide expedited transport to the hospital, with oxygen administration and IV access as necessary.

7. Describe the assessment, care, and emotional support of the sexual assault patient. pp. 650–652

Sexual assault victims are unique patients with unique needs. The psychological care of these patients is as important, if not more so, than the physical care they may need. Confine your questions to the physical injuries that the patient may have received. Unless your patient is unconscious, do not touch the patient, even to take vital signs, without her permission. Explain what's going to be done before initiating any treatment. Avoid touching the patient other than to take vital signs or to examine other physical injuries. Do not examine the external genitalia of the sexual assault victim unless there is life-threatening hemorrhage. Consider the patient to be a crime scene and protect that scene; handle clothing as little as possible, collect all bloody articles as potential evidence, do not allow the patient to change clothes or bathe and do not clean wounds if possible. Be sure to document the treatment of the sexual assault victim carefully, thoroughly, and objectively.

8. Given several preprogrammed gynecological patients, provide the appropriate assessment, management and transportation. p. 637–652

Throughout your classroom, clinical, and field training, you will encounter a variety of real and simulated gynecologic patients. Use the information provided in this chapter of your text, as well as the application of this information as demonstrated by your instructors, preceptors, and mentors to enhance your ability to assess, manage, and transport these patients. Keep in mind that gynecological emergencies are likely to be a very stressful situations for your patients, and they will appreciate your gentle, considerate care and professionalism.

CASE STUDY REVIEW

Reread the case study on pages 635 and 636 in Paramedic Care: Medical Emergencies *before reading the discussion below.*

This case study draws attention to the assessment and management of a sexual assault patient in the prehospital setting. Sexual assault continues to represent the most rapidly growing violent crime in the United States, so it is likely that you will encounter these patients in the course of your career.

In this scenario, the paramedics meet their patient in the care of the park police officer that found her. Stephanie has been allowed to cover herself and afforded privacy prior to the arrival of the medics. Being mindful of the psychological aspects of her care, the medic explains every necessary procedure and asks her permission before any action is initiated. Recognizing the need to preserve potential evidence, the medic keeps the blanket around Stephanie. The initial and rapid trauma assessments revealed no significant injuries or immediate life threats. The paramedic consistently gave control to Stephanie and reassured her that she was safe now. She was transported to the hospital for evaluation by the Sexual Assault Nurse Examiner.

CONTENT SELF-EVALUATION

MULTIPLE CHOICE

_____ 1. Thickening of the endometrium in preparation for implantation of a fertilized egg is stimulated by:
  A. follicle stimulating hormone and luteinizing hormone.
  B. luteinizing hormone and estrogen.
  C. estrogen and progesterone.
  D. progesterone and follicle stimulating hormone.
  E. estrogen and follicle stimulating hormone.

_____ 2. Ovulation occurs at approximately day 14 of the menstrual cycle in response to a surge of:
  A. follicle stimulating hormone.   D. progesterone.
  B. luteinizing hormone.   E. all of the above
  C. estrogen.

_____ 3. All of the following are phases of the menstrual cycle EXCEPT the:
  A. ischemic phase.   D. excretory phase.
  B. proliferative phase.   E. menstrual phase.
  C. secretory phase.

_____ 4. The average blood loss associated with menstruation is:
  A. 5 ml.   D. 150 ml.
  B. 50 ml.   E. 250 ml.
  C. 100 ml.

_____ 5. The variety of signs and symptoms associated with the changing hormonal levels of the menstrual cycle is known as:
  A. menarche.   D. premenstrual syndrome.
  B. menstruation.   E. hormonal surge.
  C. menopause.

_____ 6. The term used to describe the number of times a woman has been pregnant is parity.
  A. True
  B. False

_____ 7. A palpable abdominal mass found midway between the symphysis pubis and the umbilicus in the lower abdomen of a 25-year-old woman is most likely to be a(n):
   A. tumor.
   B. intrauterine pregnancy of 5 months gestation.
   C. intrauterine pregnancy of 4 months gestation.
   D. intrauterine pregnancy of 3 months gestation.
   E. ovarian cyst.

_____ 8. Pelvic inflammatory disease is often most often caused by:
   A. gonorrhea and chlamydia.   D. chlamydia and streptococcus.
   B. streptococcus and staphylococcus. E. HIV and staphylococcus.
   C. gonorrhea and HIV.

_____ 9. Mid-cycle abdominal pain associated with ovulation is known as:
   A. endometriosis.   D. cystitis.
   B. PID.   E. mittelschmerz.
   C. a miscarriage.

_____ 10. Endometriosis is an infection of the uterine lining.
   A. True
   B. False

_____ 11. The most effective means to control vaginal hemorrhage is to apply direct pressure to the perineum.
   A. True
   B. False

_____ 12. All of the following signs and symptoms are associated with endometritis EXCEPT:
   A. history of gynecologic procedure.   D. bradycardia.
   B. severe abdominal pain.   E. bloody, foul-smelling discharge.
   C. fever.

_____ 13. All of the following signs and symptoms are associated with a ruptured ovarian cyst EXCEPT:
   A. dyspareunia.   D. delayed menstrual period.
   B. severe abdominal pain. E. irregular bleeding.
   C. fever.

_____ 14. If a female patient presents with severe unilateral abdominal pain that radiates to the shoulder on one side, a missed menstrual period, and vaginal bleeding, you should suspect:
   A. mittelschmerz.   D. endometriosis.
   B. ectopic pregnancy. E. cystitis.
   C. PID.

_____ 15. The prehospital priorities for care of the sexual assault victim include all of the following EXCEPT:
   A. examining for perineal tears.
   B. determining if life-threatening injuries exist.
   C. providing emotional support.
   D. preserving evidence.
   E. protecting patient's privacy.

LABEL THE DIAGRAM

In the spaces provided write the names of the organs of the female reproductive system marked A through E on the diagram below.

A. _____

B. _____

C. _____

D. _____

E. _____

A
B
Urinary bladder
Symphysis pubis
Urethra
Clitoris
Labium major
Labium minor

C
D
E
Rectum

SPECIAL PROJECT

Problem Solving—Abdominal Pain

You are dispatched for "woman with abdominal pain." Your patient is a 26-year-old female who looks acutely ill and complains of severe abdominal pain.

1. Given this information, what would you attempt to determine when gathering a focused history?

_____   _____

_____   _____

_____   _____

_____   _____

Having obtained the history, you perform a physical exam. Your findings include the following:

- tachypnea
- tachycardia
- pale, cool, diaphoretic skin
- narrowed pulse pressure
- vaginal bleeding or discharge
- abdominal exam: masses, distention, guarding, localized tenderness, rebound

2. Based on this information, provide a differential diagnosis for this patient.

_____   _____

_____   _____

_____   _____

CHAPTER 14

✳

Obstetrics

Review of Chapter Objectives

After reading this chapter, you should be able to:

1. **Describe the anatomic structures and physiology of the reproductive system during pregnancy.**   **pp. 656–661**

The primary "organ of pregnancy" is the placenta, which arises from the site on the uterine wall where the blastocyst (fertilized egg) implants. This temporary, blood-rich structure serves as a lifeline for the developing fetus via the umbilical cord. Its functions include the transfer of heat while exchanging oxygen and carbon dioxide, delivering nutrients, and removing waste. The placenta also serves as an endocrine gland throughout the pregnancy, secreting hormones necessary for fetal survival as well as the estrogen and progesterone required to maintain the pregnancy. The placenta is also a protective barrier against harmful substances that might cross the placental barrier to the fetus.

    The fetus develops within the amniotic sac, a thin-walled membranous covering containing amniotic fluid, which surrounds and protects the fetus during intrauterine life.

2. **Identify the normal events of pregnancy.**   **pp. 661–664**

Fetal development begins at the moment of conception (fertilization). Normally, the duration of pregnancy is 40 weeks after the date of the mother's last menstrual period or 280 days. This is comparable to 10 lunar months or 9 calendar months. This time period is divided into trimesters, each of 3 calendar months duration.

    Implantation of the fertilized egg into the uterine wall occurs during the pre-embryonic stage that lasts approximately 14 days. The embryonic stage begins at day 15 and ends at approximately 8 weeks, by which time all of the body systems have been formed. It is midway through this stage that the fetal heart begins to beat. The period from 8 weeks gestation until delivery is known as the fetal stage. The gender of the infant can usually be determined by 16 weeks, and by the 20th week, fetal heart tones are audible by stethoscope. The mother usually feels fetal movement (quickening) by the 24th week. By the 38th week, the baby is considered to be full term.

3. **Describe how to assess an obstetrical patient.**   **pp. 664–667**

The initial assessment for an obstetric patient is the same as for any other patient. Utilization of the SAMPLE history will allow you to obtain specific information about the pregnancy. Ask about gravidity, parity, length of gestation, and EDC (estimated date of confinement or due date). You should also obtain information about past OB/GYN history (e.g., c-section) or complications as well as prenatal care. Determine current medications and any drug allergies as well. It is important to obtain the past medical history because pregnancy may aggravate pre-existing medical problems or trigger new ones such as gestational diabetes. It is possible to estimate the due date by measuring fundal height above the symphysis pubis. Continue the physical exam, which is essentially the same for any patient, while being mindful of the need for modesty and privacy.

4. Identify the stages of labor and the paramedic's role in each stage. pp. 680–683

Labor is the physiologic and mechanical process by which the baby, placenta, and amniotic sac are expelled through the birth canal. The three stages of labor are dilatation, expulsion, and placental. The first stage (dilatation stage) begins with the onset of true labor and ends with the complete dilatation and effacement of the cervix. The second stage (expulsion stage) begins with the complete dilatation of the cervix and ends with the delivery of the baby. The third and final stage of labor (placental stage) begins immediately after the birth of the baby and ends with the delivery of the placenta. The role of the paramedic during labor is to assist in the delivery and to recognize and treat life-threatening problems for the mother or baby.

5. Differentiate between normal and abnormal delivery. pp. 683–696

Normally, most infants present from the birth canal in a headfirst, face down position (vertex presentation), which allows the infant to be delivered vaginally. Abnormal delivery situations generally preclude vaginal delivery and are likely to require caesarean section, so transport must be expedited. These situations include: breech presentation (buttocks present first), prolapsed cord (umbilical cord protrudes from the birth canal), limb presentation (baby's arm or leg protrudes from the birth canal) or occiput posterior presentation (baby's brow is facing forward).

6. Identify and describe complications associated with pregnancy and delivery. pp. 669–679, 687–696

Medical complications of pregnancy include ectopic pregnancy, bleeding problems, supine hypotensive syndrome, gestational diabetes, and hypertensive disorders. Ectopic pregnancy refers to the implantation of the fertilized egg outside of the uterus. Abdominal pain and evidence of intra-abdominal and/or vaginal bleeding usually herald this event. Bleeding is generally differentiated as painful or painless. Vaginal bleeding, accompanied by cramping abdominal pain, prior to the 20th week of gestation is almost always associated with a spontaneous abortion. Painless bleeding is most commonly associated with placenta previa where, due to abnormal implantation of the placenta on the uterine wall, labor is accompanied by bleeding. Painful bleeding is the hallmark of abruptio placenta or the premature separation of the placenta from the uterine wall. It poses an immediate life threat to mother and child.

Supine hypotensive syndrome occurs most commonly in the third trimester as a result of compression of the inferior vena cava by the gravid uterus. Insulin resistance and decreased glucose tolerance characterize gestational diabetes, occurring in the last 20 weeks of pregnancy. Hypertensive disorders of pregnancy (formerly called toxemia) include preeclampsia or eclampsia and chronic and transient hypertension. Major motor seizures are the hallmark of eclampsia, which is the most serious of the hypertensive disorders, posing a life threat to the mother and child.

Some of complications associated with delivery are discussed in objective 5 above. Other problems can occur after delivery. One of these is postpartum hemorrhage, which is the loss of 500 cc or more of blood immediately following delivery. A common cause of the condition is lack of uterine muscle tone, and it occurs most frequently in the multigravida, with multiple births, and with the births of large infants. Uterine rupture is another complication of delivery. It can result from blunt abdominal trauma, prolonged uterine contractions, or a surgically scarred uterus. Uterine rupture presents with a patient in excruciating abdominal pain and often in shock. Uterine inversion occurs when the uterus turns inside out after delivery and extends through the cervix. Blood loss from 800 to 1,800 cc occurs, and the patient often experiences profound shock. Pulmonary embolism can also occur after pregnancy as a result of venous thromboembolism. It often presents with sudden dyspnea accompanied by sharp chest pain and a sense of impending doom.

7. Identify predelivery emergencies. pp. 669–679

Recognition of a predelivery emergency is based on information obtained from the focused history and physical exam that relates to the reported abnormality, such as pain, discomfort, or bleeding. While any of the complications listed above has potential to be an emergency, the most likely are abruptio placenta and eclampsia, both of which pose potential life threats to mother and child and require prompt and appropriate intervention.

8. State indications of an imminent delivery. pp. 681–682

Increasing frequency and duration of contractions and the sensation of needing to move one's bowels (urge to push) are all signs of impending delivery. However, crowning is the definitive sign that birth is imminent.

9. Identify the contents of an obstetrical kit and explain the use of each item. pp. 683–686

Commercially prepared OB kits are available from a variety of sources and contain the following items for use in the event of a field delivery: toweling or drape material, bulb syringe, two plastic umbilical clamps, and scissors. The toweling is used for draping the patient to minimize contamination of the baby during the birth. A bulb syringe is necessary for suctioning the baby's mouth and nose, while the cord clamps and scissors are used when separating the infant from its mother by clamping and cutting the umbilical cord.

10. Differentiate the management of a patient with predelivery emergencies from a normal delivery. pp. 667–679

Management of predelivery emergencies requires that the paramedic correctly recognize their presence based on information obtained from the focused history and physical exam and then expedite transport while anticipating the development of shock and maintaining adequate oxygenation, fluid resuscitation as necessary, and, if appropriate, pharmacological intervention. Most of the time, the mother will be transported in the left lateral recumbent position.

11. State the steps in the predelivery preparation of the mother. p. 683

The first priority is to provide the mother with privacy. Then, time permitting, administer oxygen via a nasal cannula and establish vascular access. Position the mother on her back with knees and hips flexed and buttocks slightly elevated, or the mother may prefer squatting or to be in a semi-Fowler position with knees and hips flexed. Drape the mother's perineum to minimize contamination of the infant during delivery.

12. Establish the relationship between body substance isolation and childbirth. p. 683

Normally, preparation for childbirth in the prehospital setting would entail thoroughly washing hands and forearms before donning a gown, in addition to sterile gloves and goggles. Body substance isolation for childbirth generally includes draping the mother to minimize contamination of the baby during delivery.

13. State the steps to assist in the delivery of a newborn. pp. 683–686

Key EMS actions during a routine (normal) delivery are primarily supportive, but you should remain vigilant to signs of impending problems. Providing gentle support to the perineum as the delivery progresses decreases the likelihood of an explosive delivery causing vaginal tears and the potential for neonatal head trauma. While supporting the head, gently slide your finger along the head and neck to ensure that the cord is not wrapped around the baby's head and neck. As the head emerges from the vaginal opening, suction the airway (mouth first, then nose) to insure that the airway is clear prior to the neonate taking his first breath. It may be necessary to tear the amniotic sac to release the amniotic fluid and permit the baby to breathe.

Gently guide the baby's head downward to allow delivery of the upper shoulder. Do not pull! Then gently guide the baby's body upward to allow delivery of the lower shoulder. Once the shoulders are delivered, the rest of the body will be quickly delivered. Keep the baby at the level of the mother's hips until the cord has been clamped and cut. Once the body has fully emerged from the birth canal, the baby should again be suctioned until the airway is clear. After clamping the umbilical cord at 10 cm and 15 cm from the baby and cutting in between, carefully dry the baby and wrap in a warming blanket to prevent hypothermia.

14. **Describe how to care for the newborn.**   pp. 686–689

The essential emergency care of the newborn includes the establishment and maintenance of adequate airway and breathing status and the prevention of heat loss. Support the infant's head and torso, using both hands. Maintain warmth, repeat suctioning of the mouth and nose as needed until the airway is clear, and then assess using the APGAR score. Do not delay resuscitation or transport to perform APGAR scoring.

15. **Describe how and when to cut the umbilical cord.**   pp. 683, 686

Once the baby's body has been delivered, suction the airway until clear while keeping the baby at the level of the mother's hips until the cord has been clamped and cut. Do not "milk" the cord. Supporting the baby's body, place the first umbilical clamp approximately 10 cm from the baby and the second clamp at 15 cm and carefully cut in between.

16. **Discuss the steps in the delivery of the placenta.**   p. 686

Following delivery of the baby, the vaginal opening will continue to ooze blood. Do not pull on the umbilical cord! Eventually, the cord will appear to lengthen indicating separation of the placenta from the uterine wall. Once the placenta is expelled through the vaginal opening, it should be placed in a biohazard bag and be transported to the hospital for examination.

17. **Describe the management of the mother post-delivery.**   pp. 686, 694–696

The mother should receive fundal massage to control postpartum bleeding and the perineum should be inspected for tears. Continuously monitor vital signs. If not accomplished prior to delivery, vascular access should be established should fluid resuscitation become necessary.

18. **Summarize neonatal resuscitation procedures.**   pp. 688–689

If the infant's respirations are below 30 per minute and tactile stimulation does not increase the rate to a normal range (30–60), immediately assist ventilations using a pediatric bag-valve mask with high-flow oxygen. If the heart rate is below 80 and does not increase in response to ventilations, initiate chest compressions. Transport to a facility with neonatal intensive care capabilities.

19. **Describe the procedures for handling abnormal deliveries,**
    complications of pregnancy, and maternal complications
    of labor.   pp. 668–679, 681–683, 689–696

Management of abnormal deliveries or complications of pregnancy and labor require that the paramedic correctly recognize the problem and expedite transport while anticipating the development of shock and maintaining adequate oxygenation, fluid resuscitation as necessary and, if appropriate, pharmacological intervention. Most of the time, the mother will be transported in the left lateral recumbent position. When the baby's position (breech presentation, prolapsed cord, or limb presentation) dictates, the mother should be placed on oxygen and then assisted in assuming the knee-chest position. Additionally, in the management of prolapsed cord, two gloved fingers should be placed inside the vagina to prevent the baby's weight from compressing the cord and inhibiting oxygen delivery to the baby.

20. **Describe special considerations when meconium is present in amniotic fluid**
    or during delivery.   p. 694

The presence of meconium (fetal fecal matter) in the amniotic fluid is indicative of a fetal hypoxic incident. The thicker and darker the color of the meconium staining in the amniotic fluid, the higher the risk of fetal morbidity. Once the head has emerged from the birth canal, suction the mouth and nose thoroughly while still on the perineum. However, if the meconium is thick, visualize the glottis and use an endotracheal tube to suction the hypopharynx and trachea until clear. Failure to suction will cause the meconium to be pushed further down the trachea and into the lungs.

21. **Describe special considerations of a premature baby.** pp. 678–679

Premature infants are ill suited for extrauterine life, particularly with regard to their pulmonary function. All of the concerns about caring for a neonate are exaggerated when the neonate is less than 38 weeks gestation. Of greatest concern are airway maintenance, ventilatory support, and oxygen delivery. These critically ill neonates should be taken immediately to a facility with neonatal intensive care capabilities.

22. **Given several simulated delivery situations, provide the appropriate assessment, management, and transport for the mother and child.** pp. 656–696

Throughout your training, you will encounter a variety of real and simulated obstetric patients. Use the information provided in this chapter, as well as the application of this information as demonstrated by your instructors, preceptors, and mentors to enhance your ability to assess, manage, and transport these patients. Keep in mind that this is likely to be a stressful situation for your patient, and she will appreciate your kind, considerate care and professionalism.

CASE STUDY REVIEW

Reread the case study on pages 655 and 656 in Paramedic Care: Medical Emergencies *before reading the discussion below.*

This case study draws attention to the management of childbirth in the prehospital setting. In most cases, the role of the EMS provider in a childbirth situation is merely supportive, as often no "emergency" care is needed.

As is often the case, a great deal of information about the imminence of delivery can be obtained prior to physically examining the patient. This patient reveals that she has had six pregnancies, a good indicator that this delivery may proceed very quickly. The urge to move the bowels is a sign that the cervix is fully effaced and the child is moving down the birth canal. Lastly, when exam of the perineum displays crowning this indicates that the cervix is fully dilated and that delivery is imminent.

Normally, preparation for delivery would entail thoroughly washing hands and forearms before donning a gown, in addition to the gloves and goggles that were used by the EMTs. Body substance isolation for childbirth generally includes draping the patient to minimize contamination of the baby during delivery. In this situation, there is no time to open the OB kit or provide for the mother's privacy.

Key EMS actions during a routine delivery are primarily supportive, but you should remain vigilant to signs of impending problems. Providing gentle support to the perineum as the delivery progresses decreases the likelihood of an explosive delivery causing vaginal tears and the potential for neonatal head trauma. As the head emerges from the vaginal opening, the EMT suctions the airway to insure that the airway is clear prior to the neonate taking her first breath. The paramedics arrive in time to assist the EMT in cutting the cord, after placing clamps at 10 cm and 15 cm from the baby and cutting in between, and then drying and wrapping the baby in a warming blanket to prevent hypothermia. The mother receives fundal massage to control postpartum bleeding. Vascular access is established should fluid resuscitation become necessary. The baby is assessed and APGAR scores are identified en route to the hospital.

Childbirth is one "emergency" which almost always has a positive outcome. It is common for EMS agencies to celebrate and acknowledge such calls. Rest assured that this delivery is one the EMT will remember for the balance of his career, even without a stork painted on his window.

CONTENT SELF-EVALUATION

MULTIPLE CHOICE

_____ 1. Thickening of the uterine lining in anticipation of implantation of the fertilized egg is stimulated by:
   A. estrogen.
   B. progesterone.
   C. follicle-stimulating hormone.
   D. luteinizing hormone.
   E. oxytocin.

_____ 2. All of the following are placental functions EXCEPT:
   A. acting as the "organ of pregnancy."
   B. production of hormones.
   C. serving as a protective barrier.
   D. providing fertilization.
   E. providing a means of heat transfer.

_____ 3. The normal duration of pregnancy is:
   A. 40 weeks.
   B. 280 days.
   C. 10 lunar months.
   D. 9 calendar months.
   E. all of the above

_____ 4. Blood volume increases by what percentage during pregnancy?
   A. 10%
   B. 25%
   C. 30%
   D. 45%
   E. 60%

_____ 5. The fetus receives its blood from the placenta by means of the:
   A. umbilical vein.
   B. umbilical artery.
   C. inferior vena cava.
   D. superior vena cava.
   E. aorta.

_____ 6. Fetal circulation changes to normal circulation with the:
   A. onset of labor.
   B. expulsion from the birth canal.
   C. baby's first breath.
   D. clamping of the umbilical cord.
   E. dilation and effacement of the cervix.

_____ 7. When performing a focused history on a pregnant patient, which of the following questions would be appropriate?
   A. Are you experiencing any pain or discomfort?
   B. Have you had any vaginal discharge or bleeding?
   C. When is your due date?
   D. Have you ever been pregnant before?
   E. all of the above

_____ 8. All of the following are common signs or symptoms of a predelivery emergency EXCEPT:
   A. abdominal pain or trauma.
   B. vaginal bleeding or discharge.
   C. painful deformed extremities.
   D. altered mental status or seizures.
   E. hypertension or hypotension.

_____ 9. All of the following are causes of bleeding during pregnancy EXCEPT:
   A. abortion.
   B. ovarian cyst.
   C. ectopic pregnancy.
   D. placenta previa.
   E. abruptio placenta.

_____ 10. Treatment of a female patient who is 16 weeks pregnant, is complaining of cramping abdominal pain, and has bright red vaginal bleeding should include all of the following EXCEPT:
   A. packing the vagina to control bleeding.
   B. treating for shock if indicated.
   C. maintaining oxygenation.
   D. providing emotional support.
   E. saving any tissue and clots for evaluation.

_____ 11. You suspect the patient in the situation described in question 10 is having a(n):
  A. abortion.   D. placenta previa.
  B. ovarian cyst.   E. abruptio placenta.
  C. ectopic pregnancy.

_____ 12. Pelvic inflammatory disease, endometriosis, and tubal ligation are predisposing factors for:
  A. abortion.   D. placenta previa.
  B. ovarian cyst.   E. abruptio placenta.
  C. ectopic pregnancy.

_____ 13. You find that your patient is 36 weeks pregnant, has an altered mental status, and is reported to have had a major motor seizure, which you suspect is due to:
  A. placenta previa.   D. abruptio placenta.
  B. eclampsia.   E. supine hypotensive syndrome.
  C. epilepsy.

_____ 14. Care of the patient in question 13 should include all of the following EXCEPT:
  A. administering high-flow oxygen via a nonrebreather mask.
  B. protecting the patient from injury if seizures recur.
  C. minimizing noise and light to prevent seizure activity.
  D. administering magnesium sulfate per protocol.
  E. transporting on right side to protect airway.

_____ 15. All of the following are signs and symptoms of an imminent delivery EXCEPT:
  A. the presence of crowning.
  B. contractions occurring every 1–2 minutes.
  C. passage of "bloody show."
  D. sensation of an urge for bowel movement.
  E. rupture of membranes.

_____ 16. The stage of labor that begins with complete cervical dilatation and ends with the delivery of the fetus is called the dilatation stage.
  A. True
  B. False

_____ 17. Your patient has just delivered a healthy baby boy. Following the delivery of the placenta, her vaginal bleeding seems to increase. Which of the following best describes what you should do provide emergency care for this patient?
  A. Massage the uterus and position your patient on her right side.
  B. Administer oxygen and firmly massage the uterus.
  C. Massage the uterus and pack the vagina to control bleeding
  D. Administer oxygen and pack the vagina with sanitary napkins.
  E. Provide fluid resuscitation and position patient on her right side.

_____ 18. Meconium-stained amniotic fluid should first be managed by:
  A. immediate transport to the hospital for physician evaluation.
  B. administration of oxygen to the mother to resolve fetal distress.
  C. suctioning of the mouth and nose before the infant takes his first breath.
  D. stimulation of the infant to encourage coughing to clear meconium from airway.
  E. expediting completion of delivery to decrease fetal distress.

_____ 19. Management of a limb presentation should include all of the following EXCEPT:
  A. administration of high-flow oxygen to the mother.
  B. immediate transport to the hospital.
  C. attempting to push the limb back into the vagina.
  D. positioning the mother with her head down and pelvis elevated.
  E. providing reassurance to the mother.

_____ 20. The administration of an IV fluid bolus to control premature labor is based on increasing intravascular volume and thus causing inhibition of:
  A. antidiuretic hormone.
  B. progesterone.
  C. estrogen.
  D. luteinizing hormone.
  E. follicle-stimulating hormone.

_____ 21. Elements of the APGAR assessment include appearance, pulse, grimace, activity and respirations.
  A. True
  B. False

_____ 22. Acrocyanosis in the neonate is always a sign of inadequate oxygenation.
  A. True
  B. False

_____ 23. You have just assisted with the delivery of a baby girl. She has shallow, gasping respirations and a heart rate that is less than 100 beats per minute. Which of the following best describes your emergency care for this patient?
  A. administering "blow by" oxygen and monitoring her pulse for 60 seconds
  B. assisting ventilations with a BVM and reassessing in 30 seconds
  C. administering high-flow oxygen with a nonrebreather mask
  D. assisting ventilations with a BVM and beginning chest compressions
  E. continuing to monitor and expedite transport

_____ 24. Shoulder dystocia is commonly associated with diabetic or obese mothers and:
  A. prematurity.
  B. hormonal excesses.
  C. post-term pregnancy.
  D. hormonal deficits.
  E. fetal distress.

_____ 25. If the uterus protrudes from the vaginal opening following the delivery of the placenta, you should:
  A. wrap it tightly in dry towels.
  B. wrap it in dextrose-soaked dressings.
  C. make no more than 3 attempts to replace it.
  D. make no more than 1 attempt to replace it.
  E. cover it with plastic wrap.

MATCHING

Write the letter of the definition in the space provided next to the term it describes.

_____ 26. amniotic sac

_____ 27. ovulation

_____ 28. fetus

_____ 29. placenta

_____ 30. umbilical cord

_____ 31. effacement

_____ 32. Braxton-Hicks contractions

_____ 33. parity

_____ 34. tocolysis

_____ 35. puerperium

  A. Unborn infant from the third month of pregnancy to birth
  B. Fetal lifeline, a placental extension through which the child is nourished
  C. Organ of pregnancy for the exchange of oxygen and waste products
  D. Transparent membrane forming the sac which holds the fetus
  E. Release of an egg from the ovary
  F. The time period surrounding the birth of the fetus
  G. Thinning and shortening of the cervix during labor
  H. Number of pregnancies carried to term
  I. Process of stopping labor
  J. Painless, irregular uterine contractions

SPECIAL PROJECT

Understanding the Physiologic Changes of Pregnancy

Complete the table below, identifying the physiologic changes of pregnancy by system and their associated EMS implications.

	Physiologic Changes	EMS Implications
Reproductive system		
Respiratory system		
Cardiovascular system		
Gastrointestinal system		
Urinary system		
Musculoskeletal system		

MEDICAL EMERGENCIES
Content Review

CONTENT SELF-EVALUATION

Chapter 1: Pulmonology

_____ 1. Place the structures of the respiratory system in order of inspiration.
1. alveoli
2. bronchi
3. nasal cavity
4. pharynx
5. larynx
6. trachea
7. lungs

A. 1, 7, 2, 6, 5, 4, 3   D. 3, 4, 5, 6, 2, 7, 1
B. 3, 5, 4, 2, 6, 7, 1   E. 7, 2, 4, 5, 6, 1, 3
C. 3, 4, 5, 2, 6, 7, 1

_____ 2. How long is the trachea?
A. 11 cm   D. 8 inches
B. 8 cm   E. 7 cm
C. 11 inches

_____ 3. The carina is located in the:
A. pharynx.   D. thyroid cartilage.
B. larynx.   E. division of the bronchi.
C. soft palate.

_____ 4. Aspirated material may pass into the right lung due to:
A. a straighter right mainstem bronchus.
B. an ineffective gag reflex.
C. atelectasis.
D. peristalsis that occurs in the esophagus.
E. the pleura.

_____ 5. The bronchioles are approximately 1 mm thick and contain primarily which type of muscle?
A. cardiac   D. voluntary
B. smooth   E. contractile
C. striated

_____ 6. Which pleura surrounds the lungs and does not contain nerve fibers?
A. alveolar   D. pulmonary
B. bronchial-lobar   E. visceral
C. parietal

_____ 7. The _____ pleura lines the thoracic cavity and contains nerve fibers.
A. alveolar   D. pulmonary
B. bronchial-lobar   E. visceral
C. parietal

_____ 8. The _____ muscles aid in respiration and connect each rib.
   A. accessory   D. tracheal
   B. diaphragmatic   E. sternal
   C. intercostal

_____ 9. Which nerve innervates the diaphragm?
   A. cardiac plexus   D. vagus
   B. iliac   E. thoracic
   C. phrenic

_____ 10. The chest's ability to expand during ventilation is known as:
   A. airway resistance.   D. visceral pleura elasticity.
   B. rebound.   E. compliance.
   C. transthoracic resistance.

_____ 11. Which of the following conditions most likely is occurring in an emphysema patient who is experiencing dyspnea?
   A. increased lung compliance   D. decreased airway resistance
   B. decreased lung compliance   E. bronchospasm
   C. increased airway resistance

_____ 12. Decreasing lung compliance in the elderly is best attributed to:
   A. a decrease in nerve cells.
   B. a loss of elasticity of intercostal muscles.
   C. enlargement of the chest wall.
   D. weight loss.
   E. weight gain.

_____ 13. The air that remains in the alveoli at all times is referred to as:
   A. expiratory reserve volume.   D. residual volume.
   B. functional reserve capacity. E. inspiratory reserve volume.
   C. vital capacity.

_____ 14. Average residual volume is approximately:
   A. 500 ml.   D. 3000 ml.
   B. 1200 ml.   E. 3600 ml.
   C. 2000 ml.

_____ 15. Average vital capacity is approximately:
   A. 2400 ml.   D. 5200 ml.
   B. 3600 ml.   E. 6000 ml.
   C. 4800 ml.

_____ 16. The primary portion of the brain that controls ventilation is the:
   A. cerebellum.   D. vagus nerve.
   B. frontal lobe. E. pons.
   C. medulla.

_____ 17. The medulla transmits impulses to the primary muscles of respiration through the _____ nerves.
   A. brachial plexus   D. vestibulocochlear
   B. phrenic   E. cranial
   C. vagus

_____ 18. The normal pH for the body is:
   A. 7.15–7.25.   D. 7.45–7.55.
   B. 7.25–7.35.   E. 7.55–7.60.
   C. 7.35–7.45.

_____ 19. Elevated CO_2 in the blood stream results in:
  A. acidosis.   D. hyponatremia.
  B. alkalosis.   E. glycolosis.
  C. hypernatremia.

_____ 20. Scenario: You are called to the scene of a 64-year-old male with a history of bronchitis
  and pneumonia. He takes Theodur, Atrovent, Solu-Medrol, and Lasix on a daily basis.
  He is breathing at a rate of 42, shallow and regular, and is complaining of shortness of
  breath. Most likely the patient's PCO_2 is:
  A. 35–45 mmHg.   D. 80–100 mmHg.
  B. less than 35 mmHg.   E. greater than 100 mmHg.
  C. greater than 45 mmHg.

_____ 21. One of the factors on which lung perfusion depends is:
  A. adequate blood volume.   D. intact cerebral capillaries.
  B. adequate supply of carbon dioxide. E. hyperventilation.
  C. homeostasis.

_____ 22. Under NORMAL conditions, how much oxygen is transported dissolved in plasma?
  A. 2 percent   D. 65 percent
  B. 30 percent   E. 98 percent
  C. 40 percent

_____ 23. The greatest amount of carbon dioxide is transported in the body to the lungs in the
  form of:
  A. bicarbonate ions.   D. carboxyhemoglobins.
  B. water molecules.   E. erythrocytes.
  C. plasma.

_____ 24. For inhalation to occur, the:
  A. bronchi must dilate.
  B. chest cavity must create a negative pressure.
  C. diaphragm must relax.
  D. intercostal muscles must contract down and inward.
  E. chest cavity must create a positive pressure.

_____ 25. The respiratory pattern with deep rapid breaths that result as a corrective measure from
  a metabolic acidosis condition is known as:
  A. apneustic.   D. Cheyne-Stokes.
  B. Biot's.   E. Kussmaul's.
  C. central neurogenic hyperventilation.

_____ 26. The respiratory pattern with deep, rapid respirations caused by a stroke or brainstem
  lesion and that may result in respiratory alkalosis is known as:
  A. apneustic.   D. Cheyne-Stokes.
  B. Biot's.   E. Kussmaul's.
  C. central neurogenic hyperventilation.

_____ 27. The respiratory pattern characterized by repeated episodes of irregular gasping
  ventilations separated by periods of apnea is known as:
  A. apneustic.   D. Cheyne-Stokes.
  B. Biot's.   E. Kussmaul's.
  C. Cheyne-Stokes breathing.

_____ 28. Which of the following is an alveoli perfusion disorder?
  A. hypernatremia   D. hypoxemia
  B. hyponatremia   E. hyperkalemia
  C. hypovolemia

_____ 29. All of the following clues at the scene would indicate that the patient has an underlying respiratory disorder EXCEPT:
   A. a cigarette pack.
   B. a bronchodilation inhaler.
   C. an oxygen tank.
   D. a prescription bottle of Prozac.
   E. a nebulizer.

_____ 30. Vibration felt in the chest during speaking is known as:
   A. crepitus.
   B. pleurisy.
   C. subcutaneous emphysema.
   D. tactile fremitus.
   E. rales.

_____ 31. Which of the following conditions would you expect to discover with a hollow sound when percussing the chest?
   A. emphysema
   B. hemothorax
   C. pneumonia
   D. pulmonary edema
   E. bronchitis

_____ 32. A dull sound when percussing the chest indicates:
   A. ascites.
   B. emphysema.
   C. hemothorax.
   D. pneumothorax.
   E. bronchitis.

_____ 33. A high-pitched whistling sound due to bronchoconstriction is known as:
   A. pleural friction rub.
   B. rales.
   C. rhonchi.
   D. wheezing.
   E. stridor.

_____ 34. A harsh, high-pitched sound heard on inspiration and characteristic of an upper-airway obstruction is:
   A. rales.
   B. snoring.
   C. pleural friction rub.
   D. wheezing.
   E. stridor.

_____ 35. A patient in respiratory distress has clubbing of the fingers. This condition's most likely pathophysiology is:
   A. carbon monoxide poisoning.
   B. carpopedal spasms.
   C. persistent hypoxemia.
   D. respiratory alkalosis.
   E. pneumonia.

_____ 36. Scenario: Your patient is breathing at 32 times per minute. This is known as:
   A. bradypnea.
   B. eupnea.
   C. hyperventilation.
   D. tachypnea.
   E. Kussmaul's respirations.

_____ 37. Which of the following conditions will have an accurate pulse oximetry reading?
   A. carbon monoxide poisoning
   B. hyperventilation syndrome
   C. hypothermia
   D. shock
   E. sepsis

_____ 38. Capnography evaluates the amount of:
   A. carbon dioxide expired in relation to inspired.
   B. carbon dioxide inspired in relation to expired.
   C. oxygen expired in relation to inspired.
   D. oxygen inspired in relation to expired.
   E. oxygen in relation to carbon dioxide.

_____ 39. A patient developing ARDS may have all of the following conditions EXCEPT:
   A. hyperthermia.
   B. pancreatitis.
   C. respiratory burns.
   D. sepsis.
   E. hypothermia.

_____ **40.** An excellent means to maintain patency of the alveoli in a patient who has adult respiratory distress syndrome is:
  A. endotracheal intubation.
  B. furosemide.
  C. peak expiratory flow rate device.
  D. positive end expiratory pressure.
  E. use of digoxin.

_____ **41.** Patients with COPD have a _____ chance of dying within 10 years of diagnosis.
  A. 28 percent
  B. 42 percent
  C. 50 percent
  D. 65 percent
  E. 80 percent

_____ **42.** Approximately _____ of patients who die from asthma do so before reaching the hospital.
  A. 50 percent
  B. 45 percent
  C. 40 percent
  D. 35 percent
  E. 30 percent

_____ **43.** With which other symptoms of emphysema is a 20 pack/year history best associated?
  A. atrophy of the respiratory accessory muscles
  B. obesity and cyanosis
  C. polycythemia
  D. pulmonary edema
  E. hyperkinesia

_____ **44.** Which of the following diseases has a normal to decreased residual volume and a decreased vital capacity?
  A. asthma
  B. bronchitis
  C. emphysema
  D. pneumonia
  E. ARDS

_____ **45.** The earliest sign of an asthma attack is:
  A. coughing.
  B. dyspnea.
  C. stridor.
  D. wheezing.
  E. rales.

_____ **46.** An early sign of respiratory problems is:
  A. agitation.
  B. an increased respiratory rate.
  C. cyanosis.
  D. dyspnea.
  E. a decreased respiratory rate.

_____ **47.** In patients who are experiencing status asthmaticus, the EMS provider should recognize that respiratory arrest is imminent and:
  A. be prepared for endotracheal intubation.
  B. immediately administer a beta-agonist inhaled medication.
  C. encourage the patient to cough forcefully to avoid alveolar collapse.
  D. remember that quiet breathing is a sign that the patient is improving.
  E. immediately establish IV access.

_____ **48.** Upper respiratory infections include all of the following EXCEPT:
  A. bronchiolitis.
  B. epiglottitis.
  C. otitis media.
  D. pharyngitis.
  E. rhinitis.

_____ **49.** Carbon monoxide poisoning is dangerous because it:
  A. binds to hemoglobin more readily than oxygen.
  B. leads to cellular alkalosis.
  C. causes the over-absorption of oxygen into the blood plasma.
  D. causes respiratory alkalosis.
  E. causes respiratory alkalemia.

_____ 50. Risk factors associated with pulmonary embolisms include all of the following EXCEPT:
A. pneumonia.
B. recent surgery.
C. sickle cell anemia.
D. venous pooling during pregnancy.
E. long bone fractures.

Chapter 2: Cardiology

_____ 51. The single largest killer of Americans is:
A. adult respiratory distress syndrome.
B. cancer.
C. coronary heart disease.
D. diabetes.
E. hypotension.

_____ 52. The apex of the heart is located at the:
A. bottom.
B. left atrium.
C. right atrium.
D. top.
E. hilum.

_____ 53. Pericardial fluid reduces friction as the heart beats and is encased between the parietal pericardium and the:
A. endocardium.
B. epicardium.
C. mesentery.
D. myocardium.
E. exocardium.

_____ 54. The innermost layer of the cardiac muscle is the:
A. endocardium.
B. epicardium.
C. myocardium.
D. pericardium.
E. mesentery.

_____ 55. Which chamber of the heart receives blood from the pulmonary circulation?
A. left atrium
B. left ventricle
C. right atrium
D. right ventricle
E. none of the above

_____ 56. Identify in order the flow of blood through the heart, beginning with the superior vena cava.
1. aortic semilunar valve
2. mitral valve
3. right ventricle
4. pulmonary artery
5. left atrium
6. ascending aorta
A. 1, 4, 5, 3, 2, 6
B. 2, 3, 4, 5, 1, 6
C. 3, 4, 5, 2, 1, 6
D. 5, 2, 3, 4, 1, 6
E. 1, 3, 5, 2, 4, 6

_____ 57. The structure that provides blood supply to the right atrium, right ventricle, and part of the cardiac conduction system is the:
A. anterior descending artery.
B. circumflex artery.
C. left coronary artery.
D. right coronary artery.
E. sternal artery.

_____ 58. During diastole, which of the following valves is open?
A. aortic semilunar
B. Heimlich's
C. pulmonary semilunar
D. tricuspid
E. Einthoven's

_____ 59. The resistance against which the ventricles contract is known as:
A. afterload.
B. end-diastolic volume.
C. preload.
D. pulse pressure.
E. cardioinhibitory pressure.

_____ 60. Calculate cardiac output, if the average stroke volume is 70 ml and the heart rate is 80 beats per minute.
A. 2800 ml/min
B. 2800 ml/hr
C. 5600 ml/min
D. 5600 ml/hr
E. none of the above

_____ 61. An increase in peripheral vascular resistance results in:
A. decreased afterload.
B. increased cardiac output.
C. increased preload.
D. increased stroke volume.
E. decreased stroke volume.

_____ 62. The sympathetic nervous system innervates the heart through the:
A. brachial plexus.
B. cardiac plexus.
C. cervical plexus.
D. vagus nerve.
E. median nerve.

_____ 63. Hypokalemia in the myocardium results in:
A. increased automaticity and conduction.
B. increased conduction.
C. increased contractility.
D. increased irritability.
E. increased elasticity.

_____ 64. The ability of all cardiac muscle cells to contract simultaneously is known as:
A. action potential.
B. depolarization.
C. dromotropy.
D. transference.
E. syncytium.

_____ 65. The term that pertains to the speed of impulse transmission through the myocardium is:
A. chronotropy.
B. dromotropy.
C. inotropy.
D. syncytium.
E. entropy.

_____ 66. The normal electrical state of cardiac cells is:
A. the action potential.
B. depolarization.
C. repolarization.
D. the resting potential.
E. stasis.

_____ 67. For the cardiac cell to repolarize, which ion is moved back into the cell?
A. calcium
B. magnesium
C. potassium
D. sodium
E. chromium

_____ 68. The ability of muscle cells to shorten is:
A. automaticity.
B. conductivity.
C. contractility.
D. excitability.
E. intercalatability.

_____ 69. The ability of cardiac cells to respond to an electrical stimulus is:
A. automaticity.
B. conductivity.
C. contractility.
D. excitability.
E. intercalatability.

_____ 70. The _____ has an intrinsic rate of 15–40 beats per minute.
A. AV node
B. bundle of His
C. Purkinje system
D. SA node
E. left bundle branch

_____ 71. For Lead I, placement of the leads is on the:
   A. left arm, left leg.
   B. left arm, right leg.
   C. right arm, left arm.
   D. right arm, left leg.
   E. right arm, right leg.

_____ 72. The ECG component that represents atrial depolarization is the:
   A. P wave.
   B. QRS complex.
   C. T wave.
   D. U wave.
   E. S-T segment.

_____ 73. Ventricular repolarization is indicated on the ECG tracing by the:
   A. P wave.
   B. QRS complex.
   C. T wave.
   D. U wave.
   E. S-T segment.

_____ 74. The time necessary for ventricular depolarization is represented by the:
   A. P-R interval.
   B. QRS interval.
   C. QT interval.
   D. S-T segment.
   E. QRS complex.

_____ 75. A delay in the AV node is indicated by a P-R interval:
   A. between 0.1 and 0.20 second.
   B. between 0.04 and 0.12 second.
   C. greater than 0.40 second.
   D. less than 0.12 second.
   E. greater than 0.20 second.

_____ 76. The total duration of ventricular depolarization is represented by the:
   A. P-R interval.
   B. QRS duration.
   C. QT interval.
   D. S-T segment.
   E. QRS interval.

_____ 77. With a heart rate of 180 beats per minute, you would expect the QT interval to be:
   A. approximately 0.40 second.
   B. between 0.33 and 0.42 second.
   C. greater than 0.42 second.
   D. less than 0.33 second.
   E. none of the above

_____ 78. The duration from the beginning of the P wave to the beginning of the QRS complex is the:
   A. P-R interval.
   B. QRS duration.
   C. absolute refractory period.
   D. relative refractory period.
   E. U wave.

_____ 79. A PVC falling on which part of the ECG tracing can result in immediate conversion to VF or VT?
   A. absolute refractory period
   B. relative refractory period
   C. P-R interval
   D. QT interval
   E. P wave

_____ 80. A significant Q wave has a:
   A. duration of at least 0.02 second.
   B. duration of at least 0.04 second.
   C. negative deflection at least one-fourth the height of the QRS complex.
   D. positive deflection at least one-half the height of the QRS complex.
   E. deflection equal to the height of the P wave.

_____ 81. Which of the following ECG lead combinations can be used to evaluate the anterior and lateral walls of the left ventricle?
   A. aVR and V_1
   B. V_1 and V_2
   C. V_3 and V_4
   D. V_5 and V_6
   E. V_1 and V_6

_____ 82. The _____ method of calculating heart rate counts the number of complexes in a 6-second strip.
   A. P-P interval
   B. R-R interval
   C. 6-second
   D. triplicate
   E. hexagonal

_____ 83. Which of the following is characteristic of an abnormal sinus rhythm?
   A. irregular rhythm
   B. P-R interval of 0.16 second
   C. QRS duration of 0.08 second
   D. rate of 60–100
   E. P wave before the QRS complex

_____ 84. The passive transfer of pacemaker sites from the SA node to other latent pacemaker sites in the atria or AV junction is:
   A. atrial tachycardia.
   B. premature atrial contractions.
   C. premature junctional contractions.
   D. premature ventricular contractions.
   E. atrial fibrillation.

_____ 85. Scenario: A 24-year-old female is complaining of chest pain and difficulty breathing. She has been up for 3 days studying for finals and has been taking ephedrine supplements to help her stay awake and alert. She also admits to drinking 12 Mountain Dew sodas in the past day. Vitals are BP 90/50, pulse 180, and respirations 42. Placing her on the ECG monitor, you notice a wave preceding the normal QRS complex, but you cannot discern P or T waves. You interpret this ECG as:
   A. accelerated junctional tachycardia.
   B. atrial fibrillation.
   C. atrial flutter.
   D. paroxysmal supraventricular tachycardia.
   E. first-degree AV block.

_____ 86. Scenario: Your patient is complaining of shortness of breath with a respiratory rate of 36, pulse of 76, and blood pressure of 118/64. The ECG in Lead II shows P-P intervals of 0.20 second and R-R intervals of 0.80 second. The rhythm is regular, and conduction appears to be 4:1. The BEST treatment for this patient is:
   A. cardioversion at 50 joules.
   B. diltiazem.
   C. oxygen via nonrebreather.
   D. procainamide.
   E. dextrose.

_____ 87. Scenario: A patient experiencing atrial fibrillation is being transported for a hip fracture. The patient has no complaints of chest pain or shortness of breath and is hemodynamically stable. You establish an IV and administer nitrous oxide for pain relief. Your management for her atrial fibrillation should include:
   A. cardioversion at 50 joules.
   B. Cardizem.
   C. no further treatment.
   D. verapamil.
   E. a precordial thump.

_____ 88. The cardiac rhythm that is characterized by an irregularly irregular rhythm with an atrial rate of 350–750 and normal QRS complexes is:
   A. atrial fibrillation.
   B. atrial flutter.
   C. sinus dysrhythmia.
   D. ventricular fibrillation.
   E. right bundle branch block.

_____ 89. The ECG that presents with a regular rhythm, no P waves, and a normal QRS duration at a rate of 50 is:
   A. atrial fibrillation.
   B. accelerated idioventricular rhythm.
   C. supraventricular tachycardia.
   D. ventricular tachycardia.
   E. junctional escape rhythm.

_____ 90. A rhythm in which every third beat is a PVC is known as:
  A. galloping.   D. trigeminy.
  B. triplication.   E. palpitation.
  C. salvos.

_____ 91. Which of the following antidysrhythmic agents is considered a Class IIb medication, is indicated in recurrent ventricular fibrillation and hemodynamically unstable ventricular tachycardia, and is contraindicated in cardiogenic shock and high-degree heart blocks?
  A. adenosine   D. verapamil
  B. bretylium   E. azithromycin
  C. amiodarone

_____ 92. Which of the following antidysrhythmics is a calcium channel blocker?
  A. adenosine   D. verapamil
  B. bretylium   E. azithromycin
  C. amiodarone

_____ 93. Which of the following is an adrenergic medication?
  A. atropine   D. morphine sulfate
  B. bretylium   E. aztemizole
  C. epinephrine

_____ 94. All of the following occur with beta-receptor stimulation EXCEPT:
  A. bronchodilation.
  B. negative dromotropic effects.
  C. positive chronotropic effects.
  D. positive inotropic effects.
  E. all occur with beta-receptor stimulation.

_____ 95. Scenario: You are managing a 100 kg semiconscious patient with a heart rate of 120, blood pressure of 80/40, and respirations of 12. He called EMS because of chest pain. Which of the following medications and dosages is correct for this patient?
  A. 4 mg of norepinephrine in 1000 ml infused at 1 ml/min
  B. 4 mg of norepinephrine in 1000 ml infused at 100 ml/hr
  C. 800 mg of dopamine in 500 cc of D_5W infused at 7.5 gtt/min
  D. 800 mg of dopamine in 250 ml infused at 7.5 ml/hr
  E. 200 mg of amiodarone slow IV

_____ 96. Which of the following thrombolytic agents is given over 2 minutes and repeated 30 minutes later?
  A. Activase   D. Retavase
  B. alteplase   E. Nubain
  C. aspirin

_____ 97. Which formula is used to calculate joules?
  A. amperage × (resistance ÷ duration)   D. watts × duration
  B. resistance × watts × time delivered E. resistance ÷ watts
  C. watts ÷ amperage

_____ 98. Which of the following disorders is not cardiac related but may mimic the signs and symptoms of angina?
  A. pneumonia   D. costochondritis
  B. dyspepsia   E. all of the above
  C. pancreatitis

_____ 99. Scenario: A patient is experiencing dyspnea, blood-tinged sputum, rales, and cyanosis. The most likely cause is:
  A. _cor pulmonale._   D. right ventricular failure.
  B. left ventricular failure.   E. aneurysm.
  C. pulmonary embolism.

_____ 100. Depriving the cardiac muscle of oxygen and other nutrients results in:
  A. myocardial infarction.
  B. myocardial injury.
  C. myocardial ischemia.
  D. subendocardial infarction.
  E. myocardial contractility.

Chapter 3: Neurology

_____ 101. The somatic nervous system primarily innervates:
  A. cardiac muscle.
  B. glands.
  C. skeletal muscle.
  D. smooth muscle.
  E. the respiratory system.

_____ 102. The _____ nervous system is mediated by epinephrine and norepinephrine.
  A. afferent
  B. parasympathetic
  C. somatic
  D. sympathetic
  E. central

_____ 103. Acetylcholine is the neurotransmitter of which nervous system?
  A. adrenergic
  B. afferent
  C. parasympathetic
  D. sympathetic
  E. central

_____ 104. The space between the pia mater and the arachnoid membrane is the:
  A. epiarachnoid space.
  B. epidural space.
  C. subarachnoid space.
  D. subdural space.
  E. cerebral space.

_____ 105. This portion of the brain connects the two hemispheres of the cerebrum:
  A. cerebellum.
  B. cerebral cortex.
  C. corpus callosum.
  D. midbrain.
  E. diencephalon.

_____ 106. The area of the brain responsible for emotions, hormone production, and autonomic functions is the:
  A. hypothalamus.
  B. pituitary gland.
  C. pons.
  D. thalamus.
  E. medulla oblongata.

_____ 107. The area of the brain that relays sensory information to the cerebellum and controls involuntary somatic and visceral functions is the:
  A. cerebrum.
  B. midbrain.
  C. pituitary gland.
  D. pons.
  E. medulla oblongata.

_____ 108. This portion of the brain regulates cardiovascular, respiratory, and digestive system activities:
  A. cerebellum.
  B. hypothalamus.
  C. pons.
  D. thalamus.
  E. medulla oblongata.

_____ 109. The _____ lobe of the brain is responsible for speech.
  A. frontal
  B. occipital
  C. parietal
  D. temporal
  E. semiparietal

_____ 110. The _____ system is responsible for consciousness and stimuli response.
  A. carotid
  B. limbic
  C. vertebrobasilar
  D. reticular activating
  E. cephalic

_____ 111. Which efferent fibers carry impulses to the skeletal muscles?
  A. somatic motor
  B. somatic sensory
  C. visceral motor
  D. visceral sensory
  E. visceral lymphatic

_____ 112. Which cranial nerve controls movement of the tongue?
  A. I
  B. III
  C. VI
  D. X
  E. XII

_____ 113. Which afferent cranial nerve is responsible for equilibrium?
  A. II
  B. IV
  C. VI
  D. VIII
  E. IX

_____ 114. If the patient is able to smile, frown, and wrinkle forehead muscles, which cranial nerve is intact?
  A. I
  B. V
  C. VII
  D. XI
  E. XII

_____ 115. The first "I" in AEIOU-TIPS means:
  A. infarction.
  B. impairment.
  C. insulin.
  D. infection.
  E. irritability.

_____ 116. A condition characterized by loss of memory and disorientation and is associated with chronic alcohol intake and a diet deficient in thiamine is:
  A. Korsakoff's psychosis.
  B. Wernicke's syndrome.
  C. Lein's psychosis.
  D. Esselstyne's syndrome.
  E. Makynen seizure.

_____ 117. The type of stroke caused by a ruptured cerebral artery is:
  A. occlusive.
  B. embolic.
  C. thrombotic.
  D. hemorrhagic.
  E. aneural.

_____ 118. The phase of a seizure in which a patient experiences alternating contraction and relaxation of the muscles is:
  A. tonic.
  B. clonic.
  C. aural.
  D. hypertonic.
  E. postictal.

_____ 119. All of the following are characteristics of a complex partial seizure EXCEPT:
  A. auditory hallucinations.
  B. a sense of deja vu.
  C. localized tonic-clonic movement of one extremity.
  D. unusual odors.
  E. strange tastes.

_____ 120. A disease that is chronic and is characterized by progressive motor disorder with tremor, rigidity, bradykinesia, and postural instability is:
  A. Alzheimer's.
  B. Reed-Sternberg's.
  C. Parkinson's.
  D. Lou Gehrig's.
  E. Bell's palsy.

Chapter 4: Endocrinology

_____ 121. An _____ gland secretes chemical substances to nearby tissues through a duct.
A. endocrine
B. endocyte
C. exocrine
D. exocyte
E. exophyll

_____ 122. The tendency of the body to keep the internal environment and metabolism steady and normal is:
A. homeostasis.
B. glucogenesis.
C. metabolism.
D. steady state.
E. culdocentesis.

_____ 123. All of the following are endocrine glands EXCEPT the:
A. adrenal.
B. hypothalamus.
C. pineal.
D. salivary.
E. gonads.

_____ 124. The posterior pituitary responds to nerve impulses from the:
A. hypothalamus.
B. pancreas.
C. thalamus.
D. thyroid.
E. salivary.

_____ 125. Which of the following is a major hormone effect for the hypothalamus?
A. stimulates the increased reabsorption of water
B. stimulates production and release of milk
C. stimulates the release of thyroid-stimulating hormone
D. stimulates vasoconstriction
E. stimulates blood cell production

_____ 126. Which endocrine gland's target tissues are muscle, the liver, and the cardiovascular system?
A. adrenal cortex
B. adrenal medulla
C. ovaries
D. pineal gland
E. parathyroid

_____ 127. All of the following are androgenic hormones EXCEPT:
A. epinephrine.
B. estrogen.
C. progesterone.
D. testosterone.
E. none of the above are androgenic hormones.

_____ 128. The endocrine gland that is located in the neck on either side and anterior-inferior of the laryngeal cartilage at the level of the cricoid cartilage is the:
A. adrenal gland.
B. pituitary gland.
C. thalamus gland.
D. thyroid gland.
E. thymus gland.

_____ 129. The area of the pancreas that is considered endocrine tissue is the:
A. adrenal cortex.
B. islets of Langerhans.
C. Langerhans medulla.
D. pancreatic medulla.
E. bundle of His.

_____ 130. The hormone _____ is responsible for increasing blood glucose.
A. epinephrine
B. glucagon
C. glycogen
D. insulin
E. prolactin

_____ 131. The conversion of protein and fat to form glucose is:
A. glucogenolysis.
B. gluconeogenesis.
C. glycogenolysis.
D. glyconeogenesis.
E. glucogenesis.

_____ 132. The hormone _____ is secreted from delta cells in the pancreas and inhibits the secretion of glucagon and insulin.
A. epinephrine
B. glycogen
C. insulinlytic
D. melatonin
E. somatostatin

_____ 133. The disease marked by inadequate insulin activity in the body is:
A. "thyroid storm."
B. myxedema.
C. diabetes mellitus.
D. thyrotoxicosis.
E. nephritis.

_____ 134. Normal blood glucose level is:
A. 60–100 mg/dL.
B. 70–120 mg/dL.
C. 80–140 mg/dL.
D. 90–160 mg/dL.
E. 100–180 mg/dL.

_____ 135. Scenario: A diabetic patient presents with excessive urination. This condition is best attributed to:
A. decreased insulin.
B. decreased serum glucose.
C. elevated serum glucose.
D. elevated insulin.
E. elevated thymosin.

_____ 136. The process of excessive urination in the diabetic patient is known as:
A. anabolism.
B. glycosuria.
C. ketosis.
D. anuria.
E. polyuria.

_____ 137. With which of the following signs or symptoms will the patient experiencing diabetic ketoacidosis present?
A. acetone breath odor
B. apathy
C. diplopia
D. drooling
E. diaphoresis

_____ 138. Kussmaul's respirations are seen in which of the following conditions?
A. diabetic ketoacidosis
B. hyperglycemic hyperosmolar nonketotic coma
C. hypoglycemia
D. insulin shock
E. thyrotoxicosis

_____ 139. This disorder's signs and symptoms include prominent weight gain in the trunk, face, and neck, with accumulation of fat on the upper back and easily bruised, translucent skin.
A. Addison's disease
B. Cushing's syndrome
C. Graves' disease
D. myxedema
E. "thyroid storm"

_____ 140. This disorder's signs and symptoms include progressive weakness, fatigue, decreased appetite, and weight loss.
A. Addison's disease
B. Cushing's syndrome
C. Graves' disease
D. myxedema
E. "thyroid storm"

Chapter 5: Allergies and Anaphylaxis

_____ 141. _____ is another name for a disease-producing agent or invading substance.
   A. Antigen
   B. Antibody
   C. Pathogen
   D. Toxin
   E. Endotoxin

_____ 142. The immune response in which the body's immunoglobulins (Igs) attack pathogens is:
   A. cellular immunity.
   B. humoral immunity.
   C. primary response.
   D. secondary response.
   E. tertiary response.

_____ 143. Place in order the sequence for a humoral response to an invading pathogen or antigen.
   1. secondary response
   2. release of IgG and IgM
   3. development of specific antibodies
   4. acquired immunity
   A. 1, 4, 3, 2
   B. 2, 1, 3, 4
   C. 3, 2, 4, 1
   D. 4, 2, 3, 1
   E. 1, 3, 2, 4

_____ 144. A young child is vaccinated against chickenpox. This type of immunity is known as:
   A. acquired immunity.
   B. induced active immunity.
   C. natural immunity.
   D. passive immunity.
   E. induced immunity.

_____ 145. An unexpected and exaggerated reaction to a particular antigen is termed:
   A. allergic reaction.
   B. anaphylaxis.
   C. hypersensitivity.
   D. sensitization.
   E. hyperallergenic crisis.

_____ 146. Scenario: Upon returning home after hiking in the woods for three days, Bill discovers he has a rash on both of his forearms. This is an example of:
   A. anaphylaxis.
   B. repressed hypersensitivity.
   C. immediate hypersensitivity.
   D. sensitization.
   E. delayed hypersensitivity.

_____ 147. This substance is released when an allergen binds to IgE attached to basophils and mast cells.
   A. dopamine
   B. epinephrine
   C. histamine
   D. norepinephrine
   E. pheromone

_____ 148. Which of the following occurs with the release of histamine during an allergic reaction?
   A. bronchodilation
   B. increased intestinal motility
   C. decreased vascular permeability
   D. vasoconstriction
   E. increased red cell production

_____ 149. All of the following insects are of the order _Hymenoptera_ EXCEPT:
   A. fire ants.
   B. honey bees.
   C. scorpions.
   D. wasps.
   E. yellow jackets.

_____ 150. Which of the following do the H_2 receptors mediate when they are stimulated?
   A. decreased secretion of gastric acids
   B. bronchoconstriction
   C. intestinal contraction
   D. peripheral vasodilation
   E. bronchodilation

_____ 151. Which principal body system is NOT affected during anaphylaxis?
  A. auditory
  B. cardiovascular
  C. gastrointestinal
  D. respiratory
  E. all are affected

_____ 152. All of the following findings are common in anaphylaxis EXCEPT:
  A. facial edema.
  B. laryngeal edema.
  C. neck edema.
  D. pedal edema.
  E. pharyngeal edema.

_____ 153. Scenario: A patient is experiencing anaphylaxis. You might also administer all of the following medications EXCEPT:
  A. diphenhydramine.
  B. epinephrine.
  C. furosemide.
  D. Solu-Medrol.
  E. Benadryl.

_____ 154. Which of the following antihistamine medications is the most potent for reducing symptoms due to excessive histamine release?
  A. Atarax
  B. diphenhydramine
  C. promethazine
  D. Vistaril
  E. cromolyn sodium

_____ 155. For allergic reaction, the recommended dose of subcutaneous epinephrine is:
  A. 1:100.
  B. 1:1000.
  C. 1:10,000.
  D. 1:100,000.
  E. none of the above

Chapter 6: Gastroenterology

_____ 156. Dull and poorly localized pain that originates in the walls of hollow organs is:
  A. parietal pain.
  B. referred pain.
  C. somatic pain.
  D. visceral pain.
  E. parenteral pain.

_____ 157. All of the following mechanisms are known to cause pain EXCEPT:
  A. distention.
  B. inspiration.
  C. inflammation.
  D. ischemia.
  E. all of the above cause pain.

_____ 158. Inflammation of the peritoneum is:
  A. peritoneal abscess.
  B. peritonism.
  C. peritonitis.
  D. peritonomy.
  E. periocentesis.

_____ 159. The acronym OPQRST-ASPN is useful when evaluating the history of a patient complaining of abdominal pain. The "T" stands for:
  A. temporary.
  B. time.
  C. transient.
  D. Trendelenburg.
  E. trending.

_____ 160. The terms _dull, sharp, constant,_ and _intermittent_ are used in which of the following components of history gathering?
  A. associated symptoms
  B. palliation
  C. quality
  D. region
  E. onset

_____ 161. Scenario: A 16-year-old male patient was thrown from a vehicle during a motor vehicle accident. He has Grey-Turner's sign, which indicates:
  A. abdominal fluid loss internally.
  B. colon impaction.
  C. diaphragmatic rupture.
  D. renal calculi.
  E. esophageal tearing.

_____ 162. Which of the following organs is a component of the lower GI tract?
A. colon
B. duodenum
C. esophagus
D. stomach
E. mouth

_____ 163. One reason for the high mortality rate associated with upper GI bleeding is:
A. a change in eating habits from red meat to vegetables.
B. an active lifestyle—jogging and aerobic exercise, for example.
C. many patients' treating themselves with over-the-counter remedies.
D. middle-aged patients developing GI distress.
E. lack of exercise.

_____ 164. Irritation or erosion of the lining of this organ accounts for more than 75 percent of upper GI hemorrhage.
A. colon
B. duodenum
C. ileum
D. stomach
E. esophagus

_____ 165. Mallory-Weiss syndrome is caused by:
A. colon cancer.
B. ischemia.
C. pancreatitis.
D. stomach ulcers.
E. esophageal laceration.

_____ 166. Vomiting bright red blood is known as:
A. hematochezia.
B. hematemesis.
C. melena.
D. melenin.
E. epistaxis.

_____ 167. Melena, which is dark, tarry, and foul-smelling stool, indicates partially digested:
A. bile.
B. blood.
C. fat.
D. protein.
E. carbohydrates.

_____ 168. Which of the following medications can break down mucosal surfaces of the stomach and GI tract?
A. aspirin
B. erythromycin
C. Lasix
D. Valium
E. promethazine

_____ 169. How many liters of fluid normally move through the GI tract in 24 hours?
A. 2–5
B. 3–6
C. 4–8
D. 7–9
E. 10–12

_____ 170. Scenario: A 16-month-old female has experienced nausea and diarrhea for two days. She appears pale and clammy. Which of the following signs or symptoms would you also expect?
A. bradycardia
B. bradypnea
C. hypotension
D. hypothermia
E. hypertension

_____ 171. A blocked pancreatic duct can result in duodenal ulcers. This is because the pancreas secretes _____ , which neutralizes chyme.
A. bicarbonate ions
B. glucagon
C. glycol
D. insulin
E. oxytocin

_____ 172. Chronic and non-exsanguinating hematochezia is due to bleeding in the:
A. kidneys.
B. lower GI tract.
C. pancreas.
D. upper GI tract.
E. stomach.

_____ 173. The pathogenesis of appendicitis is best attributed to:
    A. distal colitis.
    B. diverticulosis.
    C. obstruction of the appendiceal lumen by fecal material.
    D. proximal intestinal volvulus.
    E. inflamed varices.

_____ 174. Early appendicitis usually presents with nausea, vomiting, a low-grade fever, and:
    A. Murphy's sign.   D. periumbilical pain.
    B. Cullen's sign.   E. Battle's sign.
    C. Kerr's sign.

_____ 175. Pain associated with appendicitis is usually located in the _____ quadrant.
    A. left lower   D. right upper
    B. left upper   E. all of the above
    C. right lower

_____ 176. The cause of cholecystitis is calculi lodged in the:
    A. islets of Langerhans   D. pancreatic duct
    B. duodenum   E. common bile duct
    C. sphincter of Oddi

_____ 177. Pain associated with cholecystitis is often acute and located in the _____ abdominal quadrant.
    A. left lower   D. right upper
    B. left upper   E. all of the above
    C. right lower

_____ 178. All of the following are categories of causation of pancreatitis EXCEPT:
    A. systemic.   D. metabolic.
    B. infectious.   E. vascular.
    C. mechanical.

_____ 179. Which of the following is known as infectious hepatitis?
    A. HAV   D. HDV
    B. HBV   E. HEV
    C. HCV

_____ 180. Which of the following pathogens is spread by the oral-fecal route?
    A. HAV   D. HDV
    B. HBV   E. HEV
    C. HCV

Chapter 7: Urology and Nephrology

_____ 181. More than 250,000 Americans suffer from which disease?
    A. colitis   D. pancreatitis
    B. diabetes   E. prostatic hypertrophy
    C. end-stage renal failure

_____ 182. The group of organs that is responsible for maintaining fluid and electrolyte balance for the body is the:
    A. cardiovascular system. D. urinary system.
    B. gastrointestinal system. E. vascular system.
    C. integumentary system.

_____ 183. A primary compound secreted in urine is:
    A. bile.   D. urea.
    B. chyme.   E. sebum.
    C. glucose.

_____ 184. A common acute disorder of the urinary system that affects over 500,000 Americans is:
   A. dialysis.
   B. osmotic diuresis.
   C. prostatitis.
   D. renal calculi.
   E. prostatic hypertrophy.

_____ 185. The urinary system is comprised of the kidneys, ureters, urinary bladder, and the:
   A. bulbourethral glands.
   B. ovaries.
   C. prostate.
   D. urethra.
   E. fallopian tubes.

_____ 186. The inner tissue of the kidney is the:
   A. glomerulus.
   B. hilum.
   C. medulla.
   D. papilla.
   E. nephron.

_____ 187. Which of the following processes are involved in urine formation?
   A. glomerular assemblage
   B. reabsorption
   C. retention
   D. diaphoresis
   E. all of the above

_____ 188. As blood passes through the glomerular capillaries, water and chemical materials are filtered out of the blood and into the:
   A. Bowman's capsule.
   B. collecting duct.
   C. loop of Henle.
   D. pyramidal tracts.
   E. bundle of His.

_____ 189. The random movement of molecules from an area of high concentration to an area of lower concentration is:
   A. active transport.
   B. facilitated diffusion.
   C. osmosis.
   D. simple diffusion.
   E. facilitated osmosis.

_____ 190. A solution whose concentration is higher than that of a second substance is:
   A. hyperosmolar.
   B. hypo-osmolar.
   C. isotonic.
   D. ultraosmolar.
   E. none of the above

_____ 191. The movement of a molecule through a cell from an area of lower concentration to an area of higher concentration that requires cellular energy is:
   A. facilitated osmosis.
   B. diuresis.
   C. facilitated diffusion.
   D. osmosis.
   E. active transport.

_____ 192. The dominant cation in intracellular fluid is:
   A. Cl^-.
   B. H^+.
   C. K^+.
   D. Na^+.
   E. Fe^+.

_____ 193. The release of antidiuretic hormone results in:
   A. decreased reabsorption of Cl^-.
   B. increased reabsorption of Na^+.
   C. increased reabsorption of water.
   D. increased secretion of H^+.
   E. none of the above

_____ 194. A waste product of metabolism within muscle cells is:
   A. creatinine.
   B. myoglobin.
   C. plasminogen.
   D. troponin.
   E. plasmin.

_____ 195. Angiotensin II is produced by the interaction of angiotensin converting enzyme and angiotensin I. Angiotensin II results in:
A. decreased secretion of aldosterone from adrenal cells.
B. hypotension.
C. increased arterial blood pressure.
D. release of epinephrine.
E. decreased arterial blood pressure.

_____ 196. The duct that carries urine from the bladder to the exterior of the body is the:
A. collecting duct.   D. urethra.
B. Henle duct.   E. anus.
C. ureter.

_____ 197. The kidneys are protected relatively well against injury, due to their location in the:
A. chest cavity.   D. retroperitoneal space.
B. RLQ.   E. LLQ.
C. pelvic region.

_____ 198. Pain arising in hollow organs such as the ureter and bladder is known as:
A. parietal pain.   D. visceral pain.
B. referred pain.   E. parenteral pain.
C. somatic pain.

_____ 199. Pain that occurs when afferent nerve fibers carrying the pain message merge with other pain-carrying fibers at the junction with the spinal cord is:
A. parietal pain.   D. visceral pain.
B. referred pain.   E. parenteral pain.
C. somatic pain.

_____ 200. Lloyd's sign, which is an indication of pyelonephritis, is associated with:
A. pain on percussion of the costovertebral angle.
B. pain on palpation of the anterior costal margin.
C. periumbilical tenderness.
D. rebound pain at the level of the umbilicus.
E. pain on inhalation.

_____ 201. Hyperkalemia is identified on the ECG by:
A. a decrease in QRS duration.
B. a depression of the S-T segment.
C. an erratic U wave.
D. an increase in P-R interval.
E. an elevation of the T wave greater than two-thirds the diameter of the QRS.

_____ 202. Reduced nephron mass can cause all of the following EXCEPT:
A. chronic anemia.   D. loss of glucose.
B. hyperkalemia.   E. isosthenuria.
C. hyponatremia.

_____ 203. All of the following may be complications related to hemodialysis or peritoneal dialysis EXCEPT:
A. chest pain.   D. seizure.
B. dyspnea.   E. infection.
C. hypertension.

_____ 204. Which of the following types of renal calculi is found more often in women than in men?
A. calcium stones   D. uric acid stones
B. cystine stones   E. oxalate stones
C. struvite stones

_____ 205. The pathophysiology of urinary tract infections is due primarily to:
   A. bacterial infections.
   B. decreases in sexual intercourse.
   C. sexually transmitted disease infections.
   D. urinary tract lesions.
   E. viral infections.

Chapter 8: Toxicology and Substance Abuse

_____ 206. The MOST common portal of entry for toxic exposure is:
   A. absorption.   D. injection.
   B. ingestion.   E. osmosis.
   C. inhalation.

_____ 207. For which of the following ingested substances is flumazenil an antidote?
   A. arsenic   D. ethylene glycol
   B. benzodiazepines   E. methyl alcohol
   C. cyanide

_____ 208. All of the following are respiratory signs or symptoms of a toxic inhalation exposure
   EXCEPT:
   A. bradycardia.   D. tachypnea.
   B. chest tightness.   E. dizziness.
   C. cough.

_____ 209. All of the following are signs or symptoms of cyanide toxicity EXCEPT:
   A. burning sensation in mouth.   D. pulmonary edema.
   B. confusion.   E. tachycardia.
   C. early hypotension and bradycardia.

_____ 210. All of the following are signs or symptoms of carbon monoxide poisoning EXCEPT:
   A. arousal.   D. tachypnea.
   B. headache.   E. confusion.
   C. nausea.

_____ 211. Scenario: A patient has spilled a large quantity of an unknown acid on his skin.
   Treatment should consist of:
   A. contacting poison control for instructions.
   B. covering the area with activated charcoal.
   C. diluting the acid with bicarbonate.
   D. irrigation with copious amounts of water.
   E. irrigation with copious amounts of milk.

_____ 212. Ingestion of alkalis usually results in:
   A. immediate and intense pain.
   B. bradycardia.
   C. local burns to the mouth and throat.
   D. ulceration and perforation of the stomach lining.
   E. liquefaction necrosis.

_____ 213. All of the following procedures are appropriate for hydrofluoric acid exposure
   EXCEPT:
   A. immersing the injured part in iced water with sodium bicarbonate.
   B. irrigating the affected area with copious amounts of water.
   C. protecting rescue personnel from exposure.
   D. removing exposed clothing.
   E. initiating supportive measures.

_____ 214. All of the following are hydrocarbons EXCEPT:
  A. turpentine.   D. naphtha.
  B. benzene.   E. ammonia.
  C. kerosene.

_____ 215. All of the following are tricyclic antidepressant medications EXCEPT:
  A. doxepin.   D. Zoloft.
  B. Elavil.   E. imipramine.
  C. nortriptyline.

_____ 216. Scenario: A patient has attempted suicide by overdosing on amitriptyline and alcohol.
  You might expect all of the following signs or symptoms EXCEPT:
  A. hypertension.   D. widened QRS complex.
  B. respiratory depression.   E. hallucinations.
  C. tachycardia.

_____ 217. Which of the following medications can be useful in tricyclic antidepressant overdoses?
  A. activated charcoal   D. sodium bicarbonate
  B. atropine   E. dextrose
  C. flumazenil

_____ 218. Monoamine oxidase inhibitors (MAOIs) function by:
  A. increasing the availability of norepinephrine and dopamine.
  B. increasing the release of serotonin.
  C. inhibiting the breakdown of norepinephrine and dopamine.
  D. inhibiting the release of serotonin.
  E. releasing endorphins.

_____ 219. All of the following medications are selective serotonin re-uptake inhibitors EXCEPT:
  A. Elavil.   D. Zoloft.
  B. Luvox.   E. Paxil.
  C. Prozac.

_____ 220. Signs of lithium toxicity include:
  A. hyperactivity.   D. tachycardia.
  B. moist mucous membranes.   E. constipation.
  C. muscle twitching.

_____ 221. An overdose of aspirin at greater than 300 mg/kg results in:
  A. metabolic acidosis.   D. respiratory alkalosis.
  B. metabolic alkalosis.   E. respiratory arrest.
  C. respiratory acidosis.

_____ 222. All of the following are expected signs or symptoms of a salicylate overdose EXCEPT:
  A. abdominal pain.   D. pulmonary edema.
  B. cardiac dysrhythmia.   E. confusion.
  C. hypothermia.

_____ 223. An overdose of Tylenol at which level is considered toxic?
  A. 100 mg/kg   D. 300 mg/kg
  B. 150 mg/kg   E. 350 mg/kg
  C. 200 mg/kg

_____ 224. Scenario: A patient has accidentally overdosed on his theophylline medication. He is
  experiencing PVCs, palpitations, and nausea and vomiting. Which of the following
  medications can be used to manage the theophylline overdose?
  A. activated charcoal   D. phenergan
  B. lidocaine   E. digoxin
  C. morphine

_____ 225. Chronic ingestion of and exposure to which of the following metals can result in memory disturbances, abdominal pain, confusion, agitation, and tremors?
A. copper
B. iron
C. lead
D. magnesium
E. aluminum

_____ 226. Exposure to contaminated food that has this bacteria, which is the world's most toxic poison, results in respiratory distress or arrest.
A. *Clostridium botulinum*
B. *E. coli*
C. *Salmonella*
D. *Shigella*
E. Scombroid

_____ 227. The pathophysiology of an anaphylactic reaction resulting from a *Hymenoptera* sting involves:
A. decreased release of adrenergics.
B. decreased release of endorphins in the body.
C. excessive release of catecholamines.
D. increased production of beta blockers.
E. excessive release of histamine.

_____ 228. Scenario: Your patient has been bitten by a rattlesnake. He is tachypneic, is nauseated, has vomited once, and has weakness in his extremities. You would also expect all of the following EXCEPT:
A. altered mental status.
B. dyspnea.
C. hypertension.
D. localized pain.
E. thirst.

_____ 229. Routine emergency care of a pit viper bite includes which of the following?
A. applying ice to the bite site
B. encouraging the patient to walk to reduce the concentration of the venom
C. immobilizing the limb with a splint
D. using a constricting band to reduce venous circulation
E. applying a mild electrical shock to reverse the spread of venom

_____ 230. The condition that occurs when a patient's body reacts severely when deprived of an abused substance is:
A. addiction.
B. habituation.
C. tolerance.
D. delirium.
E. withdrawal.

_____ 231. Alcohol is a(n):
A. depressant.
B. narcotic.
C. opiate.
D. stimulant.
E. oxidant.

_____ 232. All of the following are signs of someone who has taken too much phenobarbital EXCEPT:
A. coma.
B. hypertension.
C. lethargy.
D. respiratory depression.
E. bradycardia.

_____ 233. Scenario: A patient is extremely anxious and complaining of euphoria and a very dry mouth. Your assessment reveals only dilated pupils. The patient states that he smoked "grass" tonight with his friends and this was his first time. Management of this patient should consist of:
A. gentle reassurance.
B. IV therapy.
C. Phenergan 12.5 mg.
D. Valium 5 mg.
E. Decadron.

_____ **234.** Signs and symptoms associated with amphetamine usage include all of the following EXCEPT:
    A. constricted pupils.
    B. exhilaration.
    C. hypertension.
    D. psychosis.
    E. tremors.

_____ **235.** Which of the following is NOT a sign or symptom of a Xanax overdose?
    A. altered mental status
    B. slurred speech
    C. hypotension
    D. respiratory depression
    E. tachycardia

Chapter 9: Hematology

_____ **236.** All of the following organs are part of the hematopoietic system EXCEPT the:
    A. heart.
    B. kidneys.
    C. liver.
    D. spleen.
    E. bone marrow.

_____ **237.** A 75 kg person has approximately how many liters of blood?
    A. 5
    B. 6
    C. 7
    D. 8
    E. 9

_____ **238.** The hormone responsible for red blood cell production is:
    A. aldosterone.
    B. cytokine.
    C. calcitonin.
    D. renin.
    E. erythropoietin.

_____ **239.** The phenomenon in which a decrease in pCO_2/acidity causes an increase in the quantity of oxygen that binds with hemoglobin and in which an increase in pCO_2/acidity causes hemoglobin to release oxygen is known as:
    A. the Bohr effect.
    B. Boyle's law.
    C. the Fick principle.
    D. the Frank-Starling law.
    E. the Clauser principle.

_____ **240.** Which of the following will REDUCE hemoglobin's affinity for oxygen?
    A. a decrease in 2,3-diphosphoglycerate (2,3-DPG)
    B. decreased exercise
    C. increased erythrocyte production
    D. pyrexia
    E. mild hypothermia

_____ **241.** Erythropoietin is secreted when these cells sense hypoxia.
    A. heart
    B. liver
    C. kidney
    D. spleen
    E. bone marrow

_____ **242.** Hemoglobin is usually expressed as the number of grams per deciliter of whole blood. The normal concentration for men is:
    A. 10.5–14.0 g/dL.
    B. 12.0–15.0 g/dL.
    C. 13.5–17.0 g/dL.
    D. 15.0–20.0 g/dL.
    E. 20.0–22.0 g/dL.

_____ **243.** White blood cells originate from which hematopoietic component?
    A. bone marrow
    B. kidney
    C. liver
    D. spleen
    E. all of the above

_____ 244. All of the following are functions of monocytes EXCEPT:
   A. attacking tumor cells.   D. stimulating the release of cytokine.
   B. repairing tissue.   E. secreting growth factors.
   C. removing foreign matter.

_____ 245. Which type of granulocytes mediates an acute allergic response by inactivating chemical mediators?
   A. basophils   D. phagocytes
   B. eosinophils   E. monocytes
   C. neutrophils

_____ 246. Which white blood cell contains antigen-specific surface receptor sites that can initiate an immune response?
   A. basophil   D. neutrophil
   B. lymphocyte   E. monocyte
   C. eosinophil

_____ 247. Cellular immunity is mediated through which type of lymphocyte?
   A. A cell   D. T cell
   B. B cell   E. I cell
   C. M cell

_____ 248. The normal number of platelets ranges from:
   A. 90,000 to 120,000 / mcL.   D. 250,000 to 550,000 / mcL.
   B. 120,000 to 250,000 / mcL.   E. 300,000 to 600,000 / mcL.
   C. 150,000 to 450,000 / mcL.

_____ 249. The primary cell from which thrombocytes are formed is the:
   A. lymphocyte.   D. thombophil.
   B. megakaryocyte.   E. leukocyte.
   C. neutrophil.

_____ 250. The process of breaking down or dismantling a clot is known as:
   A. delamination.   D. thrombolysis.
   B. platelet degradation.   E. fibrinolysis.
   C. prothrombinlysis.

_____ 251. The rarest blood type in the U.S. is:
   A. A.   D. O.
   B. AB.   E. none of the above
   C. B.

_____ 252. The universal donor blood type is:
   A. A.   D. O.
   B. AB.   E. none of the above
   C. B.

_____ 253. Lymphatic signs associated with hematologic disorders include:
   A. enlarged lymph nodes.   D. shrunken spleen.
   B. hematuria.   E. jaundice.
   C. petechiae.

_____ 254. Which disease may result in slower blood clotting?
   A. AIDS   D. pancreatitis
   B. cholecystitis   E. malaria
   C. cirrhosis

_____ 255. Patients who have sickle cell disease typically have complete infarction of the:
   A. heart.   D. spleen.
   B. liver.   E. gallbladder.
   C. pancreas.

_____ **256.** The condition in which patients with hemophilia develop swollen, discolored, and painful joints with minimal trauma is:
   A. leukotaxis.
   B. dysthralgia.
   C. ecchymotic arthralgia.
   D. hemarthrosis.
   E. arthralgia.

_____ **257.** A deficiency of _____ is linked to anemia.
   A. calcium
   B. copper
   C. iron
   D. potassium
   E. magnesium

_____ **258.** Hemophilia is acquired through:
   A. defective genetic code.
   B. excessive NSAIDs dosing.
   C. transfusion reaction.
   D. viral infection.
   E. bacterial infection.

_____ **259.** Patients with hemophilia A are deficient in blood clotting factor:
   A. VII.
   B. VIII.
   C. IX.
   D. X.
   E. XII.

_____ **260.** The disease referred to as consumption coagulation is often caused by any of the following EXCEPT:
   A. hemolytic transfusion reactions.
   B. hypertension.
   C. obstetrical complications.
   D. sepsis.
   E. hypotension.

Chapter 10: Environmental Emergencies

_____ **261.** The process of heat transfer via currents in liquids or gases is:
   A. conduction.
   B. convection.
   C. evaporation.
   D. radiation.
   E. respiration.

_____ **262.** At normal room temperature, an unclothed person loses approximately 60 percent of total body heat through:
   A. conduction.
   B. convection.
   C. evaporation.
   D. radiation.
   E. respiration.

_____ **263.** Which of the following locations indicates a patient's core temperature?
   A. axillary
   B. forehead
   C. popliteal
   D. tympanic
   E. carotid

_____ **264.** The body temperature at which temperature regulation is significantly impaired is greater than _____ and less than _____ .
   A. 100°F, 96°F
   B. 102°F, 96°F
   C. 103°F, 93°F
   D. 104°F, 94°F
   E. 106°F, 95°F

_____ **265.** For each liter of fluid lost due to sweating, a patient will lose approximately:
   A. 20–50 mEq of potassium.
   B. 20–50 mEq of sodium.
   C. 5–20 mEq of potassium.
   D. 5–20 mEq of sodium.
   E. 10–15 mEq of potassium.

_____ **266.** _____ is (are) a usually mild, acute reaction to heat exposure.
   A. Heat cramps
   B. Heat exhaustion
   C. Heatstroke
   D. Hyperpyrexia
   E. Hot flashes

_____ 267. _____ commonly presents with chronic illness and an increased core temperature due to thermoregulatory insufficiency.
  A. Classic heat exhaustion
  B. Classic heatstroke
  C. Exertional heatstroke
  D. Climactic heatstroke
  E. Excitational heat cramps

_____ 268. Dehydration often accompanies hyperthermic conditions because it inhibits:
  A. negative chronotropic effects.
  B. positive inotropic effects.
  C. thermogenesis.
  D. vasodilation.
  E. metabolism.

_____ 269. All of the following are signs of dehydration EXCEPT:
  A. abdominal distress.
  B. decreased blood pressure.
  C. decreased urine output.
  D. increased skin turgor.
  E. vision disturbances.

_____ 270. Which of the following disease processes can predispose a patient to hypothermia?
  A. duodenal ulcers
  B. hyperthyroidism
  C. hypoglycemia
  D. cirrhosis
  E. Cushing's syndrome

_____ 271. At what temperature will the body shiver the most in order to compensate for heat loss?
  A. 96.8°F
  B. 95.0°F
  C. 93.2°F
  D. 89.6°F
  E. 88.8°F

_____ 272. The ECG wave that is prominent in a patient with severe hypothermia is the:
  A. J wave.
  B. P wave.
  C. Q wave.
  D. U wave.
  E. S wave.

_____ 273. A patient with severe hypothermia will:
  A. be hypotensive.
  B. display tachycardia and tachypnea.
  C. have decreased coordination.
  D. have increased shivering.
  E. lack coordination.

_____ 274. The MOST common presenting dysrhythmia seen in the hypothermic patient with a core temperature above 86°F is:
  A. atrial fibrillation.
  B. atrial tachycardia.
  C. ventricular fibrillation.
  D. ventricular tachycardia.
  E. atrial flutter.

_____ 275. Which type of active rewarming may be used in the prehospital setting for a patient in mild hypothermia?
  A. massage of the affected extremity
  B. heat lights
  C. warm peritoneal dialysis
  D. walking the patient around
  E. blankets and heat packs at key circulatory points

_____ 276. Ventricular fibrillation in the hypothermic patient may be minimized by:
  A. increasing the patient's exposure to the environment.
  B. avoiding aggressive or rough handling of the patient.
  C. providing active rewarming if the patient is less than 5 minutes from the hospital.
  D. stimulating the patient with caffeinated beverages.
  E. using alcohol as a general system depressant.

_____ 277. Which of the following ALS interventions can be performed in the field on a patient in severe hypothermia who is pulseless?
  A. intubation
  B. lidocaine 2 mg/kg
  C. sodium bicarbonate 1 meq/kg
  D. warm peritoneal lavage
  E. precordial thump

_____ 278. Wet drowning occurs in approximately _____ of drowning patients.
  A. 10 percent
  B. 50 percent
  C. 62 percent
  D. 75 percent
  E. 90 percent

_____ 279. During saltwater drowning:
  A. atelectasis occurs.
  B. hemodilution occurs.
  C. pulmonary edema is present.
  D. surfactant is lost.
  E. cardiac dysrhythms develop.

_____ 280. Atmospheric pressure at sea level is:
  A. 12.2 psi.
  B. 14.7 psi.
  C. 17.0 psi.
  D. 34.6 psi.
  E. 43.2 psi.

_____ 281. _____ states that a volume of gas is inversely proportional to its pressure if its temperature remains constant.
  A. Boyle's law
  B. Dalton's law
  C. Henry's law
  D. Starling's law
  E. Joule's law

_____ 282. _____ states that the total pressure of a mixture of gases is equal to the sum of the partial pressures of the individual gases.
  A. Boyle's law
  B. Dalton's law
  C. Henry's law
  D. Starling's law
  E. Joule's law

_____ 283. The pressure of air at sea level is:
  A. 160 mmHg.
  B. 250 mmHg.
  C. 500 mmHg.
  D. 760 mmHg.
  E. 840 mmHg.

_____ 284. At what depth do two atmosphere absolutes (ata) occur?
  A. 33 feet
  B. 66 feet
  C. 99 feet
  D. 132 feet
  E. 165 feet

_____ 285. Oxygen and inert gases comprise 22 percent of the gases in the air at sea level. The pressure of nitrogen at sea level is:
  A. 4 mmHg.
  B. 160 mmHg.
  C. 593 mmHg.
  D. 760 mmHg.
  E. 880 mmHg.

_____ 286. _____ states that the amount of gas dissolved in a given volume of fluid is proportional to the pressure of the gas above it.
  A. Boyle's law
  B. Dalton's law
  C. Henry's law
  D. Starling's law
  E. Joule's law

_____ 287. Which gas tends to dissolve in the blood and tissues in the greatest quantities when a person descends below sea level?
  A. argon
  B. helium
  C. nitrogen
  D. oxygen
  E. carbon dioxide

_____ 288. The law that BEST describes the increasing dissolution of gases in the bloodstream as a person dives deeper in water is:
A. Boyle's law.
B. Dalton's law.
C. Henry's law.
D. Starling's law.
E. Joule's law.

_____ 289. Which demographic group is the MOST susceptible to high altitude pulmonary edema?
A. adult men
B. adult women
C. children
D. elderly women
E. diabetics

_____ 290. Substances that emit ionizing radiation are known as:
A. atoms.
B. ions.
C. isotopes.
D. protons.
E. neutrons.

Chapter 11: Infectious Disease

_____ 291. The individual who first introduced an infectious agent to a population is referred to as the:
A. first incident.
B. ground zero.
C. index case.
D. infectious deliverer.
E. target case.

_____ 292. Which public health agency is responsible for setting standards and guidelines for workplace and worker safety?
A. CDC
B. DHHS
C. FEMA
D. OSHA
E. NIHD

_____ 293. Toxic waste products that are produced by living bacteria are:
A. bacterotoxins.
B. cytotoxins.
C. endotoxins.
D. exotoxins.
E. pathotoxins.

_____ 294. Which statement about viruses is correct?
A. A host is susceptible to any particular virus during multiple encounters.
B. Antibiotic therapy is the only means to treat viral infections.
C. Viruses cannot be seen under the microscope.
D. Viruses grow and reproduce only within a host cell.
E. Viruses are larger than bacteria.

_____ 295. Which type of organism is yeast?
A. bacteria
B. fungus
C. protozoa
D. virus
E. endotoxin

_____ 296. Which of the following diseases is transmitted through an airborne route?
A. gonorrhea
B. hepatitis B
C. Lyme disease
D. measles
E. trichinosis

_____ 297. _____ is the presence of an agent (pathogen) only on the surface of the host without actual infection.
A. Communication
B. Symbiosis
C. Infection
D. Virulence
E. Contamination

_____ 298. All of the following are factors in disease transmission EXCEPT:
   A. host resistance.   D. virulence.
   B. length of exposure.   E. number of organisms transmitted.
   C. mode of entry.

_____ 299. The time between a host's exposure to an infectious agent and the appearance of symptoms is the:
   A. communicable period.   D. latent period.
   B. disease period.   E. growth period.
   C. incubation period.

_____ 300. The marker on the surface of a cell that identifies it as self or nonself is an:
   A. antibody.   D. antiprion.
   B. anticell.   E. antiphon.
   C. antigen.

_____ 301. The immunoglobulin that remembers an antigen and recognizes any repeated invasions is:
   A. IgA.   D. IgM.
   B. IgE.   E. IgD.
   C. IgG.

_____ 302. The cells in the lymph system that attach to and destroy particulate matter are:
   A. killer T-cells.   D. reticuloendothelial cells.
   B. monocytes.   E. chemotactic cells.
   C. neutrophils.

_____ 303. _____ immunity develops after birth as a result of a direct exposure to a pathogen.
   A. Acquired   D. Passive
   B. Age-related   E. Active
   C. Humoral

_____ 304. Intermediate-level disinfection is accomplished by using:
   A. 1:100 water and bleach solution. D. soap and water.
   B. chemical sterilizing agents.   E. an autoclave.
   C. gas sterilization unit.

_____ 305. When should an infectious disease exposure be reported?
   A. at the end of the shift   D. within 24 hours
   B. by the beginning of the next shift E. within 72 hours
   C. immediately

_____ 306. Clinical presentation of an HIV-infected person includes all of the following signs or symptoms EXCEPT:
   A. reduced lymph nodes.
   B. general fatigue, fever, lymphadenopathy, and weight loss.
   C. _Pneumocystis carinii_ pneumonia.
   D. purplish skin lesions.
   E. enlarged spleen.

_____ 307. Which of the following medications is recommended as part of the triple therapy following HIV exposure?
   A. TCP   D. IDG
   B. AZT   E. MVC
   C. HBV

_____ 308. The mode of transmission of hepatitis A is:
   A. contact with fecal matter to mucous membranes or nonintact skin.
   B. direct blood contact.
   C. saliva.
   D. vaginal secretions.
   E. through the air.

_____ 309. For which of the following diseases is the health care worker at the GREATEST risk of exposure?
A. hepatitis B
B. HIV
C. meningitis
D. tuberculosis
E. pneumonia

_____ 310. Hepatitis C is transmitted primarily through:
A. blood transfusions.
B. the fecal-oral route.
C. household contact.
D. IV drug abuse.
E. contaminated food.

_____ 311. The mode of transmission for tuberculosis is:
A. bloodborne.
B. cutaneous contact.
C. fecal-oral.
D. respiratory.
E. gastrointestinal.

_____ 312. Which of the following precautions BEST reduces the emergency responder's risk of tuberculosis exposure?
A. administering oxygen via a nasal cannula
B. a NIOSH-approved respirator
C. placing a mask over the patient's face
D. opening the ambulance's patient compartment windows
E. gloves and standard mask

_____ 313. All of the following significantly increase a patient's risk for developing pneumonia EXCEPT:
A. a transplanted kidney.
B. gastroenteritis.
C. sickle cell disease.
D. a splenectomy.
E. diabetes mellitus.

_____ 314. Which virus causes chickenpox?
A. herpes zoster
B. influenza zoster
C. streptococcus zoster
D. varicella zoster
E. Klebsiella zoster

_____ 315. A prophylactic postexposure medication for meningitis is:
A. Wymox.
B. cyclosporin.
C. erythromycin.
D. Zithromax.
E. Cipro.

_____ 316. Which patient group is MOST susceptible to influenza?
A. teenagers
B. young adults
C. middle-aged adults
D. the elderly
E. children

_____ 317. The most life-threatening sequela of measles in children who are not immunized is:
A. encephalitis.
B. eye damage.
C. myocarditis.
D. pneumonia.
E. cardiovascular damage.

_____ 318. The _____ phase of pertussis is characterized by a deep, high-pitched cough similar to a "whoop."
A. catarrhal
B. convalescent
C. entry
D. paroxysmal
E. virulent

_____ 319. The MOST common sign of herpes simplex virus type 1 infection is:
A. conjunctivitis.
B. Epstein-Barr syndrome.
C. herpetic whitlow.
D. HSV labialis.
E. a rash.

_____ 320. All of the following are among the "four Ds" associated with epiglottitis EXCEPT:
A. drooling.
B. dyspepsia.
C. dysphagia.
D. dysphonia.
E. distress.

_____ 321. A viral illness in children characterized by inspiratory and expiratory stridor and seal-bark-like cough is:
A. croup.
B. epiglottitis.
C. pertussis.
D. pharyngitis.
E. variola.

_____ 322. All of the following complications may result from gastroenteritis EXCEPT:
A. dehydration.
B. diarrhea and emesis.
C. dysuria.
D. electrolyte imbalance.
E. hypovolemic shock.

_____ 323. Urban rabies is transmitted through:
A. foxes.
B. raccoons.
C. skunks.
D. unimmunized domestic dogs.
E. rats.

_____ 324. An acute bacterial infection of the central nervous system that presents with muscle rigidity near the injury site and pain and stiffness of the jaw muscles is:
A. meningitis.
B. mumps.
C. rickettsia.
D. tetanus.
E. variola.

_____ 325. Gonorrhea presentation in men is characterized by:
A. impotence.
B. priapism.
C. purulent urethral discharge.
D. scrotum enlargement.
E. facial sores.

_____ 326. The stage of syphilis that is known as the "great imitator" may result in all of the following EXCEPT:
A. aortic aneurysms.
B. deep lesions with sharp borders on skin and bones.
C. increased sensation of pain and temperature.
D. progressive dementia.
E. enlargement of the lymph nodes.

_____ 327. All of the following are transmission routes for chlamydia EXCEPT:
A. hand-to-hand transfer of eye secretions.
B. oral intercourse.
C. sexual intercourse.
D. respiratory route.
E. use of infected linens.

_____ 328. A parasitic infection of the skin, scalp, trunk, or pubic area is:
A. impetigo.
B. lice.
C. psoriasis.
D. scabies.
E. roundworm.

_____ 329. Infection of the skin by staphylococci or streptococci is:
A. impetigo.
B. lice.
C. psoriasis.
D. scabies.
E. roundworm.

_____ 330. Infections acquired while in the hospital are referred to as:
A. social.
B. administrative.
C. nosocomial.
D. pathologic.
E. opportunistic.

Chapter 12: Psychiatric and Behavioral Disorders

_____ 331. Normal behavior varies based on culture, ethnic group, and:
  A. affective attitude.
  B. interpersonal characteristics.
  C. personal interpretation.
  D. religious beliefs.
  E. financial status.

_____ 332. Psychological disorders that arise from interactions within society include all of the following EXCEPT:
  A. economic problems.
  B. dysfunctional families.
  C. social isolation.
  D. witnessing the victimization of another.
  E. clashes of values.

_____ 333. Psychosocial conditions are related to a patient's personality style and:
  A. crisis management methods.
  B. personal values.
  C. social habits.
  D. socioeconomic status.
  E. use of drugs.

_____ 334. A state of being unclear or unable to make a decision easily is:
  A. affect.
  B. ambivalence.
  C. fear.
  D. posture.
  E. confusion.

_____ 335. A feeling of alarm and discontentment in the expectation of danger is:
  A. anxiety.
  B. confusion.
  C. depression.
  D. fear.
  E. angst.

_____ 336. A condition characterized by the rapid onset of widespread disorganized thought is:
  A. delirium.
  B. delusions.
  C. dementia.
  D. dysphasia.
  E. dysfunction.

_____ 337. All of the following diseases typically may cause dementia EXCEPT:
  A. Alzheimer's disease.
  B. Bell's palsy.
  C. head trauma.
  D. Parkinson's disease.
  E. AIDS.

_____ 338. Impaired ability to recognize objects or stimuli despite intact sensory function is:
  A. aphasia.
  B. delirium.
  C. flat affect.
  D. agnosia.
  E. catatonia.

_____ 339. Scenario: You are called to the scene of a patient threatening suicide. The patient is preoccupied with a sense of persecution, her speech is very disorganized, and she's exhibiting peculiar movements. The best management for this condition is to:
  A. tell the patient you hear the same voices that she hears.
  B. present a calm and reassuring demeanor.
  C. reinforce the patient's hallucinations.
  D. restrain the patient.
  E. ignore the patient's speech and just do your job.

_____ 340. Scenario: A student is preparing to take an exam and suddenly begins to feel palpitations, sweating, shaking, and abdominal distress. These symptoms are BEST characterized as:
  A. anxiety.
  B. panic attack.
  C. phobia.
  D. posttraumatic stress.
  E. delirium.

_____ 341. Displaying hostility or rage to compensate for an underlying feeling of anxiety is:
  A. depression.
  B. anger.
  C. paranoia.
  D. phobia.
  E. catatonia.

_____ 342. A patient who is preoccupied with physical symptoms most likely has _____ disorder.
  A. conversion
  B. pain
  C. body dysmorphic
  D. somatization
  E. affective

_____ 343. In which of the following disorders does the patient avoid stress by separating from his core personality?
  A. bipolar
  B. dissociative
  C. factitious
  D. somatoform
  E. affective

_____ 344. Which of the following disorders is a dissociative disorder?
  A. anorexia
  B. conversion
  C. depersonalization
  D. factitious
  E. hypochondriasis

_____ 345. A patient with recurrent episodes of binge eating and purging most likely has:
  A. fugue state.
  B. bulimia nervosa.
  C. conversion disorder.
  D. anorexia nervosa.
  E. hypochondriasis.

_____ 346. _____ behavior involves a pattern of excessive emotions and attention seeking.
  A. Codependent
  B. Histrionic
  C. Narcissistic
  D. Paranoiac
  E. Antisocial

_____ 347. Kleptomania, pyromania, trichotillomania, gambling, and intermittent explosive disorder are all types of _____ disorders.
  A. anxiety
  B. impulse control
  C. mood
  D. somatoform
  E. factitious

_____ 348. The MOST common method of committing suicide is:
  A. cutting.
  B. drowning.
  C. poisoning.
  D. strangulation.
  E. gunshot wound.

_____ 349. Which of the following usually would be MOST appropriate when caring for a child experiencing an emotional crisis?
  A. Separate the child from the parent.
  B. Explain in detail what you are doing.
  C. Have the child bring a favorite blanket or toy.
  D. Discourage the child from crying.
  E. Maintain an authoritative distance from the child.

_____ 350. Which statement regarding restraining a patient is NOT true?
  A. Preferably three or four people should restrain the patient, but more may be used if the patient is extremely large or combative.
  B. Combative patients should be hog-tied and placed on the stretcher, then transported to the local hospital.
  C. Restrained patients should be placed supine on the stretcher with one arm extended and restrained above the head and the other arm adducted and restrained next to the body.
  D. The patient's mental status and ABCs should be constantly reevaluated during transport.
  E. Commercial leather restraints, jacket restraints, and soft restraints are optimal.

Chapter 13: Gynecology

_____ 351. Which of the following structures is part of the external female genitalia?
A. ovary
B. perineum
C. uterus
D. vagina
E. fallopian tube

_____ 352. An elastic canal that connects the internal and external female genitalia is the:
A. ureter.
B. urethra.
C. vagina.
D. vulva.
E. fallopian tube.

_____ 353. The distance from the symphysis pubis to the fundus can be used to calculate:
A. duration of premenstrual cycle.
B. gestational length in weeks.
C. length of menses.
D. time since menopause.
E. age of the patient.

_____ 354. The layer of the uterine wall where the fertilized egg implants is the:
A. dermametrium.
B. cyclometrium.
C. myometrium.
D. perimetrium.
E. endometrium.

_____ 355. Which of the following hormones is released by the ovaries?
A. estrogen
B. follicle-stimulating hormone
C. gonadotropin
D. luteinizing hormone
E. thymosin

_____ 356. The menstrual cycle generally lasts:
A. 2 weeks.
B. 28 days.
C. 7 days.
D. 9 months.
E. 3 weeks.

_____ 357. The onset of ovulation that establishes female sexual maturity is known as:
A. menarche.
B. menopause.
C. menses.
D. menstruation.
E. menacme.

_____ 358. The _____ phase of the menstrual cycle terminates with ovulation.
A. ischemic
B. menstrual
C. proliferative
D. secretory
E. fallow

_____ 359. Which process occurs during the proliferative phase of the menstrual cycle?
A. drop in estrogen level
B. rupture of small endometrial blood vessels
C. shedding of the endometrium
D. thickening of the endometrium
E. the endometrium becomes pale

_____ 360. The age range in which menopause generally occurs is:
A. 35–40 years.
B. 40–55 years.
C. 45–55 years.
D. 50–60 years.
E. 60–65 years.

_____ 361. Which of the following questions is LEAST likely to get an accurate response from a female who is complaining of abdominal pain?
A. Are you currently menstruating?
B. Are you sexually active?
C. Could you be pregnant?
D. Have you ever experienced this pain before during menses?
E. Have you experienced dizziness?

_____ 362. The term used to describe the number of times a woman has been pregnant is:
A. *gravida.*
B. *gravity.*
C. *paridy.*
D. *parita.*
E. *completa.*

_____ 363. The easiest means by which an EMS provider can estimate menstrual flow is:
A. cervical palpation.
B. the testimony of the patient.
C. direct observation.
D. the saturation of one tampon or pad.
E. the number of tampons or pads used in the past hour.

_____ 364. The most common cause of nontraumatic abdominal pain is:
A. cystitis.
B. mittelschmerz.
C. pelvic inflammatory disease.
D. ruptured ovarian cyst.
E. endometriosis.

_____ 365. Scenario: A female patient reports frequent urination and dysuria. This is probably due to:
A. cholecystitis.
B. cystitis.
C. dysmenorrhea.
D. dyspareunia.
E. endometritis.

_____ 366. Severe abdominal pain associated with ovulation is:
A. cystitis.
B. endometriosis.
C. endometritis.
D. cholecystitis.
E. mittelschmerz.

_____ 367. A condition in which endometrial tissue is found outside the uterus is:
A. ectopic pregnancy.
B. endometriosis.
C. endometritis.
D. eschar.
E. mittelschmerz.

_____ 368. Which condition often mimics signs and symptoms of severe PID?
A. endometriosis
B. endometritis
C. mittelschmerz
D. ruptured ovarian cyst
E. cholecystitis

_____ 369. Scenario: A female reports that during aggressive intercourse she felt a sudden and sharp tearing sensation. She is now bleeding from the external genitalia, although the bleeding is minimal. Management should include:
A. asking the woman to hold a dressing over the area and apply direct pressure.
B. establishing an IV and beginning fluid resuscitation regardless of blood loss.
C. packing the vagina with sterile dressings.
D. palpating the interior of the vagina to determine the extent of bleeding.
E. securing a hot pack over the vaginal opening with tape.

_____ 370. The BEST management for a victim of a sexual assault is:
A. aggressive questioning and management.
B. discouraging the patient from dressing since this may taint evidence.
C. examining the genitalia.
D. psychological and emotional support.
E. prompt summoning of law enforcement officials.

Chapter 14: Obstetrics

_____ 371. Fertilization of the ovum usually occurs in the:
A. cervix.
B. fallopian tubes.
C. ovaries.
D. uterus.
E. perineum.

_____ 372. A change in the reproductive system during pregnancy is that:
   A. mammary glands decrease in number.
   B. secretion of estrogen causes sloughing of the endometrial lining.
   C. the uterus contains about 16 percent of the total maternal blood volume.
   D. uterine connective tissue stiffens to allow for support of the fetus.
   E. dissolution of a mucous plug in the cervix.

_____ 373. The normal duration of pregnancy is _____ from the first day of the mother's last menstrual period.
   A. 36 weeks   D. 44 weeks
   B. 40 weeks   E. 48 weeks
   C. 42 weeks

_____ 374. Fetal heart tones can be detected by the _____ week of gestation.
   A. eighth   D. twentieth
   B. twelfth   E. twenty-eighth
   C. sixteenth

_____ 375. By which week of gestation is a baby is considered term?
   A. twentieth   D. thirty-eighth
   B. twenty-fifth   E. fortieth
   C. thirty-second

_____ 376. Which structure allows for mixing of blood between the right and left atria?
   A. ductus arteriosus   D. umbilical vein
   B. ductus venosus   E. umbilical artery
   C. foramen ovale

_____ 377. The ductus arteriosus connects which two structures?
   A. inferior vena cava and aorta
   B. pulmonary artery and aorta
   C. pulmonary vein and aorta
   D. superior vena cava and aorta
   E. superior vena cava and pulmonary artery

_____ 378. All of the following are typical causes of vaginal bleeding during pregnancy EXCEPT:
   A. abortion.   D. placenta previa.
   B. abruptio placentae. E. prolapsed umbilical cord.
   C. ectopic pregnancy.

_____ 379. A naturally occurring expulsion of the fetus prior to viability, generally due to chromosomal abnormalities, that may occur before the twelfth week of gestation is:
   A. inevitable abortion.   D. threatened abortion.
   B. missed abortion.   E. term abortion.
   C. spontaneous abortion.

_____ 380. Which sign or symptom differentiates eclampsia from preeclampsia?
   A. chronic hypertension   D. supine hypotensive disorder
   B. gestational diabetes   E. none of the above
   C. seizure

_____ 381. One way to minimize supine hypotension in the pregnant patient is to:
   A. allow her to sit in the semi-Fowler's position.
   B. place her in a full Trendelenburg position.
   C. position her tilted slightly to the right.
   D. sit her upright with feet dangling.
   E. place her in the left lateral recumbent position.

_____ 382. All of the following may cause preterm labor EXCEPT:
       A. exercise.
       B. infection.
       C. multiple gestation.
       D. placenta previa.
       E. diabetes.

_____ 383. Which of the following medications is considered a tocolytic for preterm labor?
       A. magnesium sulfate
       B. oxytocin
       C. Pitocin
       D. racemic epinephrine
       E. dextran

_____ 384. Crowning of the fetus occurs during the _____ stage.
       A. dilatation
       B. expulsion
       C. placental
       D. puerperium
       E. postpartal

_____ 385. After the infant's head has delivered through the birth canal, the paramedic should:
       A. NOT pull the umbilical cord from around the infant's neck.
       B. pull the child out of the canal.
       C. push the baby's head down to facilitate delivery of the shoulders.
       D. suction the mouth and then the nose of the infant.
       E. suction the nose and then the mouth of the infant.

_____ 386. Immediate care of the newborn should include all of the following EXCEPT:
       A. assessing the neonate using APGAR scoring.
       B. drying the infant.
       C. immediately ventilating the infant with 100% oxygen.
       D. repeated suctioning of the mouth and nose.
       E. covering the infant with a dry receiving blanket.

_____ 387. Which of the following is considered a normal delivery?
       A. breech presentation
       B. occiput posterior
       C. prolapsed cord
       D. vertex position
       E. limb presentation

_____ 388. Management of breech presentation delivery includes all of the following EXCEPT:
       A. gently pulling on the infant's legs to facilitate delivery of the head.
       B. inserting a gloved hand into the vagina to allow for unrestricted respirations.
       C. placing the mother in supine position with legs flexed.
       D. supporting the infant's trunk.
       E. rotating the infant's body so that the shoulders are in anterior-posterior position.

_____ 389. The proper position for the expectant mother in the event of a limb presentation is:
       A. flat prone.
       B. prone in a knee to chest fashion.
       C. supine with legs flat and forced together.
       D. supine with legs flexed.
       E. the Trendelenburg position.

_____ 390. The most common cause of postpartum hemorrhage is:
       A. uterine atony.
       B. uterine hypertrophy.
       C. uterine inversion.
       D. uterine rupture.
       E. uterine abscess.

WORKBOOK ANSWER KEY

Note: Throughout Answer Key, textbook page references are shown in italic.

CHAPTER 1: Pulmonology

Part 1

CONTENT SELF-EVALUATION

MULTIPLE CHOICE

1. C	*p. 5*	13. E	*p. 22*	25. D	*p. 26*
2. D	*p. 5*	14. B	*p. 22*	26. D	*p. 29*
3. E	*p. 8*	15. A	*p. 22*	27. D	*p. 28*
4. E	*p. 9*	16. C	*p. 24*	28. B	*p. 29*
5. A	*p. 11*	17. B	*p. 24*	29. E	*p. 30*
6. A	*p. 11*	18. A	*p. 24*	30. B	*p. 30*
7. D	*p. 16*	19. B	*p. 25*	31. E	*p. 31*
8. E	*p. 17*	20. A	*p. 25*	32. D	*p. 31*
9. C	*p. 19*	21. C	*p. 26*	33. C	*p. 31*
10. D	*p. 20*	22. A	*p. 26*	34. A	*p. 31*
11. B	*p. 21*	23. A	*p. 26*	35. C	*p. 33*
12. B	*p. 21*	24. E	*p. 26*		

LABEL THE DIAGRAMS

p. 6

36. J	39. C	42. B	45. I	48. O
37. H	40. E	43. A	46. M	49. K
38. G	41. F	44. D	47. N	50. L

p. 9

51. B	52. E	53. D	54. C	55. A

SPECIAL PROJECT: Evaluating Abnormal Breathing Patterns
pp. 19–21

A. Apneustic respirations
B. Cheyne-Stokes respirations
C. Central neurogenic hyperventilation
D. Kussmaul's respirations
E. Ataxic (Biot's) respirations

Suggested Responses to Scenarios

Scenario 1: *Breathing pattern:* Cheyne-Stokes; *Probable cause:* terminal illness

Scenario 2: *Breathing pattern:* Ataxic (Biot's); *Probable cause:* hemorrhagic stroke. (The ataxic breathing is a clue that the stroke is hemorrhagic rather than obstructive because ataxic breathing typically results from a build-up of intracranial pressure as would be caused by bleeding into the brain.) Other possibilities include intracranial bleeding caused by a blow to the head when the patient fell. A brain infection or tumor could also cause increased intracranial pressure and ataxic breathing, but the sudden onset and severe headache are more indicative of a stroke.

Scenario 3: *Breathing pattern:* Kussmaul's; *Probable cause:* diabetic ketoacidosis (A variety of medical emergencies can result from diabetes. The clue to acidosis is the deep, rapid breathing, which is a compensatory mechanism that rids the body of excess CO_2 to alleviate the acidic condition. The cause in this case is that the patient has not been taking her insulin. Insulin is

necessary to help glucose enter the body cells. When insulin is absent, the cells turn to metabolism of fats instead of the normal glucose metabolism. A by-product of fat metabolism is ketones, which result in acidosis.)

CHAPTER 1: Pulmonology

Part 2

CONTENT SELF-EVALUATION

MULTIPLE CHOICE

1. E	*pp. 42, 43*	14. A	*p. 54*
2. C	*pp. 36, 37*	15. B	*p. 54*
3. A	*p. 39*	16. A	*pp. 54, 55*
4. A	*p. 40*	17. A	*p. 55*
5. B	*p. 42*	18. D	*p. 55*
6. B	*p. 43*	19. C	*p. 56*
7. B	*p. 44*	20. A	*p. 57*
8. D	*p. 45*	21. A	*p. 58*
9. D	*p. 45*	22. A	*p. 59*
10. B	*p. 49*	23. C	*p. 55*
11. B	*p. 50*	24. B	*p. 53*
12. A	*p. 49*	25. D	*p. 50*
13. B	*p. 52*		

MATCHING

26. C	*p. 38*	30. G	*p. 52*
27. F	*p. 42*	31. B	*p. 53*
28. A	*p. 45*	32. D	*pp. 55, 56*
29. E	*p. 48*		

SPECIAL PROJECT: Assessing Respiratory Emergencies

pp. 22–60
Scenario 1: *Probable cause:* asthma
Scenario 2: *Probable cause:* pneumonia; *Underlying probable cause:* emphysema (COPD)
Scenario 3: *Probable cause:* pulmonary embolism

CHAPTER 2: Cardiology

Part 1

CONTENT SELF-EVALUATION

MULTIPLE CHOICE

1. C	*p. 71*	11. A	*pp. 127, 129*
2. A	*p. 75*	12. E	*p. 131*
3. D	*pp. 79, 80*	13. A	*p. 131*
4. A	*p. 80*	14. C	*pp. 132, 133*
5. B	*p. 84*	15. D	*p. 133*
6. B	*p. 93*	16. B	*pp. 140, 141*
7. E	*pp. 97, 98*	17. E	*p. 145*
8. C	*p. 101*	18. C	*p. 143*
9. D	*p. 111*	19. D	*p. 149*
10. B	*p. 125*	20. A	*p. 151*

MATCHING

LABEL THE DIAGRAMS

Figure 1 *p. 72*   **Figure 2** *p. 83*

43. D	47. F	49. C	53. E
44. A	48. E	50. D	54. B
45. B		51. F	55. A
46. C		52. G	

Figure 3 *p. 89*

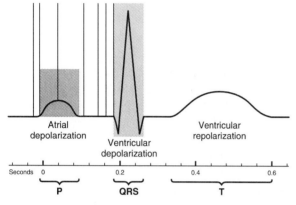

FILL-IN-THE-BLANKS

56. atrioventricular, semilunar *p. 73 (order must be exact for this question)*
57. excitability, conductivity, automaticity, contractility *p. 83 (any order)*
58. Lead II *p. 86*
59. 25 mm/sec (25 millimeters per second) *p. 87*
60. two (2) *p. 87*
61. 0.04 sec, 0.20 sec *p. 87 (order must be exact for this question)*
62. 3.0 sec *p. 88*
63. hypokalemia *p. 157*

SPECIAL PROJECT: ECG Interpretation

pp. 84–157

ECG #1
Rate: roughly 150 bpm
Rhythm: regular
P waves: always present, upright, normal shape
P-R interval: approx. 0.10–0.12 sec
QRS complexes: normal appearance, approx. 0.08–0.10 second
Overall rhythm (or Dysrhythmia): Sinus tachycardia

ECG #2
Rate: roughly 100 bpm
Rhythm: irregularly irregular
P waves: none detected: fibrillation (f) waves are visible
P-R interval: none (because of absence of P waves)

QRS complexes: normal appearance, approx. 0.10–0.12 sec
Overall rhythm (or Dysrhythmia): Atrial fibrillation

ECG #3
Rate: roughly 90 bpm
Rhythm: ventricular rhythm is roughly regularly irregular
P waves: normal in appearance, two are not followed by a QRS complex
P-R interval: widens over five beats, then comes apparent missed beat
QRS complexes: inverted, approx. 0.10 sec
Overall rhythm (or Dysrhythmia): Type I second-degree AV block

ECG #4
Rate: roughly 60 bpm or less
Rhythm: slow, roughly regular except for premature beat (last shown on strip)
P waves: normal in appearance, precede all but last beat on strip
QRS complexes: abnormal shape, S-T segment abnormal and lengthened, T waves peaked, somewhat tall?
Overall rhythm (or dysrhythmia): Sinus bradycardia, one premature ventricular contraction (PVC). Possible hyperkalemia?

ECG #5
Rate: impossible to determine
Rhythm: irregular, disorganized rhythm
P waves: not clearly discernible
QRS complexes: not discernible
Overall rhythm (or dysrhythmia): ventricular fibrillation

CHAPTER 2: Cardiology

Part 2

CONTENT SELF-EVALUATION

MULTIPLE CHOICE

MATCHING

FILL-IN-THE-BLANKS

37. transmural *p. 196*
38. dysrhythmias *p. 197*
39. 6 hours *p. 199*
40. pulmonary edema *p. 202*
41. Labored breathing *p. 205*
42. 1 hour *p. 212*
43. pallor, pain, pulselessness, paralysis, paresthesias *p. 220*
44. greater *p. 204*
45. nitroglycerin *p. 178*

CHAPTER 2: Cardiology

Part 3

CONTENT SELF-EVALUATION

MULTIPLE CHOICE

1.	A	*p. 223*	5.	C	*p. 229*
2.	B	*p. 223*	6.	D	*p. 229*
3.	A	*p. 223*	7.	C	*p. 234*
4.	D	*p. 224*	8.	E	*p. 255*

MATCHING

9.	C	*pp. 226, 227*	18.	E	*p. 238*
10.	A	*p. 226*	19.	C	*pp. 245, 246*
11.	B	*p. 228*	20.	A	*p. 247*
12.	A	*p. 238*	21.	D	*p. 248*
13.	G	*p. 238*	22.	G	*p. 249*
14.	F	*p. 238*	23.	E	*p. 250*
15.	C	*p. 238*	24.	B	*p. 250*
16.	B	*p. 238*	25.	F	*p. 250*
17.	D	*p. 238*			

SPECIAL PROJECT: Interpreting an ECG

pp. 80–258

1. The QRS complexes are widened and have a notched appearance that is readily apparent in Leads I, II, aVL, V_5, III, aVF, and V_6. In addition, there are deep S waves in Leads V_1, V_2, and V_3 and relatively tall R waves in Leads I, aVL, V_5, and V_6. This strongly suggests left bundle branch block.

2. The tracing shows significant S-T segment depression and inverted T waves in Leads aVL, V_5, and V_6, which suggests myocardial ischemia in the anterolateral part of the heart. However, you know that left bundle branch block can produce these changes in the absence of any ischemia, so the ECG is not useful in detecting or localizing ischemia or an acute MI.

   NOTE: Although the ECG is not useful in this instance, the presence of left bundle branch block in no way negates the possibility of myocardial ischemia or infarction in the patient, and you should treat and transport accordingly.

   You should give the tracing to the emergency team when you deliver Mr. Benon so they can compare the tracing with previous ECGs and any ECGs that may be taken while he is at the hospital.

CHAPTER 3: Neurology

CONTENT SELF-EVALUATION

MULTIPLE CHOICE

1.	A	*p. 271*	7.	C	*p. 293*
2.	C	*pp. 275–276*	8.	B	*pp. 295, 298*
3.	B	*p. 276*	9.	B	*p. 298*
4.	E	*p. 285*	10.	A	*p. 299*
5.	C	*p. 288*	11.	C	*p. 300*
6.	A	*pp. 292–293*	12.	E	*p. 308*

FILL-IN-THE-BLANKS

13. heart rate, bronchioles, pupils *p. 263*
14. temporal, cerebrum *p. 269*
15. involuntary *p. 263*
16. smooth, cardiac *p. 263*
17. thalamus, hypothalamus, limbic *p. 268*
18. dendrites *p. 264*
19. somatic nervous system, autonomic nervous system *p. 263*
20. central nervous system, peripheral nervous system *p. 263*
21. meninges *p. 265*
22. axon *p. 264*
23. heart rate, bronchioles, pupils *p. 263*
24. mesencephalon, pons, medulla oblongata *p. 269*
25. cerebrospinal fluid (CSF) *p. 265*
26. consciousness, stimuli *p. 269*
27. occipital, cerebrum *p. 269*
28. frontal, cerebrum *p. 269*
29. voluntary, conscious *p. 263*
30. synapse, neurotransmitter *p. 264*
31. brain, spinal cord *p. 263*

LABEL THE DIAGRAM

p. 268

32. Thalamus, H
33. Hypothalamus, E
34. Pituitary gland, G
35. Midbrain, B
36. Pons, D
37. Medulla Oblongata, C
38. Cerebrum, F
39. Cerebellum, A

MATCHING

40. B, G *p. 281 (and Objective 9)*
41. E, H *p. 282*
42. A, D *p. 282*
43. C, I *p. 282*
44. F, J *p. 282*
45. A, D *p. 290*
46. C, E *p. 291*
47. C, F *p. 290*
48. B, C *p. 291*

LISTING

49. A, alert and oriented to surroundings; V, responsive to verbal stimuli; P, responsive to painful stimuli; U, unresponsive to all
50. M, mood; T, thought processes; P, perception of surroundings; J, judgment in context of situation; MA, memory and attention *pp. 278, 279*
51. increased blood pressure, decreased pulse, decreased respirations, increased temperature *p. 285*

52. A, acidosis or alcohol; E, epilepsy; I, infection; O, overdose; U, uremia; T, trauma, toxin, or tumor; I, insulin (either hypoglycemia or ketoacidosis); P, psychosis or poison; S, stroke or seizure *pp. 287–288*
53. Thrombotic, embolic *p. 290*
54. Intracerebral, subarachnoid *p. 291*
55. tremor, rigidity, bradykinesia, postural instability *p. 305*
56. occulta, meningocele, myelomeningocele *p. 306* (*order DOES matter for this question*)
57. migraine, cluster *p. 300*

SPECIAL PROJECT: Distinguishing Different Conditions in the Field

Scenario 1 *p. 285*

Vital Signs	Shock	Increased ICP
Blood pressure	Decreased	Increased
Pulse	Increased	Decreased
Respirations	Increased	Decreased
Level of Consciousness	Decreased	Decreased

Scenario 2 *p. 297*

Trait	Syncope	Tonic-Clonic Seizure
Starting position	Usually begins in standing position	May begin in any position
Warning?	Patient usually remembers warning of fainting	May or may not have warning; may be preceded by aura
Jerking motions?	Jerking motions usually not present	Jerking motions present while unconscious
Return of consciousness	Consciousness returns almost immediately on becoming supine	Patient unconscious during seizure and drowsy during postictal period

CHAPTER 4: Endocrinology

CONTENT SELF-EVALUATION

MULTIPLE CHOICE

1. C *p. 315*	11. E *p. 323*	21. E *p. 331*
2. C *p. 315*	12. C *p. 327*	22. A *p. 331*
3. B *p. 317*	13. B *p. 323*	23. C *p. 333*
4. B *p. 320*	14. C *p. 324*	24. E *p. 333*
5. A *p. 320*	15. A *p. 324*	25. A *p. 333*
6. B *p. 320*	16. A *p. 324*	26. B *p. 338*
7. B *p. 322*	17. A *p. 325*	27. A *p. 338*
8. D *p. 323*	18. E *p. 326*	28. E *p. 339*
9. B *p. 323*	19. B *p. 329*	29. A *p. 340*
10. B *p. 323*	20. D *p. 331*	30. B *p. 341*

MATCHING

31. J *p. 341*	35. G *p. 322*	39. B *p. 315*
32. C *p. 327*	36. D *p. 327*	40. A *p. 315*
33. E *p. 320*	37. F *p. 320*	
34. H *p. 323*	38. I *p. 323*	

SPECIAL PROJECT: Label the Diagram

pp. 316, 318–319

A. pineal gland: melatonin
B. hypothalamus: growth hormone releasing hormone, growth hormone inhibiting hormone, corticotropin releasing hormone, thyrotropin releasing hormone, gonadotropin releasing hormone, prolactin releasing hormone, prolactin inhibiting hormone
C. pituitary gland: antidiuretic hormone, oxytocin, growth hormone, adrenocorticotropic hormone, thyroid-stimulating hormone, follicle-stimulating hormone, luteinizing hormone, prolactin
D. thyroid gland: thyroxine, triiodothyronine, calcitonin
E. parathyroid gland: parathyroid hormone
F. thymus: thymosin
G. pancreas: glucagon, insulin, somatostatin
H. adrenal glands: epinephrine, norepinephrine, glucocorticoids (cortisol), mineralocorticoids (aldosterone), androgenic hormones (estrogen, progesterone, testosterone)
I. gonads (ovaries): estrogen, progesterone, (testosterone from testes)

CHAPTER 5: Allergies and Anaphylaxis

CONTENT SELF-EVALUATION

MULTIPLE CHOICE

1. B *p. 347*	6. A *p. 346*	11. A *p. 353*
2. D *p. 347*	7. C *p. 350*	12. B *p. 353*
3. B *p. 347*	8. C *p. 350*	13. C *p. 354*
4. C *p. 348*	9. C *p. 350*	14. D *p. 354*
5. D *p. 348*	10. B *p. 351*	15. D *p. 354*

MATCHING

16. E *p. 355*	19. B *p. 354*
17. C *p. 355*	20. A *p. 355*
18. D *p. 355*	

SPECIAL PROJECT: Completing Tables

Part A *p. 352*
Skin: flushing, itching, hives, swelling, cyanosis
Respiratory: respiratory difficulty, sneezing, coughing, wheezing, stridor, laryngeal edema, laryngospasm, bronchospasm
Cardiovascular: vasodilation, increased heart rate, decreased blood pressure
Gastrointestinal: nausea and vomiting, abdominal cramping, diarrhea
Nervous system: dizziness, headache, convulsions, tearing

Part B *pp. 354–355*
Albuterol: beta agonist, reverses bronchospasm and laryngeal edema
Diphenhydramine: blocks histamine receptors
Dopamine: potent vasopressor to support blood pressure (vasoconstrictors)
Epinephrine: sympathetic agonist that increases heart rate, increases cardiac contractile force, increases peripheral vasoconstriction, and reverses much of the capillary permeability caused by histamine
Methylprednisolone: suppresses the inflammatory response

CHAPTER 6: Gastroenterology

CONTENT SELF-EVALUATION

MULTIPLE CHOICE

1.	D	*p. 363*	15.	B	*p. 388*
2.	A	*p. 363*	16.	C	*p. 363*
3.	B	*p. 367*	17.	E	*p. 364*
4.	E	*p. 368*	18.	A	*p. 363*
5.	A	*pp. 368, 369*	19.	B	*p. 363*
6.	C	*p. 369*	20.	A	*p. 364*
7.	D	*p. 369*	21.	E	*p. 364*
8.	B	*pp. 369, 373*	22.	A	*pp. 363, 364*
9.	A	*pp. 372, 373*	23.	D	*p. 366*
10.	E	*pp. 374, 389*	24.	D	*p. 389*
11.	B	*pp. 374, 387*	25.	A	*p. 388*
12.	A	*p. 378*	26.	B	*p. 381*
13.	C	*pp. 377, 381*	27.	C	*p. 388*
14.	D	*p. 382*			

FILL-IN-THE-BLANKS

28. Symptoms; Allergies; Medications; Past medical history; Last oral intake; Events *p. 365*
29. Six hours *p. 368*
30. ligament of Treitz *p. 369*

SPECIAL PROJECT: History Taking

Question types (in sequence) are Severity, Associated Symptoms, Time, Quality, Region, Onset, Provocation/Palliation, Pertinent Negatives *pp. 365–366*

Probable field diagnosis: Appendicitis (probably ruptured, with peritonitis) *pp. 385, 386*

CHAPTER 7: Urology and Nephrology

CONTENT SELF-EVALUATION

MULTIPLE CHOICE

1.	B	*p. 395*	9.	A	*p. 409*
2.	A	*p. 401*	10.	C	*p. 413*
3.	D	*p. 402*	11.	D	*p. 415*
4.	B	*p. 402*	12.	A	*p. 414*
5.	C	*p. 403*	13.	E	*p. 420*
6.	E	*pp. 405–406*	14.	B	*p. 420*
7.	B	*p. 407*	15.	C	*p. 421*
8.	A	*p. 409*			

MATCHING

16.	A	*p. 395*	19.	C	*p. 410*	22.	D	*p. 422*
17.	B	*p. 395*	20.	A	*p. 410*	23.	A	*p. 421*
18.	B	*p. 410*	21.	C	*p. 421*	24.	B	*p. 422*

FILL-IN-THE-BLANKS

25. proximal tubule, descending loop of Henle, ascending loop of Henle, distal tubule *p. 398*
26. Bowman's capsule, filtrate *p. 398*
27. water, sodium and chloride ions *p. 400*
28. secretion *p. 398*
29. Onset, Provocation/Palliation, Quality, Region, Severity, Time *p. 405*
30. semipermeable membrane, dialysate *p. 417*
31. semipermeable membrane *p. 418*
32. artificial graft connecting an artery and vein, arteriovenous fistula *p. 417*
33. Infection *pp. 417, 418*

LABEL THE DIAGRAMS

pp. 396, 397

34.	D	38.	D	42.	G
35.	C	39.	A	43.	E
36.	B	40.	C	44.	F
37.	A	41.	B		

SPECIAL PROJECT: Making a Call

1. The external portion of the indwelling catheter is visible above the skin. Beneath the skin, the catheter tunnels through the abdominal wall and into the peritoneal cavity. *p. 418*
2. infection *p. 418*
3. The skin and subcutaneous tissues, the muscle of the abdominal wall, and the peritoneal membrane itself. Peritonitis is unlikely given history of pain, so infection probably has not spread as far as the peritoneal membrane. *p. 418*
4. You already know that the patient has had either vascular (shift in blood pressure?) or neurologic (because of change in chemical milieu for the brain) complications because of the fainting episode. You should be prepared for rapid evolution of physiologic instability (as in all patients with chronic renal failure/end-stage renal failure), with treatment during transport including close monitoring and support of ABCs with high-flow oxygen, constant monitoring of ECG, establishment of IV access. The risks/benefits of peritoneal lavage may be discussed with medical direction. Talking quietly with patient helps to monitor mental status. Monitoring of BP may pick up development of hypotension. *pp. 416, 418*

CHAPTER 8: Toxicology and Substance Abuse

CONTENT SELF-EVALUATION

MULTIPLE CHOICE

1.	C	*p. 429*	15.	A	*p. 441*
2.	A	*p. 430*	16.	B	*pp. 442–443*
3.	D	*pp. 430–431*	17.	A	*p. 443*
4.	B	*p. 431*	18.	C	*pp. 445, 447*
5.	A	*p. 432*	19.	E	*pp. 448–449*
6.	B	*p. 430*	20.	A	*p. 446*
7.	E	*p. 432*	21.	B	*p. 447*
8.	B	*p. 433*	22.	D	*pp. 450–451*
9.	B	*p. 434*	23.	E	*p. 446*
10.	C	*p. 435*	24.	A	*p. 452*
11.	A	*p. 435*	25.	A	*p. 454*
12.	D	*p. 436*	26.	C	*pp. 462–463*
13.	B	*pp. 437–438*	27.	B	*p. 467*
14.	E	*p. 439*			

MATCHING

28.	B	*p. 431*	34.	G	*p. 445*	40.	K	*p. 462*
29.	H	*p. 461*	35.	P	*p. 430*	41.	D	*p. 464*
30.	N	*p. 428*	36.	F	*p. 467*	42.	C	*p. 462*
31.	M	*p. 430*	37.	L	*p. 451*	43.	E	*p. 461*
32.	A	*p. 428*	38.	I	*p. 432*			
33.	O	*p. 461*	39.	J	*p. 431*			

44. ingestion, inhalation, surface absorption, injection
    p. 430
45. organophosphates *p. 437*

SPECIAL PROJECT: Analyzing an Emergency Scene

pp. 429–468

1. This probably represents an accidental ingestion overdose involving multiple medications of unknown type(s). This is not an uncommon call; you will see this kind of situation.
2. As in all other cases involving a potentially unstable patient, the first priority is support of the ABCs: After checking that the airway is clear, high-flow oxygen should be started and attention paid on an ongoing basis that the airway remains clear (suspect possible vomiting and aspiration; intubate if necessary). Ventilation does not appear to need support at the moment, but you are aware that ventilation can decompensate quickly. Circulation clearly is impaired based on the peripheral pulses. Prepare for ECG monitoring and for pulse oximetry. If it looks like IV access can be established easily, it may be done at this point.
3. Transport of this unstable, elderly man with unclear toxic ingestion and underlying medical conditions is the first priority. Contact with Medical Control can be made en route as the focused physical is done and evaluation of vitals and patient condition continues. Poison Control is not useful until you have some idea of the medications involved in the ingestion.
4. Take the pill case. If there are any empty or partially full glasses/cups around, check for signs of alcohol or coffee or tea (which might contain caffeine). Look for opened bottles of over-the-counter medications such as aspirin. If one team partner has time while en route, he/she can inspect the medications to see if any are definitively recognizable.

CHAPTER 9: Hematology

CONTENT SELF-EVALUATION

MULTIPLE CHOICE

1. C	*p. 473*	8. B	*p. 479*	15. D	*p. 488*
2. B	*p. 473*	9. A	*p. 479*	16. E	*p. 489*
3. C	*p. 474*	10. B	*p. 480*	17. A	*p. 490*
4. A	*p. 474*	11. E	*p. 480*	18. C	*p. 494*
5. D	*p. 475*	12. D	*p. 481*	19. E	*p. 496*
6. A	*p. 476*	13. B	*p. 484*	20. D	*p. 497*
7. E	*p. 478*	14. C	*p. 476*		

MATCHING

21. C	*p. 476*	26. G	*p. 493*	31. B	*p. 477*
22. J	*p. 483*	27. I	*p. 489*	32. H	*p. 482*
23. L	*p. 484*	28. E	*p. 492*	33. M	*p. 497*
24. N	*p. 488*	29. A	*p. 473*	34. O	*p. 499*
25. D	*p. 492*	30. K	*p. 495*	35. F	*p. 481*

SPECIAL PROJECT: Completing a Table

pp. 492–499

Hematological Disorder	Common Signs and Symptoms	Prehospital Management
Anemia	dyspnea, tachycardia, fatigue, syncope, diaphoresis, pallor, hypotension	oxygen control bleeding volume replacement expedite transport
Hemophilia	bleeding	oxygen control bleeding volume replacement analgesia expedite transport
Leukemia	bleeding, fever, weakness, anorexia, weight loss, abdominal pain, fatigue	oxygen control bleeding volume replacement analgesia expedite transport
Lymphoma	fatigue, night sweats, anorexia and weight loss, pruritis	oxygen control bleeding volume replacement analgesia expedite transport
Sickle Cell Anemia	abdominal or joint pain, pulmonary problems, renal infarction, priapism	oxygen control bleeding volume replacement analgesia expedite transport

CHAPTER 10: Environmental Emergencies

CONTENT SELF-EVALUATION

MULTIPLE CHOICE

1. C	*p. 505*	11. E	*p. 524*
2. A	*p. 505*	12. B	*p. 526*
3. E	*pp. 506–507*	13. D	*pp. 527–528*
4. B	*p. 510*	14. C	*p. 529*
5. B	*p. 511*	15. C	*p. 528*
6. A	*p. 515*	16. B	*p. 528*
7. B	*p. 516*	17. E	*p. 535*
8. D	*p. 517*	18. D	*p. 535*
9. A	*p. 520*	19. C	*p. 539*
10. C	*pp. 520, 522*	20. B	*p. 542*

MATCHING

21. F	*p. 508*	35. J	*p. 512*
22. A	*p. 507*	36. D	*p. 524*
23. H	*p. 511*	37. E	*p. 539*
24. G	*p. 506*	38. K	*p. 520*
25. B	*p. 507*	39. G	*p. 538*
26. D	*p. 508*	40. I	*p. 512*
27. C	*p. 508*	41. F	*p. 534*
28. E	*p. 510*	42. H	*p. 535*
29. E	*p. 509*	43. A	*p. 512*
30. B	*p. 509*	44. C	*pp. 532–533*
31. A	*p. 509*	45. B	*pp. 538–539*
32. F	*p. 509*	46. A	*p. 511*
33. C	*p. 509*	47. C	*pp. 536–537*
34. D	*p. 509*	48. B	*p. 518*

Listing

49. Work-induced thermogenesis, thermoregulatory thermogenesis, diet-induced thermogenesis *p. 506*

50. Sweating, vasodilation *p. 508*
51. Shivering, vasoconstriction *p. 508*

CHAPTER 11: Infectious Disease

CONTENT SELF-EVALUATION

MULTIPLE CHOICE

1.	B	*p. 551*	16.	C	*p. 565*
2.	E	*p. 554*	17.	E	*p. 568*
3.	B	*p. 550*	18.	D	*p. 575*
4.	C	*p. 553*	19.	A	*p. 572*
5.	D	*p. 555*	20.	A	*p. 574*
6.	A	*p. 556*	21.	B	*p. 576*
7.	E	*pp. 556–557*	22.	D	*p. 580*
8.	C	*p. 557*	23.	C	*p. 581*
9.	B	*p. 557*	24.	D	*p. 583*
10.	E	*p. 558*	25.	E	*p. 601*
11.	A	*p. 558*	26.	A	*p. 584*
12.	D	*p. 559*	27.	E	*p. 584*
13.	C	*p. 559*	28.	B	*p. 591*
14.	B	*p. 560*	29.	A	*p. 592*
15.	B	*p. 567*	30.	C	*pp. 596–598*

SPECIAL PROJECT: Decontamination Procedures

pp. 566–567

Low-level disinfection
Agent: EPA-registered disinfectant
Indication: routine housekeeping/cleaning and removing visible body fluids
Effectiveness: destroys most bacteria and some viruses and fungi

Intermediate-level disinfection
Agent: 1:10 to 1:100 dilution of water and chlorine bleach, hard surface germicide, EPA-registered disinfectant/chemical germicide
Indication: all equipment that has been in contact with intact skin
Effectiveness: destroys *Mycobacterium tuberculosis*, most viruses, fungi

High-level disinfection
Agent: EPA-approved chemical sterilizing agent, hot water (176–212°F) immersion
Indication: reusable devices that have been in contact with mucous membranes
Effectiveness: destroys all forms of microorganisms except certain bacterial spores

Sterilization
Agent: autoclave (pressurized steam or ethylene-oxide gas), EPA-approved chemical sterilizing agent (prolonged immersion)
Indication: contaminated invasive instruments
Effectiveness: destroys all microorganisms

CHAPTER 12: Psychiatric and Behavioral Disorders

CONTENT SELF-EVALUATION

MULTIPLE CHOICE

1.	B	*p. 609*	6.	D	*p. 613*	11.	C	*p. 615*
2.	B	*p. 609*	7.	E	*p. 616*	12.	A	*p. 615*
3.	C	*p. 611*	8.	C	*p. 618*	13.	A	*p. 620*
4.	C	*p. 612*	9.	C	*p. 618*	14.	B	*p. 628*
5.	B	*p. 613*	10.	A	*p. 614*	15.	B	*p. 631*

MATCHING

16.	J	*p. 621*	20.	E	*p. 615*	24.	G	*p. 616*
17.	A	*p. 615*	21.	H	*p. 619*	25.	B	*p. 615*
18.	D	*p. 615*	22.	F	*p. 615*			
19.	I	*p. 622*	23.	C	*p. 615*			

SPECIAL PROJECT: Crossword Puzzle

CHAPTER 13: Gynecology

CONTENT SELF-EVALUATION

MULTIPLE CHOICE

1.	C	*p. 641*	6.	B	*p. 644*	11.	B	*p. 649*
2.	B	*p. 642*	7.	C	*p. 646*	12.	D	*p. 648*
3.	D	*p. 642*	8.	A	*p. 647*	13.	C	*p. 648*
4.	B	*p. 643*	9.	E	*p. 648*	14.	B	*p. 649*
5.	D	*p. 643*	10.	B	*p. 648*	15.	A	*p. 651*

LABELING THE DIAGRAM

pp. 638–639

A. Ovary
B. Fallopian tube
C. Uterus
D. Cervix
E. Vagina

SPECIAL PROJECT: Problem Solving—Abdominal Pain

pp. 643–649

1. Focused history elements:
   • SAMPLE and OPQRST
   • obstetric history: gravida, parity, abortion
   • gynecologic history: past ectopic pregnancies, surgical procedures
   • history of trauma
   • last menstrual period (LMP)
   • form of birth control and regularity of use
2. Differential diagnosis possibilities:
   • PID
   • Ruptured ovarian cyst
   • Endometritis
   • Ectopic pregnancy

CHAPTER 14: Obstetrics

CONTENT SELF-EVALUATION

MULTIPLE CHOICE

1.	B	p. 657	14.	E	p. 676
2.	D	p. 657	15.	C	p. 680
3.	E	p. 661	16.	B	p. 680
4.	D	p. 659	17.	B	p. 695
5.	A	p. 663	18.	C	p. 694
6.	C	p. 663	19.	C	pp. 689–692
7.	E	p. 664	20.	A	p. 679
8.	C	p. 675	21.	A	p. 687
9.	B	p. 669	22.	B	p. 687
10.	A	p. 671	23.	B	pp. 688–689
11.	A	pp. 670–671	24.	C	p. 694
12.	C	p. 671	25.	D	pp. 695–696
13.	B	pp. 674–675			

MATCHING

26.	D	p. 658	31.	G	p. 678
27.	E	p. 656	32.	J	p. 678
28.	A	p. 661	33.	H	p. 664
29.	C	p. 657	34.	I	p. 679
30.	B	p. 658	35.	F	p. 679

SPECIAL PROJECT: Understanding the Physiologic Changes of Pregnancy

pp. 656–661

Reproductive system
Physiologic changes:
- Increased vascularity—1/6 of total blood volume
- Increased uterine size and capacity—can cause supine hypotensive syndrome and compress vena cava
- Mucus plug blocks cervix to protect fetus
- Mammary glands increase in size and number

EMS implications:
- Fetal well-being dependent on maternal well-being
- Position mother tilted slightly to the left to minimize hypotension

Respiratory system
Physiologic changes:
- Increased oxygen demand
- Progesterone causes decrease in airway resistance
- Slight increase in respiratory rate
- Rib margins flare to accommodate diaphragmatic elevation due to increased fundal height

EMS implications:
- Maintain airway
- Administer high-flow, high-concentration oxygen as needed

Cardiovascular system
Physiologic changes:
- Increased cardiac output
- Maternal blood volume increases (slightly more plasma than red blood cells, causing relative anemia)
- Maternal heart rate increases 10–15 beats/minute
- Blood pressure initially decreases in first trimester, then rises to near normal during third trimester
- Supine hypotensive syndrome due to weight of gravid uterus compressing the inferior vena cava and impaired venous return

EMS implications:
- Vital signs should be assessed with patient lying on her left side
- May suffer significant blood loss without significant change in vital signs
- Syncope is relatively common in pregnancy
- Assess amount of reported vaginal bleeding based on number of sanitary pads used (two per hour is significant)
- Anticipate shock based on chief complaint or mechanism of injury
- Overt signs of shock are late and inconsistent
- Initiate vascular access with two large-bore IVs (crystalloid fluids)

Gastrointestinal system
Physiologic changes:
- Nausea and vomiting common in first trimester
- Changed carbohydrate needs
- Peristalsis slows, causing delayed gastric emptying
- Abdominal organs compressed and compartmentalized due to enlarged uterus

EMS implications:
- MD should evaluate all complaints of abdominal pain
- Assessment is difficult due to compression of organs by uterus, thus "classic signs" of abdominal pathology may be absent or altered
- Potential for regurgitation always present in pregnant patient

Urinary system
Physiologic changes:
- Renal blood flow increases, as does renal tubular absorption
- Glucosuria may result from kidney's inability to reabsorb glucose
- Urinary bladder is displaced anteriorly and superiorly
- Urinary frequency is common due to uterine compression

EMS implications:
- Glucosuria may indicate the development of gestational diabetes—check blood glucose for any altered mental status during pregnancy
- Displacement of bladder increases risk of traumatic rupture

Musculoskeletal system
Physiologic changes:
- Pelvic joints loosen to due hormonal influence
- Postural changes compensate for anterior uterine growth

EMS Implications:
- Due to loosened joints, pelvis may appear unstable on exam
- Anterior growth may increase incidence of falls due to changed center of gravity

MEDICAL EMERGENCIES: Content Review

CONTENT SELF-EVALUATION

CHAPTER 1: Pulmonology

1. D *p. 6*	18. C *p. 16*	35. C *p. 30*
2. A *p. 8*	19. A *p. 16*	36. D *p. 32*
3. E *p. 8*	20. C *p. 16*	37. B *p. 33*
4. A *p. 8*	21. A *p. 17*	38. A *p. 34*
5. B *p. 9*	22. A *p. 17*	39. A *p. 37*
6. E *p. 11*	23. A *p. 18*	40. D *p. 38*
7. C *p. 11*	24. B *p. 19*	41. C *p. 38*
8. C *p. 12*	25. E *p. 20*	42 A *p. 43*
9. C *p. 12*	26. C *p. 20*	43. C *p. 40*
10. E *p. 13*	27. B *p. 20*	44. B *p. 42*
11. B *p. 14*	28. C *p. 21*	45. A *p. 44*
12. B *p. 14*	29. D *p. 22*	46. B *p. 45*
13. D *p. 14*	30. D *p. 28*	47. A *p. 45*
14. B *p. 14*	31. A *p. 28*	48. A *p. 49*
15. C *p. 14*	32. C *p. 28*	49. A *p. 53*
16. C *p. 15*	33. D *p. 30*	50. A *p. 54*
17. B *p. 15*	34. E *p. 30*	

CHAPTER 2: Cardiology

51. C *p. 68*	65. B *p. 80*	79. B *p. 94*
52. A *p. 70*	66. D *p. 81*	80. B *p. 95*
53. B *p. 71*	67. C *p. 82*	81. D *p. 95*
54. A *p. 71*	68. C *p. 83*	82. C *p. 96*
55. A *p. 74*	69. D *p. 83*	83. A *p. 97*
56. C *p. 74*	70. C *p. 84*	84. A *p. 109*
57. D *p. 75*	71. D *p. 85*	85. D *p. 115*
58. D *p. 77*	72. A *p. 88*	86. C *p. 119*
59. A *p. 78*	73. C *p. 89*	87. C *p. 121*
60. C *p. 78*	74. B *p. 93*	88. A *p. 121*
61. E *p. 78*	75. E *p. 93*	89. E *p. 135*
62. B *p. 79*	76. C *p. 93*	90. D *p. 142*
63. D *p. 80*	77. D *p. 93*	91. C *p. 176*
64. E *p. 80*	78. A *p. 93*	92. D *p. 176*
93. C *p. 177*	96. D *p. 179*	99. B *p. 202*
94. C *p. 177*	97. D *p. 181*	100. C *p. 232*
95. C *p. 177*	98. E *p. 194*	

CHAPTER 3: Neurology

101. C *p. 263*	108. E *p. 268*	115. D *p. 287*
102. D *p. 263*	109. D *p. 269*	116. B *p. 289*
103. C *p. 263*	110. D *p. 269*	117. D *p. 290*
104. C *p. 265*	111. A *p. 273*	118. B *p. 295*
105. C *p. 268*	112. E *p. 274*	119. C *p. 296*
106. A *p. 268*	113. D *p. 274*	120. C *p. 305*
107. D *p. 268*	114. C *p. 280*	

CHAPTER 4: Endocrinology

121. C *p. 315*	128. D *p. 321*	135. C *p. 329*
122. A *p. 315*	129. B *p. 322*	136. E *p. 329*
123. D *p. 316*	130. B *p. 323*	137. A *p. 331*
124. A *p. 317*	131. B *p. 323*	138. A *p. 331*
125. C *p. 318*	132. E *p. 324*	139. B *p. 340*
126. B *p. 319*	133. C *p. 326*	140. A *p. 341*
127. A *p. 319*	134. C *p. 328*	

CHAPTER 5: Allergies and Anaphylaxis

141. C *p. 347*	149. C *p. 351*
142. B *p. 347*	150. D *p. 351*
143. B *pp. 347–348*	151. A *p. 351*
144. B *p. 348*	152. D *p. 353*
145. C *p. 349*	153. C *p. 355*
146. E *p. 349*	154. B *p. 355*
147. C *p. 351*	155. B *p. 357*
148. B *p. 351*	

CHAPTER 6: Gastroenterology

156. D *p. 363*	165. E *p. 369*	174. D *p. 385*
157. B *p. 363*	166. B *p. 369*	175. C *p. 386*
158. C *p. 363*	167. B *p. 369*	176. E *p. 386*
159. B *p. 366*	168. A *p. 372*	177. D *p. 387*
160. C *p. 366*	169. D *p. 373*	178. A *p. 388*
161. A *p. 367*	170. C *p. 373*	179. A *p. 389*
162. B *p. 368*	171. A *p. 375*	180. A *p. 389*
163. C *p. 369*	172. B *p. 376*	
164. D *p. 369*	173. C *p. 385*	

CHAPTER 7: Urology and Nephrology

181. C *p. 395*	190. A *p. 399*	199. B *p. 404*
182. D *p. 395*	191. E *p. 399*	200. A *p. 407*
183. D *p. 395*	192. C *p. 399*	201. E *p. 412*
184. D *p. 395*	193. C *p. 400*	202. C *p. 414*
185. D *p. 396*	194. A *p. 401*	203. C *p. 418*
186. C *p. 397*	195. C *p. 401*	204. C *p. 420*
187. B *p. 398*	196. D *p. 402*	205. A *p. 421*
188. A *p. 398*	197. D *p. 403*	
189. D *p. 399*	198. D *p. 404*	

CHAPTER 8: Toxicology and Substance Abuse

206. B *p. 430*	219. A *p. 447*
207. B *p. 434*	220. C *p. 448*
208. A *p. 437*	221. A *p. 448*
209. C *pp. 438–439*	222. C *p. 448*
210. A *p. 439*	223. B *p. 449*
211. A *p. 443*	224. A *p. 450*
212. E *p. 443*	225. C *p. 451*
213. A *p. 444*	226. A *p. 451*
214. E *p. 444*	227. E *p. 454*
215. D *p. 445*	228. C *p. 459*
216. A *pp. 445–446*	229. C *p. 459*
217. D *p. 446*	230. E *p. 462*
218. C *p. 446*	231. A *p. 463*
232. B *p. 464*	234. A *p. 465*
233. A *p. 465*	235. E *p. 465*

CHAPTER 9: Hematology

236. A *p. 473*	245. B *p. 478*	254. C *p. 490*
237. B *p. 473*	246. B *p. 479*	255. D *p. 490*
238. E *p. 473*	247. D *p. 479*	256. E *p. 491*
239. A *p. 474*	248. C *p. 481*	257. C *p. 493*
240. D *p. 475*	249. B *p. 481*	258. A *p. 497*
241. C *p. 476*	250. E *p. 482*	259. B *p. 497*
242. B *p. 476*	251. B *p. 484*	260. B *p. 499*
243. A *p. 477*	252. D *p. 484*	
244. D *p. 478*	253. A *p. 490*	

CHAPTER 10: Environmental Emergencies

261.	B	*p. 506*	276.	B	*p. 522*
262.	D	*p. 506*	277.	A	*p. 523*
263.	D	*p. 508*	278.	E	*p. 525*
264.	E	*p. 509*	279.	C	*p. 526*
265.	B	*p. 513*	280.	B	*p. 528*
266.	B	*p. 513*	281.	A	*p. 529*
267.	B	*p. 514*	282.	B	*p. 529*
268.	D	*p. 515*	283.	D	*p. 529*
269.	D	*p. 515*	284.	A	*p. 529*
270.	C	*p. 517*	285.	C	*p. 529*
271.	B	*p. 519*	286.	C	*p. 529*
272.	A	*p. 520*	287.	C	*p. 529*
273.	A	*p. 520*	288.	C	*p. 530*
274.	A	*p. 520*	289.	C	*p. 538*
275.	E	*pp. 521–522*	290.	C	*p. 540*

CHAPTER 11: Infectious Disease

291.	C	*p. 549*	311.	D	*p. 577*
292.	D	*p. 550*	312.	B	*pp. 578–579*
293.	D	*p. 552*	313.	B	*p. 580*
294.	D	*pp. 552–553*	314.	D	*p. 581*
295.	B	*p. 554*	315.	E	*p. 583*
296.	D	*p. 555*	316.	D	*p. 584*
297.	E	*p. 556*	317.	A	*p. 585*
298.	B	*p. 556*	318.	D	*p. 587*
299.	C	*p. 557*	319.	D	*p. 588*
300.	C	*p. 558*	320.	B	*p. 589*
301.	C	*p. 559*	321.	A	*p. 589*
302.	D	*p. 559*	322.	C	*p. 590*
303.	E	*p. 560*	323.	D	*pp. 592–593*
304.	A	*p. 566*	324.	D	*p. 594*
305.	C	*p. 567*	325.	C	*p. 596*
306.	A	*p. 572*	326.	C	*p. 597*
307.	B	*p. 572*	327.	D	*p. 598*
308.	A	*p. 574*	328.	B	*p. 600*
309.	A	*p. 575*	329.	A	*p. 600*
310.	D	*p. 576*	330.	C	*p. 601*

CHAPTER 12: Psychiatric and Behavioral Disorders

331.	C	*p. 608*	341.	B	*p. 617*
332.	B	*p. 610*	342.	D	*p. 620*
333.	A	*p. 610*	343.	B	*p. 621*
334.	E	*p. 611*	344.	C	*p. 621*
335.	D	*p. 611*	345.	B	*p. 621*
336.	A	*p. 615*	346.	B	*p. 622*
337.	B	*p. 615*	347.	B	*p. 623*
338.	D	*p. 615*	348.	E	*p. 623*
339.	B	*p. 616*	349.	C	*p. 625*
340.	B	*p. 617*	350.	B	*pp. 628–629*

CHAPTER 13: Gynecology

351.	B	*p. 637*	361.	C	*p. 644*
352.	C	*p. 639*	362.	A	*p. 644*
353.	B	*p. 640*	363.	E	*p. 644*
354.	E	*p. 641*	364.	C	*p. 647*
355.	A	*p. 641*	365.	B	*p. 648*
356.	B	*p. 641*	366.	E	*p. 648*
357.	A	*p. 641*	367.	B	*p. 648*
358.	C	*p. 642*	368.	B	*p. 648*
359.	D	*p. 642*	369.	A	*p. 650*
360.	D	*p. 643*	370.	D	*p. 651*

CHAPTER 14: Obstetrics

371.	B	*p. 657*	381.	E	*p. 677*
372.	C	*p. 659*	382.	A	*p. 678*
373.	B	*p. 661*	383.	A	*p. 679*
374.	D	*p. 661*	384.	B	*p. 680*
375.	D	*p. 661*	385.	D	*p. 683*
376.	C	*p. 663*	386.	C	*p. 687*
377.	B	*p. 663*	387.	D	*p. 689*
378.	E	*p. 669*	388.	A	*p. 690*
379.	C	*p. 670*	389.	B	*p. 692*
380.	C	*p. 675*	390.	A	*pp. 694–695*

National Registry of Emergency Medical Technicians

PRACTICAL EVALUATION FORMS

The forms on the next pages are provided to help you identify common criteria by which you will be evaluated. It may be valuable to review your practical skills by using these sheets during your class practice sessions and as you review those skills before class, state, and any national testing. Evaluation forms will vary; however, many of the important elements of paramedic practice are common to all forms.

EMT-PARAMEDIC FORMS

The following skill instruments for the EMT-Paramedic level were developed by the National Registry of EMTs and have been approved for use in advanced level National Registry examinations.

- Bleeding Control/Shock Management
- Dual Lumen Airway Device
- Dynamic Cardiology
- Intravenous Therapy
- Oral Station
- Patient Assessment—Medical
- Patient Assessment—Trauma
- Pediatric Intraosseous Infusion
- Pediatric (less than 2 years) Ventilatory Management
- Spinal Immobilization (Seated Patient)
- Spinal Immobilization (Supine Patient)
- Static Cardiology
- Ventilatory Management—Adult

EMT-Paramedic Form

National Registry of Emergency Medical Technicians
Advanced Level Practical Examination

BLEEDING CONTROL/SHOCK MANAGEMENT

Candidate: _____ Examiner: _____

Date: _____ Signature: _____

Time Start:_____	Possible Points	Points Awarded
Takes or verbalizes body substance isolation precautions	1	
Applies direct pressure to the wound	1	
Elevates the extremity	1	
NOTE: The examiner must now inform the candidate that the wound continues to bleed.		
Applies an additional dressing to the wound	1	
NOTE: The examiner must now inform the candidate that the wound still continues to bleed. The second dressing does not control the bleeding.		
Locates and applies pressure to appropriate arterial pressure point	1	
NOTE: The examiner must now inform the candidate that the bleeding is controlled.		
Bandages the wound	1	
NOTE: The examiner must now inform the candidate that the patient is exhibiting signs and symptoms of hypoperfusion.		
Properly positions the patient	1	
Administers high concentration oxygen	1	
Initiates steps to prevent heat loss from the patient	1	
Indicates the need for immediate transportation	1	
Time End: _____ TOTAL	10	

CRITICAL CRITERIA

_____ Did not take or verbalize body substance isolation precautions
_____ Did not apply high concentration of oxygen
_____ Applied a tourniquet before attempting other methods of bleeding control
_____ Did not control hemorrhage in a timely manner
_____ Did not indicate the need for immediate transportation

You must factually document your rationale for checking any of the above critical items on the reverse side of this form.

EMT-Paramedic Form

National Registry of Emergency Medical Technicians
Advanced Level Practical Examination

DUAL LUMEN AIRWAY DEVICE (COMBITUBE® OR PTL®)

Candidate: _____ Examiner: _____

Date: _____ Signature: _____

NOTE: If candidate elects to initially ventilate with BVM attached to reservoir and oxygen, full credit must be awarded for steps denoted by "**" so long as first ventilation is delivered within 30 seconds.

	Possible Points	Points Awarded
Takes or verbalizes body substance isolation precautions	1	
Opens the airway manually	1	
Elevates tongue, inserts simple adjunct [oropharyngeal or nasopharyngeal airway]	1	
NOTE: Examiner now informs candidate no gag reflex is present and patient accepts adjunct		
**Ventilates patient immediately with bag-valve-mask device unattached to oxygen	1	
**Hyperventilates patient with room air	1	
NOTE: Examiner now informs candidate that ventilation is being performed without difficulty		
Attaches oxygen reservoir to bag-valve-mask device and connects to high flow oxygen regulator [12-15 L/minute]	1	
Ventilates patient at a rate of 10-20/minute with appropriate volumes	1	
NOTE: After 30 seconds, examiner auscultates and reports breath sounds are present and equal bilaterally and medical control has ordered insertion of a dual lumen airway. The examiner must now take over ventilation.		
Directs assistant to pre-oxygenate patient	1	
Checks/prepares airway device	1	
Lubricates distal tip of the device [may be verbalized]	1	
NOTE: Examiner to remove OPA and move out of the way when candidate is prepared to insert device		
Positions head properly	1	
Performs a tongue-jaw lift	1	

☐ USES COMBITUBE®	☐ USES PTL®		
Inserts device in mid-line and to depth so printed ring is at level of teeth	Inserts device in mid-line until bite block flange is at level of teeth	1	
Inflates pharyngeal cuff with proper volume and removes syringe	Secures strap	1	
Inflates distal cuff with proper volume and removes syringe	Blows into tube #1 to adequately inflate both cuffs	1	
Attaches/directs attachment of BVM to the first [esophageal placement] lumen and ventilates		1	
Confirms placement and ventilation through correct lumen by observing chest rise, auscultation over the epigastrium, and bilaterally over each lung		1	
NOTE: The examiner states, "You do not see rise and fall of the chest and you only hear sounds over the epigastrium."			
Attaches/directs attachment of BVM to the second [endotracheal placement] lumen and ventilates		1	
Confirms placement and ventilation through correct lumen by observing chest rise, auscultation over the epigastrium, and bilaterally over each lung		1	
NOTE: The examiner confirms adequate chest rise, absent sounds over the epigastrium, and equal bilateral breath sounds.			
Secures device or confirms that the device remains properly secured		1	
		TOTAL	**20**	

CRITICAL CRITERIA

_____ Failure to initiate ventilations within 30 seconds after taking body substance isolation precautions or interrupts ventilations for greater than 30 seconds at any time
_____ Failure to take or verbalize body substance isolation precautions
_____ Failure to voice and ultimately provide high oxygen concentrations [at least 85%]
_____ Failure to ventilate patient at a rate of at least 10/minute
_____ Failure to provide adequate volumes per breath [maximum 2 errors/minute permissible]
_____ Failure to pre-oxygenate patient prior to insertion of the dual lumen airway device
_____ Failure to insert the dual lumen airway device at a proper depth or at either proper place within 3 attempts
_____ Failure to inflate both cuffs properly
_____ **Combitube** - failure to remove the syringe immediately after inflation of each cuff
       PTL - failure to secure the strap prior to cuff inflation
_____ Failure to confirm that the proper lumen of the device is being ventilated by observing chest rise, auscultation over the epigastrium, and bilaterally over each lung
_____ Inserts any adjunct in a manner dangerous to patient

You must factually document your rationale for checking any of the above critical items on the reverse side of this form.

p304/8-003k

EMT-Paramedic Form

National Registry of Emergency Medical Technicians
Advanced Level Practical Examination

DYNAMIC CARDIOLOGY

Candidate: _____ Examiner: _____

Date: _____ Signature: _____

SET #_____

Level of Testing:　　□ NREMT-Intermediate/99　　　□ NREMT-Paramedic

Time Start:_____

	Possible Points	Points Awarded
Takes or verbalizes infection control precautions	1	
Checks level of responsiveness	1	
Checks ABCs	1	
Initiates CPR if appropriate [verbally]	1	
Attaches ECG monitor in a timely fashion or applies paddles for "Quick Look"	1	
Correctly interprets initial rhythm	1	
Appropriately manages initial rhythm	2	
Notes change in rhythm	1	
Checks patient condition to include pulse and, if appropriate, BP	1	
Correctly interprets second rhythm	1	
Appropriately manages second rhythm	2	
Notes change in rhythm	1	
Checks patient condition to include pulse and, if appropriate, BP	1	
Correctly interprets third rhythm	1	
Appropriately manages third rhythm	2	
Notes change in rhythm	1	
Checks patient condition to include pulse and, if appropriate, BP	1	
Correctly interprets fourth rhythm	1	
Appropriately manages fourth rhythm	2	
Orders high percentages of supplemental oxygen at proper times	1	

Time End: _____　　　　　　　　　　　　　　　　　　　　**TOTAL**　24

CRITICAL CRITERIA

_____ Failure to deliver first shock in a timely manner due to operator delay in machine use or providing treatments other than CPR with simple adjuncts

_____ Failure to deliver second or third shocks without delay other than the time required to reassess rhythm and recharge paddles

_____ Failure to verify rhythm before delivering each shock

_____ Failure to ensure the safety of self and others [verbalizes "All clear" and observes]

_____ Inability to deliver DC shock [does not use machine properly]

_____ Failure to demonstrate acceptable shock sequence

_____ Failure to order initiation or resumption of CPR when appropriate

_____ Failure to order correct management of airway [ET when appropriate]

_____ Failure to order administration of appropriate oxygen at proper time

_____ Failure to diagnose or treat 2 or more rhythms correctly

_____ Orders administration of an inappropriate drug or lethal dosage

_____ Failure to correctly diagnose or adequately treat v-fib, v-tach, or asystole

You must factually document your rationale for checking any of the above critical items on the reverse side of this form.

EMT-Paramedic Form

National Registry of Emergency Medical Technicians
Advanced Level Practical Examination

INTRAVENOUS THERAPY

Candidate: _____ Examiner: _____

Date: _____ Signature: _____

Level of Testing: ❑ NREMT-Intermediate/85 ❑ NREMT-Intermediate/99 ❑ NREMT-Paramedic

Time Start: _____

	Possible Points	Points Awarded
Checks selected IV fluid for: -Proper fluid (1 point) -Clarity (1 point)	2	
Selects appropriate catheter	1	
Selects proper administration set	1	
Connects IV tubing to the IV bag	1	
Prepares administration set [fills drip chamber and flushes tubing]	1	
Cuts or tears tape [at any time before venipuncture]	1	
Takes/verbalizes body substance isolation precautions [prior to venipuncture]	1	
Applies tourniquet	1	
Palpates suitable vein	1	
Cleanses site appropriately	1	
Performs venipuncture -Inserts stylette (1 point) -Notes or verbalizes flashback (1 point) -Occludes vein proximal to catheter (1 point) -Removes stylette (1 point) -Connects IV tubing to catheter (1 point)	5	
Disposes/verbalizes disposal of needle in proper container	1	
Releases tourniquet	1	
Runs IV for a brief period to assure patent line	1	
Secures catheter [tapes securely or verbalizes]	1	
Adjusts flow rate as appropriate	1	

Time End: _____   **TOTAL** 21

CRITICAL CRITERIA
_____ Failure to establish a patent and properly adjusted IV within 6 minute time limit
_____ Failure to take or verbalize body substance isolation precautions prior to performing venipuncture
_____ Contaminates equipment or site without appropriately correcting situation
_____ Performs any improper technique resulting in the potential for uncontrolled hemorrhage, catheter shear, or air embolism
_____ Failure to successfully establish IV within 3 attempts during 6 minute time limit
_____ Failure to dispose/verbalize disposal of needle in proper container

NOTE: Check here (_____) if candidate did not establish a patent IV and do not evaluate IV Bolus Medications.

INTRAVENOUS BOLUS MEDICATIONS

Time Start: _____

Asks patient for known allergies	1	
Selects correct medication	1	
Assures correct concentration of drug	1	
Assembles prefilled syringe correctly and dispels air	1	
Continues body substance isolation precautions	1	
Cleanses injection site [Y-port or hub]	1	
Reaffirms medication	1	
Stops IV flow [pinches tubing or shuts off]	1	
Administers correct dose at proper push rate	1	
Disposes/verbalizes proper disposal of syringe and needle in proper container	1	
Flushes tubing [runs wide open for a brief period]	1	
Adjusts drip rate to TKO/KVO	1	
Verbalizes need to observe patient for desired effect/adverse side effects	1	

Time End: _____   **TOTAL** 13

CRITICAL CRITERIA
_____ Failure to begin administration of medication within 3 minute time limit
_____ Contaminates equipment or site without appropriately correcting situation
_____ Failure to adequately dispel air resulting in potential for air embolism
_____ Injects improper drug or dosage [wrong drug, incorrect amount, or pushes at inappropriate rate]
_____ Failure to flush IV tubing after injecting medication
_____ Recaps needle or failure to dispose/verbalize disposal of syringe and needle in proper container

You must factually document your rationale for checking any of the above critical items on the reverse side of this form.

p309/8-003k

EMT-Paramedic Form

National Registry of Emergency Medical Technicians
Advanced Level Practical Examination

ORAL STATION

Candidate: _____ Examiner: _____

Date: _____ Signature: _____

Scenario: _____

Time Start: _____

	Possible Points	Points Awarded
Scene Management		
Thoroughly assessed and took deliberate actions to control the scene	3	
Assessed the scene, identified potential hazards, did not put anyone in danger	2	
Incompletely assessed or managed the scene	1	
Did not assess or manage the scene	0	
Patient Assessment		
Completed an organized assessment and integrated findings to expand further assessment	3	
Completed initial, focused, and ongoing assessments	2	
Performed an incomplete or disorganized assessment	1	
Did not complete an initial assessment	0	
Patient Management		
Managed all aspects of the patient's condition and anticipated further needs	3	
Appropriately managed the patient's presenting condition	2	
Performed an incomplete or disorganized management	1	
Did not manage life-threatening conditions	0	
Interpersonal relations		
Established rapport and interacted in an organized, therapeutic manner	3	
Interacted and responded appropriately with patient, crew, and bystanders	2	
Used inappropriate communication techniques	1	
Demonstrated intolerance for patient, bystanders, and crew	0	
Integration (verbal report, field impression, and transport decision)		
Stated correct field impression and pathophysiological basis, provided succinct and accurate verbal report including social/psychological concerns, and considered alternate transport destinations	3	
Stated correct field impression, provided succinct and accurate verbal report, and appropriately stated transport decision	2	
Stated correct field impression, provided inappropriate verbal report or transport decision	1	
Stated incorrect field impression or did not provide verbal report	0	

Time End: _____   **TOTAL   15**

Critical Criteria

_____ Failure to appropriately address any of the scenario's "Mandatory Actions"

_____ Performs or orders any harmful or dangerous action or intervention

You must factually document your rationale for checking any of the above critical items on the reverse side of this form.

EMT-Paramedic Form

National Registry of Emergency Medical Technicians
Advanced Level Practical Examination

PATIENT ASSESSMENT - MEDICAL

Candidate: _____ **Examiner:** _____

Date: _____ **Signature:** _____

Scenario:_____

Time Start: _____

	Possible Points	Points Awarded
Takes or verbalizes body substance isolation precautions	1	
SCENE SIZE-UP		
Determines the scene/situation is safe	1	
Determines the mechanism of injury/nature of illness	1	
Determines the number of patients	1	
Requests additional help if necessary	1	
Considers stabilization of spine	1	
INITIAL ASSESSMENT		
Verbalizes general impression of the patient	1	
Determines responsiveness/level of consciousness	1	
Determines chief complaint/apparent life-threats	1	
Assesses airway and breathing -Assessment (1 point) -Assures adequate ventilation (1 point) -Initiates appropriate oxygen therapy (1 point)	3	
Assesses circulation -Assesses/controls major bleeding (1 point) -Assesses skin [either skin color, temperature, or condition] (1 point) -Assesses pulse (1 point)	3	
Identifies priority patients/makes transport decision	1	
FOCUSED HISTORY AND PHYSICAL EXAMINATION/RAPID ASSESSMENT		
History of present illness -Onset (1 point) -Severity (1 point) -Provocation (1 point) -Time (1 point) -Quality (1 point) -Clarifying questions of associated signs and symptoms as related to OPQRST (2 points) -Radiation (1 point)	8	
Past medical history -Allergies (1 point) -Past pertinent history (1 point) -Events leading to present illness (1 point) -Medications (1 point) -Last oral intake (1 point)	5	
Performs focused physical examination [assess affected body part/system or, if indicated, completes rapid assessment] -Cardiovascular -Neurological -Integumentary -Reproductive -Pulmonary -Musculoskeletal -GI/GU -Psychological/Social	5	
Vital signs -Pulse (1 point) -Respiratory rate and quality (1 point each) -Blood pressure (1 point) -AVPU (1 point)	5	
Diagnostics [must include application of ECG monitor for dyspnea and chest pain]	2	
States field impression of patient	1	
Verbalizes treatment plan for patient and calls for appropriate intervention(s)	1	
Transport decision re-evaluated	1	
ON-GOING ASSESSMENT		
Repeats initial assessment	1	
Repeats vital signs	1	
Evaluates response to treatments	1	
Repeats focused assessment regarding patient complaint or injuries	1	

Time End: _____

CRITICAL CRITERIA   **TOTAL**   48

_____ Failure to initiate or call for transport of the patient within 15 minute time limit
_____ Failure to take or verbalize body substance isolation precautions
_____ Failure to determine scene safety before approaching patient
_____ Failure to voice and ultimately provide appropriate oxygen therapy
_____ Failure to assess/provide adequate ventilation
_____ Failure to find or appropriately manage problems associated with airway, breathing, hemorrhage or shock [hypoperfusion]
_____ Failure to differentiate patient's need for immediate transportation versus continued assessment and treatment at the scene
_____ Does other detailed or focused history or physical examination before assessing and treating threats to airway, breathing, and circulation
_____ Failure to determine the patient's primary problem
_____ Orders a dangerous or inappropriate intervention
_____ Failure to provide for spinal protection when indicated

You must factually document your rationale for checking any of the above critical items on the reverse side of this form.

EMT-Paramedic Form

National Registry of Emergency Medical Technicians
Advanced Level Practical Examination

PATIENT ASSESSMENT - TRAUMA

Candidate: _____ Examiner: _____

Date: _____ Signature: _____

Scenario # _____

Time Start: _____   NOTE: Areas denoted by "**" may be integrated within sequence of Initial Assessment

	Possible Points	Points Awarded
Takes or verbalizes body substance isolation precautions	1	
SCENE SIZE-UP		
Determines the scene/situation is safe	1	
Determines the mechanism of injury/nature of illness	1	
Determines the number of patients	1	
Requests additional help if necessary	1	
Considers stabilization of spine	1	
INITIAL ASSESSMENT/RESUSCITATION		
Verbalizes general impression of the patient	1	
Determines responsiveness/level of consciousness	1	
Determines chief complaint/apparent life-threats	1	
Airway -Opens and assesses airway (1 point) -Inserts adjunct as indicated (1 point)	2	

Breathing
  -Assess breathing (1 point)
  -Assures adequate ventilation (1 point)
  -Initiates appropriate oxygen therapy (1 point)
  -Manages any injury which may compromise breathing/ventilation (1 point)
	4	

Circulation
  -Checks pulse (1point)
  -Assess skin [either skin color, temperature, or condition] (1 point)
  -Assesses for and controls major bleeding if present (1 point)
  -Initiates shock management (1 point)
	4	

Identifies priority patients/makes transport decision	1	
FOCUSED HISTORY AND PHYSICAL EXAMINATION/RAPID TRAUMA ASSESSMENT		
Selects appropriate assessment	1	
Obtains, or directs assistant to obtain, baseline vital signs	1	
Obtains SAMPLE history	1	
DETAILED PHYSICAL EXAMINATION		

Head
  -Inspects mouth**, nose**, and assesses facial area (1 point)
  -Inspects and palpates scalp and ears (1 point)
  -Assesses eyes for PERRL** (1 point)
	3	

Neck**
  -Checks position of trachea (1 point)
  -Checks jugular veins (1 point)
  -Palpates cervical spine (1 point)
	3	

Chest**
  -Inspects chest (1 point)
  -Palpates chest (1 point)
  -Auscultates chest (1 point)
	3	

Abdomen/pelvis**
  -Inspects and palpates abdomen (1 point)
  -Assesses pelvis (1 point)
  -Verbalizes assessment of genitalia/perineum as needed (1 point)
	3	

Lower extremities** -Inspects, palpates, and assesses motor, sensory, and distal circulatory functions (1 point/leg)	2	
Upper extremities -Inspects, palpates, and assesses motor, sensory, and distal circulatory functions (1 point/arm)	2	

Posterior thorax, lumbar, and buttocks**
  -Inspects and palpates posterior thorax (1 point)
  -Inspects and palpates lumbar and buttocks area (1 point)
	2	

Manages secondary injuries and wounds appropriately	1	
Performs ongoing assessment	1	
Time End: _____ **TOTAL**	43	

CRITICAL CRITERIA

_____ Failure to initiate or call for transport of the patient within 10 minute time limit
_____ Failure to take or verbalize body substance isolation precautions
_____ Failure to determine scene safety
_____ Failure to assess for and provide spinal protection when indicated
_____ Failure to voice and ultimately provide high concentration of oxygen
_____ Failure to assess/provide adequate ventilation
_____ Failure to find or appropriately manage problems associated with airway, breathing, hemorrhage or shock [hypoperfusion]
_____ Failure to differentiate patient's need for immediate transportation versus continued assessment/treatment at the scene
_____ Does other detailed/focused history or physical exam before assessing/treating threats to airway, breathing, and circulation
_____ Orders a dangerous or inappropriate intervention

You must factually document your rationale for checking any of the above critical items on the reverse side of this form.

p301/8-003k

EMT-Paramedic Form

National Registry of Emergency Medical Technicians
Advanced Level Practical Examination

PEDIATRIC INTRAOSSEOUS INFUSION

Candidate: _____ Examiner: _____

Date: _____ Signature: _____

Time Start:_____	Possible Points	Points Awarded
Checks selected IV fluid for: -Proper fluid (1 point) -Clarity (1 point)	2	
Selects appropriate equipment to include: -IO needle (1 point) -Syringe (1 point) -Saline (1 point) -Extension set (1 point)	4	
Selects proper administration set	1	
Connects administration set to bag	1	
Prepares administration set [fills drip chamber and flushes tubing]	1	
Prepares syringe and extension tubing	1	
Cuts or tears tape [at any time before IO puncture]	1	
Takes or verbalizes body substance isolation precautions [prior to IO puncture]	1	
Identifies proper anatomical site for IO puncture	1	
Cleanses site appropriately	1	
Performs IO puncture: -Stabilizes tibia (1 point) -Inserts needle at proper angle (1 point) -Advances needle with twisting motion until "pop" is felt (1 point) -Unscrews cap and removes stylette from needle (1 point)	4	
Disposes of needle in proper container	1	
Attaches syringe and extension set to IO needle and aspirates	1	
Slowly injects saline to assure proper placement of needle	1	
Connects administration set and adjusts flow rate as appropriate	1	
Secures needle with tape and supports with bulky dressing	1	
Time End: _____ **TOTAL**	23	

CRITICAL CRITERIA

_____ Failure to establish a patent and properly adjusted IO line within the 6 minute time limit
_____ Failure to take or verbalize body substance isolation precautions prior to performing IO puncture
_____ Contaminates equipment or site without appropriately correcting situation
_____ Performs any improper technique resulting in the potential for air embolism
_____ Failure to assure correct needle placement before attaching administration set
_____ Failure to successfully establish IO infusion within 2 attempts during 6 minute time limit
_____ Performing IO puncture in an unacceptable manner [improper site, incorrect needle angle, etc.]
_____ Failure to dispose of needle in proper container
_____ Orders or performs any dangerous or potentially harmful procedure

You must factually document your rationale for checking any of the above critical items on the reverse side of this form.

EMT-Paramedic Form

National Registry of Emergency Medical Technicians
Advanced Level Practical Examination

PEDIATRIC (<2 yrs.) VENTILATORY MANAGEMENT

Candidate: _____ Examiner _____

Date: _____ Signature: _____

NOTE: If candidate elects to ventilate initially with BVM attached to reservoir and oxygen, full credit must be awarded for steps denoted by "**" so long as first ventilation is delivered within 30 seconds.

	Possible Points	Points Awarded
Takes or verbalizes body substance isolation precautions	1	
Opens the airway manually	1	
Elevates tongue, inserts simple adjunct [oropharyngeal or nasopharyngeal airway]	1	
NOTE: Examiner now informs candidate no gag reflex is present and patient accepts adjunct		
**Ventilates patient immediately with bag-valve-mask device unattached to oxygen	1	
**Hyperventilates patient with room air	1	
NOTE: Examiner now informs candidate that ventilation is being performed without difficulty and that pulse oximetry indicates the patient's blood oxygen saturation is 85%		
Attaches oxygen reservoir to bag-valve-mask device and connects to high flow oxygen regulator [12-15 L/minute]	1	
Ventilates patient at a rate of 20-30/minute and assures adequate chest expansion	1	
NOTE: After 30 seconds, examiner auscultates and reports breath sounds are present, equal bilaterally and medical direction has ordered intubation. The examiner must now take over ventilation.		
Directs assistant to pre-oxygenate patient	1	
Identifies/selects proper equipment for intubation	1	
Checks laryngoscope to assure operational with bulb tight	1	
NOTE: Examiner to remove OPA and move out of the way when candidate is prepared to intubate		
Places patient in neutral or sniffing position	1	
Inserts blade while displacing tongue	1	
Elevates mandible with laryngoscope	1	
Introduces ET tube and advances to proper depth	1	
Directs ventilation of patient	1	
Confirms proper placement by auscultation bilaterally over each lung and over epigastrium	1	
NOTE: Examiner to ask, "If you had proper placement, what should you expect to hear?"		
Secures ET tube [may be verbalized]	1	
TOTAL	**17**	

CRITICAL CRITERIA

_____ Failure to initiate ventilations within 30 seconds after applying gloves or interrupts ventilations for greater than 30 seconds at any time
_____ Failure to take or verbalize body substance isolation precautions
_____ Failure to pad under the torso to allow neutral head position or sniffing position
_____ Failure to voice and ultimately provide high oxygen concentrations [at least 85%]
_____ Failure to ventilate patient at a rate of at least 20/minute
_____ Failure to provide adequate volumes per breath [maximum 2 errors/minute permissible]
_____ Failure to pre-oxygenate patient prior to intubation
_____ Failure to successfully intubate within 3 attempts
_____ Uses gums as a fulcrum
_____ Failure to assure proper tube placement by auscultation bilaterally **and** over the epigastrium
_____ Inserts any adjunct in a manner dangerous to the patient
_____ Attempts to use any equipment not appropriate for the pediatric patient

You must factually document your rationale for checking any of the above critical items on the reverse side of this form.

EMT-Paramedic Form

National Registry of Emergency Medical Technicians
Advanced Level Practical Examination

SPINAL IMMOBILIZATION (SEATED PATIENT)

Candidate:_____Examiner:_____

Date: _____Signature:_____

Time Start: _____	Possible Points	Points Awarded
Takes or verbalizes body substance isolation precautions	1	
Directs assistant to place/maintain head in the neutral, in-line position	1	
Directs assistant to maintain manual immobilization of the head	1	
Reassesses motor, sensory, and circulatory function in each extremity	1	
Applies appropriately sized extrication collar	1	
Positions the immobilization device behind the patient	1	
Secures the device to the patient's torso	1	
Evaluates torso fixation and adjusts as necessary	1	
Evaluates and pads behind the patient's head as necessary	1	
Secures the patient's head to the device	1	
Verbalizes moving the patient to a long backboard	1	
Reassesses motor, sensory, and circulatory function in each extremity	1	

Time End: _____   **TOTAL**   12

CRITICAL CRITERIA

_____ Did not immediately direct or take manual immobilization of the head

_____ Did not properly apply appropriately sized cervical collar before ordering release of manual immobilization

_____ Released or ordered release of manual immobilization before it was maintained mechanically

_____ Manipulated or moved patient excessively causing potential spinal compromise

_____ Head immobilized to the device **before** device sufficiently secured to torso

_____ Device moves excessively up, down, left, or right on the patient's torso

_____ Head immobilization allows for excessive movement

_____ Torso fixation inhibits chest rise, resulting in respiratory compromise

_____ Upon completion of immobilization, head is not in a neutral, in-line position

_____ Did not reassess motor, sensory, and circulatory functions in each extremity after voicing immobilization to the long backboard

You must factually document your rationale for checking any of the above critical items on the reverse side of this form.

EMT-Paramedic Form

Candidate:_____ Examiner:_____

Date: _____ Signature:_____

Time Start: _____	Possible Points	Points Awarded
Takes or verbalizes body substance isolation precautions	1	
Directs assistant to place/maintain head in the neutral, in-line position	1	
Directs assistant to maintain manual immobilization of the head	1	
Reassesses motor, sensory, and circulatory function in each extremity	1	
Applies appropriately sized extrication collar	1	
Positions the immobilization device appropriately	1	
Directs movement of the patient onto the device without compromising the integrity of the spine	1	
Applies padding to voids between the torso and the device as necessary	1	
Immobilizes the patient's torso to the device	1	
Evaluates and pads behind the patient's head as necessary	1	
Immobilizes the patient's head to the device	1	
Secures the patient's legs to the device	1	
Secures the patient's arms to the device	1	
Reassesses motor, sensory, and circulatory function in each extremity	1	
Time End: _____ **TOTAL**	14	

CRITICAL CRITERIA

_____ Did not immediately direct or take manual immobilization of the head
_____ Did not properly apply appropriately sized cervical collar before ordering release of manual immobilization
_____ Released or ordered release of manual immobilization before it was maintained mechanically
_____ Manipulated or moved patient excessively causing potential spinal compromise
_____ Head immobilized to the device **before** device sufficiently secured to torso
_____ Patient moves excessively up, down, left, or right on the device
_____ Head immobilization allows for excessive movement
_____ Upon completion of immobilization, head is not in a neutral, in-line position
_____ Did not reassess motor, sensory, and circulatory functions in each extremity after voicing immobilization to the device

You must factually document your rationale for checking any of the above critical items on the reverse side of this form.

EMT-Paramedic Form

National Registry of Emergency Medical Technicians
Advanced Level Practical Examination

STATIC CARDIOLOGY

Candidate: _____ Examiner: _____

Date: _____ Signature: _____

SET #_____

Level of Testing:　　□ **NREMT-Intermediate/99**　　　　□ **NREMT-Paramedic**

Note: No points for treatment may be awarded if the diagnosis is incorrect.
　　　　Only document incorrect responses in spaces provided.

Time Start:_____

	Possible Points	Points Awarded
STRIP #1		
Diagnosis:	1	
Treatment:	2	
STRIP #2		
Diagnosis:	1	
Treatment:	2	
STRIP #3		
Diagnosis:	1	
Treatment:	2	
STRIP #4		
Diagnosis:	1	
Treatment:	2	
Time End: _____　　　　　　　　　　　**TOTAL**	12	

p307/8-003k

EMT-Paramedic Form

Candidate:_____Examiner:_____

Date: _____Signature: _____

NOTE: If candidate elects to ventilate initially with BVM attached to reservoir and oxygen, full credit must be awarded for steps denoted by "**" so long as first ventilation is delivered within 30 seconds.

	Possible Points	Points Awarded
Takes or verbalizes body substance isolation precautions	1	
Opens the airway manually	1	
Elevates tongue, inserts simple adjunct [oropharyngeal or nasopharyngeal airway]	1	
NOTE: Examiner now informs candidate no gag reflex is present and patient accepts adjunct		
**Ventilates patient immediately with bag-valve-mask device unattached to oxygen	1	
**Hyperventilates patient with room air	1	
NOTE: Examiner now informs candidate that ventilation is being performed without difficulty and that pulse oximetry indicates the patient's blood oxygen saturation is 85%		
Attaches oxygen reservoir to bag-valve-mask device and connects to high flow oxygen regulator [12-15 L/minute]	1	
Ventilates patient at a rate of 10-20/minute with appropriate volumes	1	
NOTE: After 30 seconds, examiner auscultates and reports breath sounds are present, equal bilaterally and medical direction has ordered intubation. The examiner must now take over ventilation.		
Directs assistant to pre-oxygenate patient	1	
Identifies/selects proper equipment for intubation	1	
Checks equipment for: -Cuff leaks (1 point) -Laryngoscope operational with bulb tight (1 point)	2	
NOTE: Examiner to remove OPA and move out of the way when candidate is prepared to intubate		
Positions head properly	1	
Inserts blade while displacing tongue	1	
Elevates mandible with laryngoscope	1	
Introduces ET tube and advances to proper depth	1	
Inflates cuff to proper pressure and disconnects syringe	1	
Directs ventilation of patient	1	
Confirms proper placement by auscultation bilaterally over each lung and over epigastrium	1	
NOTE: Examiner to ask, "If you had proper placement, what should you expect to hear?"		
Secures ET tube [may be verbalized]	1	
NOTE: Examiner now asks candidate, "Please demonstrate one additional method of verifying proper tube placement in this patient."		
Identifies/selects proper equipment	1	
Verbalizes findings and interpretations [compares indicator color to the colorimetric scale and states reading to examiner]	1	
NOTE: Examiner now states, "You see secretions in the tube and hear gurgling sounds with the patient's exhalation."		
Identifies/selects a flexible suction catheter	1	
Pre-oxygenates patient	1	
Marks maximum insertion length with thumb and forefinger	1	
Inserts catheter into the ET tube leaving catheter port open	1	
At proper insertion depth, covers catheter port and applies suction while withdrawing catheter	1	
Ventilates/directs ventilation of patient as catheter is flushed with sterile water	1	
TOTAL	**27**	

CRITICAL CRITERIA

_____ Failure to initiate ventilations within 30 seconds after applying gloves or interrupts ventilations for greater than 30 seconds at any time
_____ Failure to take or verbalize body substance isolation precautions
_____ Failure to voice and ultimately provide high oxygen concentrations [at least 85%]
_____ Failure to ventilate patient at a rate of at least 10/minute
_____ Failure to provide adequate volumes per breath [maximum 2 errors/minute permissible]
_____ Failure to pre-oxygenate patient prior to intubation and suctioning
_____ Failure to successfully intubate within 3 attempts
_____ Failure to disconnect syringe **immediately** after inflating cuff of ET tube
_____ Uses teeth as a fulcrum
_____ Failure to assure proper tube placement by auscultation bilaterally **and** over the epigastrium
_____ If used, stylette extends beyond end of ET tube
_____ Inserts any adjunct in a manner dangerous to the patient
_____ Suctions the patient for more than 15 seconds
_____ Does not suction the patient

You must factually document your rationale for checking any of the above critical items on the reverse side of this form.

p303/8-003k